Mentoring and Supervision in Healthcare

7224 7853

⑤SAGE | 50 YEARS

SAGE was founded in 1965 by Sara Miller McCune to support the dissemination of usable knowledge by publishing innovative and high-quality research and teaching content. Today, we publish more than 750 journals, including those of more than 300 learned societies, more than 800 new books per year, and a growing range of library products including archives, data, case studies, reports, conference highlights, and video. SAGE remains majority-owned by our founder, and after Sara's lifetime will become owned by a charitable trust that secures our continued independence.

Los Angeles | London | Washington DC | New Delhi | Singapore

Third Edition

Mentoring and Supervision in Healthcare

Neil Gopee

Los Angeles | London | New Delhi
Singapore | Washington DC

Los Angeles | London | New Delhi
Singapore | Washington DC

SAGE Publications Ltd
1 Oliver's Yard
55 City Road
London EC1Y 1SP

SAGE Publications Inc.
2455 Teller Road
Thousand Oaks, California 91320

SAGE Publications India Pvt Ltd
B 1/l 1 Mohan Cooperative Industrial Area
Mathura Road
New Delhi 110 044

SAGE Publications Asia-Pacific Pte Ltd
3 Church Street
#10-04 Samsung Hub
Singapore 049483

Editor: Becky Taylor
Associate editor: Emma Milman
Production editor: Katie Forsythe
Copyeditor: Roza I.M. El-Eini
Proofreader: William Baginsky
Marketing manager: Tamara Navaratnam
Cover design: Wendy Scott
Typeset by: C&M Digitals (P) Ltd, Chennai, India
Printed by CPI Group (UK) Ltd, Croydon, CR0 4YY

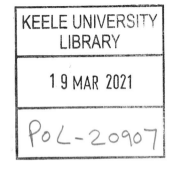
First edition published 2007. Reprinted in 2008 twice, 2009 and 2010.
Second edition published 2011. Reprinted in 2011.

This 3rd edition first published 2015

Library of Congress Control Number: 2014945226

British Library Cataloguing in Publication data

A catalogue record for this book is available from the British Library

ISBN 978-1-4739-0246-6
ISBN 978-1-4739-0247-3 (pbk)

At SAGE we take sustainability seriously. Most of our products are printed in the UK using FSC papers and boards. When we print overseas we ensure sustainable papers are used as measured by the Egmont grading system. We undertake an annual audit to monitor our sustainability.

Contents

List of Boxes, Templates, Figures and Tables

Boxes

Templates

Figures

Tables

About the Author

I am currently employed as Lecturer at the Faculty of Health and Life Sciences at Coventry University, and have until recently also been Associate Lecturer at the Open University. My role as external examiner at various higher education institutions in my subject areas has further broadened my insights into the two subject areas that I teach and research: first, learning, teaching and assessment in relation to undergraduate and postgraduate students; and, second, management and leadership in healthcare settings.

I first qualified as a nurse a few decades ago and worked in general surgical nursing for a year before moving on to complete the registered mental health nurse course. Through my nursing career, a combination of clinical experiences in primary care and general intensive care nursing was also supplemented by attendance at numerous professional development short and long courses, including various workshops on writing for publication, and also completing my doctorate in continuing professional education at University of Warwick.

My first peer-reviewed article was published in 1991 based on my then nurse tutor role. The 1990s were when nurse education programmes became a part of university provision, which further opened up authoring opportunities, and I negotiated with Alison Poyner, Commissioning Editor at SAGE Publications, to write the *Mentoring and Supervision in Healthcare* book, the first edition of which was published in 2007. Along the way, I also worked with SAGE Publications to write *Leadership and Management in Healthcare* (now in its second edition) and *Practice Teaching in Healthcare* textbooks. I have also had chapters published in edited books and a range of peer-reviewed articles.

Neil Gopee, February 2015

Acknowledgements

The authors and publishers would like to thank Claire McGuinness, Lecturer and Mentorship Lead at Glasgow Caledonian University and Su Everett, Senior Lecturer, Middlesex University, for providing scenario suggestions for the companion website.

Neil: I would like to acknowledge the support and constructive comments provided by the editors at SAGE Publications, especially Emma Milman and Katie Forsythe and I am also thankful to my daughters Hema, Sheila and Neeta for their recognition of my writing.

We would also like to thank the reviewers who commented on the initial proposal for a third edition and draft chapters from the text:

Nora Cooper, Senior Lecturer, Middlesex University

Jeff Fernandez, Nurse Consultant of Islington drug and alcohol services

Joady Mitchell, Principal lecturer, Practice Learning, London South Bank University

Gil Truscott, Practice Educator, Glyndŵr University

List of Abbreviations

ACE	Accreditation of Clinical Educators
AHP	Allied health professions
BACP	British Association for Counselling and Psychotherapy
CAIPE	Centre for Advancement of Interprofessional Education
CATS	Credit accumulation and transfer scheme
CCG	Clinical commissioning group
CHEF	Care Home Education Facilitator
CINAHL	Cumulative Index to Nursing and Allied Health Literature
CIPD	Chartered Institute of Personnel and Development
CLE	Clinical learning environment
CLEI	Clinical Learning Environment Inventory
CLES+T	Clinical Learning Environment, Supervision and Nurse Teacher
CLOCS	Clinical Learning Organisational Culture Survey
CNO	Chief Nursing Officer
CODP	College of Operating Department Practitioners
COPD	Chronic Obstructive Pulmonary Disease
COT	College of Occupational Therapists
CPD	Continuing professional development
CPS	Crown Prosecution Service
CPT	Community Practice Teacher
CQC	Care Quality Commission
CSP	Chartered Society of Physiotherapy
DDA	Disability Discrimination Act
DH	Department of Health
EBHC	Evidence-based healthcare
EBM	Evidence-based medicine
EBP	Evidence-based practice
ECQ	Education Commissioning for Quality
ESC	Essential skills clusters
EWS	Early warning systems

GMC	General Medical Council
GP	General Practitioner
GROW	Goal, Reality, Options, Will/Wrap up (model)
HCPC	Health and Care Professions Council
HEE	Health Education England
HEI	Higher education institute/institution
HMSO	Her Majesty's Stationery Office
IHI	Institute of Healthcare Improvement
IPE	Interprofessional education
IPL	Interprofessional learning
LETB	Local Education and Training Boards
LSQ	Learning Style Questionnaire
MDT	Multidisciplinary team
MMP	Measuring mentorship potential
NCIHE	National Committee of Inquiry into Higher Education
NHS IQ	NHS Improving Quality
NHS KSF	NHS Knowledge and Skills Framework
NIACE	National Institute of Adult Continuing Education
NICE	National Institute for Health and Care Excellence
NMC	Nursing and Midwifery Council
NQB	England National Quality Board (NHS)
NVQ	National Vocational Qualification
OAR	Ongoing achievement record
ODP	Operating department practitioner
OPSI	Office of Public Sector Information
OSCE	Objective Structured/Simulated Clinical Examination (at times referred to as OSCA, with the substituted alphabet A signifying assessment)
PCA	Patient-controlled analgesia
PDP	Personal development plan
PDSA	Plan–Do–Study–Act
PEF	Practice education facilitator
PREP	Post-registration education and practice
QAA	Quality Assurance Agency for Higher Education
QIPP	Quality, Innovation, Productivity and Prevention
RAPSIES	Recognition, Analysis, Preparation, Strategies, Implementation, Evaluation, Sustaining (framework)
RCN	Royal College of Nursing
RCT	Randomised controlled trial
RM	Registered midwife
RN	Registered nurse
SCOPME	Standing Committee on Postgraduate Medical and Dental Education
SCPHN	Specialist community public health nurse
SEN	Special education needs

SMART	Specific, measurable, achievable, realistic and time-limited
SMS	Short message service (texting)
SOLER	Sit squarely, open posture, lean towards the other, eye contact, relax
SOM	Sign-off mentor
SOP	Standards of proficiency
STEP	Social, technological, economic and political
SURETY	Sit at an angle, uncross legs and arms, relax, eye contact, touch, your intuition
SWOT	Strengths, weaknesses, opportunities and threats
UKCC	United Kingdom Central Council for Nursing, Midwifery and Health Visiting
VARK	Visual, aural, read–write and kinaesthetic
WBL	Work-based learning

About the Companion Website

Visit the companion website at https://study.sagepub.com/gopee to find a range of materials which will support your learning, including:

Resources for student mentors

- A **video** of Neil Gopee talking about key themes in the book
- Free **SAGE journal articles** to support you in your studies and expand your knowledge. These are linked to each chapter of the book
- An **interactive glossary** that allows you to test your knowledge of important concepts
- **Weblinks** that take you directly to further resources
- A **lesson plan** for teaching a clinical skill
- Examples of evidence you can give to show you meet the **NMC Mentor Outcomes**

Resources for lecturers

- Extra **case scenarios**, not available in the book, for use in your teaching
- Commentary on how the **activities** in the book can be used in your teaching
- Videos of Neil Gopee giving his response to the case scenarios. Neil's videos are not exhaustive answers to the scenarios, and your students can discuss these in class to come up with other ideas.

Look out for the web icon in the chapters to see where the material is available.

Introduction

The Rationale and Scope of this Book

Mentoring has become a significant dimension of professional life in nursing, midwifery and other healthcare professions (and for some of us, in our personal lives), particularly in relation to supporting educational preparation of pre-registration students (see Glossary at the back of this book). Also known by other titles such as 'clinical educator' and 'clinical instructor' in other healthcare professions and in non-UK countries, formal educational preparation is required in nursing and midwifery so as to enable mentors to perform this role competently.

Several definitions of this role have evolved over the years and various research findings on mentoring in different professions have been published. Mentoring was redefined in a Department of Health (DH) (2001a) publication mainly as a result of research findings by Phillips et al. (2000), extending the role beyond the facilitation of practice-based learning during student practice placements to include the assessment of students' practice competencies. The Nursing and Midwifery Council (NMC) (2008a: 45) has retained a very similar definition in its *Standards to Support Learning and Assessment in Practice*, indicating that the mentor is a 'registrant who … facilitates learning, and supervises and assesses students in practice settings'.

Although the standards for mentors in the NMC publication are for registered nurses (RN) and registered midwives (RM) (from here on all healthcare professionals registered with the NMC or the Health and Care Professions Council (HCPC) will be referred to as 'registrants'), they are based on general principles of mentoring (or clinical education) so that they are fully applicable to the other three groups of health and social care professions, namely allied health professions (AHP), social work and medicine. In the current scene of interprofessional learning, reciprocal mentoring between health professions has already been happening, where permissible, for at least a decade.

The NMC standards also identify the criteria for becoming a mentor, and the requirements of educational preparation programmes (or courses) for registrants to qualify as mentors; and also the criteria for sign-off mentor (SOM), practice teacher and qualified teacher (for example, nurse lecturer) as other learning support roles. Furthermore, the standards provide details of the specific competencies (or outcomes) that are required to fulfil the roles of mentor, practice teacher and 'Teacher' (the term 'Teacher' refers to nurse or midwife lecturer) effectively. The requirement to maintain a local register of healthcare professionals in these learning support roles and for their continuing professional development (CPD) in these roles are also detailed by the NMC.

Mentoring is a widely taught topic and mentorship courses are provided by most universities offering healthcare courses. Furthermore, for a number of reasons, which include increased appreciation of the value of learning in practice settings for pre-registration nursing students and interprofessional learning, there is an increased demand for mentors and universities are asked to provide more diverse mentorship education programmes, for example by e-learning. This book explores in detail the standards, competence areas and outcomes for effective mentoring.

To do so, the book draws on contemporary knowledge on the dynamics of mentoring across different professions and research and current policies, and aims to enable registrants to acquire the knowledge and skills that are necessary to fulfil all NMC (2008a) standards for mentors. It thus brings together and builds on existing knowledge on principles and practices of mentoring in various arenas, and updates it to current-day mentoring requirements in health and social care. It thus constitutes a firm backdrop for healthcare professionals to further develop and enhance their mentoring expertise.

Recently qualified healthcare professionals who might not yet be functioning in a formal mentoring capacity (associate mentors, for instance) should also find this book useful, as also might more experienced qualified health professionals who either have not completed a mentoring course or who were prepared for the role through a previous 'teaching and assessing' course.

This book is a direct result of my numerous years of experience of teaching and examining on mentoring and 'teaching and assessing' courses, as well as my experience as a registered nurse in adult nursing and mental health nursing, along with the need for a textbook that reflects current policies and research findings on mentoring comprehensively. In addition to current knowledge in the field, this textbook also recognises the challenges facing both newly qualified and more experienced mentors, often doing so within resource constraints, role changes and changing healthcare workforce profile. It confronts the day-to-day and longer-term issues and challenges in mentoring, and explores potential solutions, where possible supporting them with relevant theories, frameworks and current research base. The ensuing implications with regard to responsibility and accountability are also necessarily explored.

The Structure of this Book

As just indicated, this book is firmly based on current knowledge in the field and is structured to ensure that it also addresses all NMC's (2008a) standards for mentors. These standards, which can apply to other healthcare professions as well, are based on the recognition that all RNs' and RMs' roles include teaching and supporting learning. Then, approximately a year after qualifying as a healthcare professional, they would participate in an educational preparation programme for the mentor role, some years afterwards maybe for the practice teacher role, and later perhaps for the 'Teacher' role. The NMC refers to this continuum as a developmental framework for supporting learning.

Standards for mentors and other teachers have been available for almost two decades. They have been revised a few times, and the current NMC's *Standards to Support Learning and Assessment in Practice* policy document was published in 2008. These now well-established standards are detailed under eight domains of competence and associated outcomes that are different for mentors, practice teachers and qualified teachers. Universities have been implementing these standards in their mentoring programmes since 2007. This textbook focuses on the content of the eight domain areas identified by the NMC (2008a) and the outcomes for mentors.

Chapter 1 begins by examining mentoring as a theme in its own right. It starts by identifying the exact nature of the term 'mentor', and differentiates it from other similar or overlapping roles. It thus examines role boundaries between various healthcare learning facilitation roles such as preceptors, clinical supervisors, practice teachers, link lecturers and practice education facilitators (PEF), and mentoring in allied health professions. The common aim of all these roles is to facilitate healthcare profession students and learners to acquire clinical competence and knowledge, especially during practice placements.

A range of different rationales for the mentoring role are then identified, which is followed by the factors that enable mentors to fulfil this role effectively, including the modes of communication that enable mentors to build effective working relationships with their learners. Subsequently, the necessary personal and professional attributes of effective mentors, including being role models, are explored. The nature and detrimental effects of poor or adverse mentoring are also discussed, followed by an examination of different models of effective mentoring.

After an exploration of the nature of mentoring, *Chapter 2* takes a detailed look at how learning occurs. It examines why and what learners learn, significant different perspectives on learning, teaching and education, and learning theories, styles and approaches in healthcare professions, including use of learning contracts, as well as the special education needs of students with disabilities.

Chapter 3 builds on these dimensions of the concept, and explores facilitation of learning. The chapter starts by ascertaining the range of people whom healthcare professionals teach, followed by the reasons for teaching and learning. It then focuses on various ways in which healthcare students learn patient or service user care delivery skills, and how the mentor utilises opportunities for informal teaching.

The concept facilitation of learning, as distinct from the teaching, is examined, followed by key perceptions and major views and approaches in teaching, including andragogy. The levels and stages of skill acquisition (taxonomy levels) are explored, and the types of knowledge associated with skills, for example practical knowledge and theoretical knowledge, are considered, along with levels of theory acquisition.

Steps in lesson planning for structured short teaching sessions for teaching skills and knowledge on a one-to-one level or for teaching small groups of learners or peers are then discussed. This is followed by an examination of different teaching methods and the use of different teaching aids.

Following on from facilitation of learning, *Chapter 4* focuses on the attributes that make practice settings effective learning environments, and on ways in which mentors can maintain and enhance the learning ethos. The NMC indicates that the mentor should create and develop opportunities for students to identify and undertake experiences to meet their learning needs. Students' perspectives on practice placements such as their own expectations and their practice objectives are considered, and then an examination is made of the part played by national guidelines and current policy documents on practice placements. Issues related to practice placements are also examined.

Research related to clinical learning environments, which underpins the development of the tool for annual educational audits of practice placement areas, is then examined. Educational audits include ascertaining the psychosocial ethos and the availability of learning resources (human and material) for facilitation of the acquisition of practice competencies by healthcare profession students. The utilisation of learning pathways (based on patient journeys), which can be incorporated into learning contracts and can play an important role in ensuring the success of the placement, is also explored, as well as the concept of work-based learning.

Fundamental to mentorship are safe and effective clinical practice, evidence-based practice (EBP), research implementation, practice development and management of change. Therefore, how the mentor engages with these activities constitutes the focus of *Chapter 5*, as research, and the NMC standards for mentorship, firmly indicate that the role of the mentor incorporates full awareness and close monitoring by the mentor of their own standards of patient or service user care.

It is therefore incumbent upon the mentor, especially as a role model for mentees, to practise evidence-based care, which the mentor can do by utilising various sources of evidence such as electronic databases where systematically reviewed research evidence is stored. Hierarchies of evidence are then examined in detail, along with identifying, critical evaluation, implementation and dissemination of research findings.

One of the principal purposes of mentor education programmes is to equip course participants with the capability of assessing students' clinical competence. Ongoing assessment of competence of healthcare students is a fundamental component of the mentor role, and is therefore a component of all educational programmes for skill-based healthcare professions, and this is the area that *Chapter 6* focuses on.

To fulfil this key mentor function effectively, the mentor needs to know and understand the principles and processes of assessment – i.e. what assessments are, the various reasons for assessment of competence, who assesses and when, and differing ways in which they are conducted – and also have a good understanding of the student's pre-registration programme and how to implement the approved assessment requirements (mentors may be required to assess students on a specific competency using two methods such as direct observation and questioning).

As to what assessments are, various definitions of assessment are examined, followed by the specific aims of assessments. Then, under how to assess, in addition to different methods of assessment, the chapter explores key principles of assessments, including dimensions of assessment, as well as levels and fairness of assessments. Student self-assessment and peer assessment are also explored. Validity and reliability as crucial attributes of assessments are then explored in some detail, the aim being to ascertain the assessee's fitness to practise. Furthermore, the management of assessments is explored, along with techniques for giving useful feedback and the documentation of assessments. Pass or fail criteria are examined, followed by the signing-off proficiency role.

Recent research findings have highlighted various day-to-day problems encountered by both mentors and students in relation to assessment of competence during practice placements. Therefore, the mentor needs to exercise leadership, which includes forward planning the mentee's learning and assessment and also averting problems of assessment. *Chapter 7* delves into the details of various potential problems that could occur with assessments, such as those detailed by Phillips et al. (2000) and Gainsbury (2010), and how they should be prevented or resolved. The ethical and legal implications of assessments are also examined.

The mentor's accountability, responsibility and the use of 'professional judgement' are also addressed in the context of the mentor's leadership role. In addition, supporting the student, who is generally perceived as struggling to progress with their placement learning, is examined, including the role of action plans and reassessment of the learner. Monitoring ways in which intra- and inter-mentor reliability are achieved, is also explored.

The facilitation of learning and assessment of learners' competence are therefore essential components of the mentor role. *Chapter 8* concentrates on the evaluation of these components. The nature and purpose of evaluation amount to the mentor self-monitoring the quality of their mentoring. The chapter therefore considers what evaluation is, who is involved in evaluation of learning facilitation and assessment, and how it is performed, including the use of models of evaluation. The challenges of facilitation of learning and assessment are examined, followed by an examination of the mentor's ongoing professional development, incorporating details of continuing professional development, mentor updates and triennial reviews and lifelong learning.

Each chapter in the book begins by identifying the chapter outcomes, followed by the main text, a chapter summary and suggestions for further reading. A logical combination of text, illustrations, activities, reflection points and case studies are incorporated to engage the reader fully with the material in the book.

How to Use this Book

To examine the knowledge base, skills and attitudes required for effective mentoring and the NMC's standards for mentors, this textbook adopts an analytical and interactive style throughout the book, with a clear focus on the means of application of principles and theories of mentoring to various practice settings. Therefore, through activities and reflection points, the reader is encouraged to explore and apply concepts to their own practice and roles.

The activities usually ask the reader to consider a particular point or component and make some notes, whilst reflection points ask the reader to reflect on their own experience and knowledge prior to moving on to the next theme in the text. They thus allow mentors to exercise the freedom and scope to be creative in enabling mentees' learning and assessment of their competence.

A number of case studies have been incorporated into the text as examples of situations that the mentor might encounter so that the reader can explore ways in which they can manage the situation satisfactorily. Furthermore, the information in some of the boxes, for example in Chapter 4's box titled 'Significant characteristics of learners for effective learning', is derived from a number of workshops on mentor preparation programmes. As events evolve, and because different practice settings have their own specific requirements and strengths, feel free to make further notes of your own on other components in addition to those in the boxes.

In summary:

Chapter Outcomes

These identify briefly the key theories and concepts covered in the chapter.

Activities

These ask you to consider a particular point and make some notes. They are not compulsory, but they endeavour to enable you to apply or explore the theories or concepts to mentoring in your practice setting.

Ask you to reflect on your own personal experience and potential actions, but can also be discussed with a peer or in a small group.

Text boxes

These highlight numerous aspects of a key theme.

> **Templates**
>
> These are examples of tools that you can use with your own students when you qualify as a mentor.

. . . .

Are examples of situations that you may encounter when you become a mentor, as they are based on previous actual mentoring situations.

. . . .

Chapter Summaries

These remind you of the key points addressed in the chapter that you have just read or worked through.

Further optional reading

Carefully selected learning material that will enable you to expand your knowledge further with regard to key themes in the chapter.

Companion Website
Lively presentation of further aspects of the mentor role.

The term 'healthcare professionals' is used in the text to signify all healthcare employees, medical and non-medical, including nurses and allied health professionals who hold a qualification that is recognised by either their national regulatory body (for example, the NMC) or professional body. The term 'learner' is used to refer to everyone who wants or needs to learn healthcare skills, whilst 'students' are those learners who are actually following a professional education programme leading to a university qualification. The Glossary just before the Index defines a range of other terminologies that are integral components of this book.

The UK reader is strongly advised to have a good look through the NMC's (2008a) policy document *Standards to Support Learning and Assessment in Practice*, which essentially provides a sound framework for effective mentoring.

1

Effective Mentoring

Introduction

Chapter Outcomes

On completion of this chapter, you should be able to:

1 Distinguish between mentoring and similar roles that support learning for healthcare students and learners.
2 Explain a range of reasons for requiring mentors to facilitate students' acquisition of professional competence.
3 Identify and evaluate a number of factors that can enable effective mentoring, including the characteristics and roles of effective mentors, and the ability to build sound mentor–mentee 'working' relationships.
4 Analyse the likelihood and effects of poor or adverse mentoring, and the actions that can be taken where it is likely to occur.
5 Analyse a number of approaches, guidelines and frameworks for enabling informed and systematic mentoring.

One of the key mechanisms for facilitating learning for healthcare profession students while on practice placements is mentoring. This mechanism is well established now and is indeed a very important component of pre-registration education programmes, albeit using a handful of different titles by different health and social care professions. Policy documents such as *Standards to Support Learning and Assessment in Practice* (NMC, 2008a) provide a firm indication of the criteria that healthcare professionals have to meet to use the title 'mentor' and detail the capabilities that they need to fulfil the role effectively.

The first chapter of this book focuses on mentoring as a concept in its own right, defines and differentiates it from similar and overlapping roles and titles, examines the various reasons for mentoring and explores how to mentor effectively. It also examines poor mentoring and how it can be redressed.

The chapter thus examines a wide range of perspectives on mentoring itself and also focuses on the NMC's (2008a: 50) domain 'establishing effective working relationships'. The related mentor competence is: 'Demonstrate effective relationship building skills sufficient to support learning, as part of a wider inter-professional team, for a range of students in both practice and academic learning environments'. The NMC's outcomes for this competence are:

- Demonstrate an understanding of factors that influence how students integrate into practice settings.
- Provide ongoing and constructive support to facilitate transition from one learning environment to another.
- Have effective professional and interprofessional working relationships to support learning for entry to the register.

The Concept of 'Mentoring'

'Mentoring' as a concept and practice for facilitating learning in healthcare settings has evolved consistently since the 1970s and was formally implemented in pre-registration nursing and midwifery education in the 1980s. Slightly different titles and terminologies are used by different healthcare professional groups for this role, and different definitions have been offered over time as research and expert opinions have influenced the forms in which it is currently utilised.

It is generally well documented, for example in the *Shorter Oxford English Dictionary* (Brown, 2002: 1747), that the term 'mentor' originates from the Greek classical story *The Odyssey*, in which King Odysseus called on a trusted friend named Mentor to act as the guide and advisor to his young son Telemachus when he left for another country to fight a war. The word 'mentor' also relates to the Latin word '*mens*', that is, pertaining to or occurring in the mind (Simpson and Weiner, 1989: 614). The term has gradually evolved to signify a designated person who dedicates some of their time to help individuals to learn during their developmental years, to progress towards and achieve maturity and establish their identity. It has been implemented as a formal role in nurse education to direct focus on enabling students to gain safe and effective clinical practice skills during practice placements. This section disentangles the concept of mentor from similar titles by exploring the differences and similarities between them.

Distinguishing between the mentor's and related roles

The mentor role is just one of several that support learning in practice settings and therefore there is some overlap in certain aspects of such roles, such as in the characteristics of the appropriate personnel who support learning, but there are distinct boundaries as well. For instance, a study conducted by Carnwell et al. (2007) to explore the likely differences in the roles of mentors, lecturer–practitioners and link lecturers indicate that mentors tend to focus principally on individual students, lecturer–practitioners on the 'learning environment', and link lecturers on knowledge acquisition and fulfilling course requirements.

Activity 1.1   Different education support roles and functions

To begin with, make notes on what you think are the meanings and functions of the following roles: mentor, preceptor, clinical supervisor, assessor and other similar roles that you have encountered, and the differences between them.

You are likely to have identified a variety of roles that enable or support learning for students and other learners in practice settings, which might include practice facilitators and even the university-based course director. In addition to the above roles for supporting learning, other roles such as buddy and coach are also emerging (the latter is discussed later in this chapter). All the same, although there are common elements in the definitions, scope and remit of mentor and similar roles, there are also differences. The most popular learning support roles are examined next.

Mentor

Beside the helping function during developmental years indicated by dictionary definitions of the term 'mentor', as a result of research by Phillips et al. (2000) on behalf of the then English National Board for Nursing, Midwifery and Health Visiting, the Department of Health (DH) (2001a: 6) redefined 'mentor' as 'a nurse, midwife or health visitor who facilitates learning, supervises and assesses students in the clinical setting'. Prior to this, the mentor was a registrant who facilitated learning, and the assessor was another registrant who assessed students' competencies.

Mentor is similarly defined by the NMC (2008a: 45) as a registrant (i.e. qualified nurse or midwife whose name is on the NMC's live register) who has met the outcomes of Stage 2 (being those of a qualified mentor) and who facilitates learning, and supervises and assesses students in practice settings. The DH's (2001a) definition resulted from a range of issues related to mentoring and assessing pre-registration student nurses and midwives during practice placements that had been identified by Phillips et al.'s (2000) research and contemporary smaller studies such as Spouse's (2001a), which revealed that the terms 'mentorship', 'preceptorship' and 'supervision' were being used synonymously.

Going beyond definitions of mentor, the NMC (2008a) identifies a range of day-to-day functions of the mentor in terms of 26 outcomes that are grouped under eight domains (these form the major focus of this book), which essentially is a framework for effective mentoring. The NMC's functions of mentors build on existing knowledge of the subject area such as research by Kerry and Mayes (1995) that indicates that definitions of mentor need to include:

- nurturing
- role modelling
- functioning (as teacher, sponsor, encourager, counsellor and friend)
- focusing on the professional development of the mentee and
- sustaining a caring relationship over time.

A subsequent concept analysis of the mentor role by Billay and Yonge (2004: 573) across several health, non-health and social care professions indicates that its defining attributes include 'being a role model, being a facilitator, having good communication skills, being knowledgeable about the field of expertise, and needing to understand the principles of adult education'. A more recent concept analysis of mentoring by Hodgson and Scanlan (2013) reveals that mentoring is associated with increased job satisfaction and staff retention, which is beneficial for the mentee, mentor, organisation and nursing profession, as ultimately the patient benefits. Mentoring empowers mentors and mentees, which 'enhances employees' motivation and professional development … [and] … a culture and workplace is created in which nurses want to come to work' (ibid.: 392).

It has to be noted at this point that although the term 'mentor' is clearly defined in UK policy documents, in particular by the NMC (2008a) and the DH (2001a), it is defined differently in nursing in other countries, such as in Canada (Billay and Yonge, 2004), and in various countries the term 'preceptor' is used to signify a role that in the UK is referred to as 'mentor'; and in some countries, the formal mentor role does not exist.

Even in the UK, in the medical profession (NHS England, 2014a), 'mentor' refers to qualified healthcare professionals being mentored by more experienced mutually selected colleagues. Also, in some UK professions, for instance psychologists, the term 'protégé' is used when referring to the mentee (for example, Barnett, 2008).

Preceptor

In the UK, the term 'preceptor' is identified by the NMC (2006a) as a first-level registrant who has had at least 12 months' (or equivalent) experience within the same area of practice as the practitioner requiring support, and will normally have completed a mentor or practice teacher educational preparation programme. The NMC indicates that the preceptor and the preceptee should agree between themselves about the nature of their working relationship and the specific desired outcomes. It should be noted, however, that preceptorship is not clinical supervision, which in the UK refers to structured peer support for, and by, registrants during their careers.

The preceptor role emerged from the realisation that for newly qualified nurses, the transition from being a student to becoming a registered healthcare professional is a major leap in responsibility and accountability. It is partly based on an earlier study by Kramer (1974) who found that the first few months after qualifying were often marked by dramatically conflicting value systems, between the aims of pre-registration education and the reality of day-to-day nursing. This led to high attrition rates among newly qualified nurses. Various studies reveal such concerns even today (e.g. Marks-Maran et al., 2013).

The NMC (2006a) recommends preceptorship for all newly qualified registrants, for RNs changing their area of practice and for qualified nurses from other European Economic Area states and other countries. It indicates that for preceptorship to be effective it should last approximately four months, and recommends that the preceptor should:

- facilitate the transition of the 'new registrant' from student to a registrant who is confident, effective and up to date with their practice and knowledge
- provide feedback to the preceptee on those nursing or midwifery interventions that they are performing safely and effectively, and those that they are not (if any)
- facilitate the preceptee to achieve the standards, competencies or objectives set by the employer for new registrants.

Structured preceptorship programmes are devised locally by trusts or their departments and are normally of four to six months' duration, and often include the specialism-specific competencies in the induction programmes for the particular practice setting, which, when achieved, the preceptee can incorporate into their professional portfolio.

Lately, drawing partly on the successful implementation of preceptorship in Scotland through the *Flying Start* (NHS Education for Scotland, 2014a) pilot schemes, which started in 2006, the DH (2010a: 11) redefines preceptorship as:

> A period of structured transition for the newly registered practitioner during which he or she will be supported by a preceptor, to develop their confidence as an autonomous professional, refine skills, values and behaviours and to continue on their journey of lifelong learning.

It identifies a preceptor as: 'a registered practitioner who has been given a formal responsibility to support a newly registered practitioner through preceptorship' (DH, 2010a: 6). The DH presents a framework for effective preceptoring, within which it also identifies the 'attributes' of an effective preceptor, which are similar to those of mentors, as discussed later in this chapter.

The College of Occupational Therapists (COT) (2013) suggests four standards for preceptors namely: (1) working with clients; (2) working with colleagues; (3) written communication; and (4) health and safety policies. Professional development needs to be achieved in conjunction with *NHS Knowledge and Skills Framework (NHS KSF)*

(DH, 2004a) dimensions along with indicators that progress through the four levels that can then form the basis for developmental activities for individual occupational therapists, which is also congruous with competencies that they will require for their future careers.

Furthermore, the NMC (2014) has been exploring the appropriateness and feasibility of whether the point of completion of the preceptorship programme can comprise the point of 'validation' for the healthcare professional when they have their name and qualification entered in the NMC's register, which can subsequently be followed up by regular revalidation (currently known as PREP: post-registration education and practice) at re-registration points.

Assessor

The term 'assessor' remains in use and is often used to denote a role similar to that of the mentor but solely with the assessment component (DH, 2001a). It usually refers to an appropriately qualified and experienced health or social care professional who has undertaken relevant educational preparation to develop skills in assessing students' level of attainment related to the stated practice competencies (for example, National Vocational Qualifications (NVQ) assessor).

Clinical educator

The role of the clinical educator is akin to mentoring and is generally used by some healthcare professions such as medicine and physiotherapy for facilitating student learning during practice placements. In physiotherapy, for instance, a clinical educator is: 'A qualified practitioner who directly supports a student's learning during clinical education/practice-based learning. Also applies to the clinician's education role in relation to other learners (for example junior staff)' (Chartered Society of Physiotherapy (CSP), 2004: 20).

Practice teacher

The title or role of practice teacher was initially specifically adopted in recognition of the additional educational preparation required for mentoring students on specialist community public health nurses (SCPHN) courses. A practice teacher is therefore: 'A registrant who has gained knowledge, skills and competence in both their specialist area of practice and in their teaching role, meeting the outcomes of stage 3, and who facilitates learning, supervises and assesses students in a practice setting' (NMC, 2008a: 46). It refers to specialist areas of practice where they support students undertaking a specialist qualification or at a level beyond initial registration.

Practice teachers therefore facilitate learning and assess post-qualifying students on their achievement of specialism-specific specialist or advanced practice competencies. However, practice teaching, practice learning and student supervision are terms that are also used for mentoring student social workers, during practice placements for instance (Parker, 2010).

Clinical supervisor and clinical supervision

Clinical supervisor is a term used in the context of clinical supervision signifying the provider of peer support to the clinical supervisee. It may be used to identify mentoring-type roles in some healthcare professions or vocations.

Clinical supervision itself refers to a peer-support role based on a clinically focused professional relationship between healthcare professionals in which one party is the clinical supervisor and the other the supervisee. The clinical supervisor undergoes educational preparation for this role and utilises clinical knowledge and experience to assist peers to develop further their own knowledge, competence, values and practices.

Waskett (2010: 12) notes that 'many nurses do not have regular, protected access to confidential conversations about the everyday challenges of their work', and amongst the various models of clinical supervision that are available for a systematic approach to this activity is Waskett's 4S model, comprising: structure, skills, support and sustainability.

Supervisor and supervision

The term 'supervisor' tends to be used in the context of management of workers to ensure designated tasks are completed, and to a specified standard, rather than in relation to the facilitation of learning. It refers to individuals in the organisation who have authority in the interest of the employer to recruit staff for specified posts, assign duties, oversee the quality of their work and take relevant professional development or disciplinary actions as appropriate.

In this book, the term 'supervision' is used in accordance with its dictionary meaning, which is to direct or oversee the performance, action or work of another, which in this instance refers to the mentor directing and overseeing the mentee's learning. The term does, however, have a very specific meaning in the field of counselling, in which it refers to counselling situations wherein one or more highly experienced counsellors help a less experienced or more junior counsellor develop their practice.

In a comprehensive exploration of the concept and applications of supervision in health and social care professions, Hawkins and Shohet (2012) refer to supervision as a joint endeavour in which the identified supervisor helps the supervisee to improve the quality of their work and continuously develop themselves and their practice. The British Association for Counselling and Psychotherapy (BACP) (2013) indicates that all counsellors, psychotherapists, supervisors and their trainers have an obligation to use regular and ongoing supervision to enhance the quality of the services they provide, and to commit to updating practice by seeking training and other opportunities for continuing professional development, which is also accessed independently of any managerial relationships. An effective interpersonal relationship is essential in both of the above-mentioned interpretations of supervision, and a thorough investigation of mentoring shows that the underpinning principles of supervision apply to mentoring as well.

Practice education facilitator and practice educator

The practice education facilitator (PEF) role in nursing and midwifery also emerged largely from the study of mentors by Phillips et al. (2000). It is defined by the DH (2001a: 6) as a 'role of the teacher of nursing, midwifery or health visiting who makes a significant contribution to education in the practice setting, coordinating student experiences and assessment of learning'. The PEF thus leads the development of practice learning and provides support and guidance to mentors and others who contribute to the student's learning in practice settings, and achievement of practice competencies (see, for example, Sykes et al., 2014). An alternative title has been implemented for PEFs who are based in non-NHS nursing homes as Care Home Education Facilitator (CHEF) (NHS Education for Scotland, 2014b).

The educational preparation for the PEF role is usually at postgraduate level, for a post that was previously funded mostly directly by the pre-2013 Strategic Health Authorities, most of whose functions were taken over by NHS England (2014b) in 2013. It generally entails practice-based teaching and supporting practice learning four days a week, and university-based work one day a week. This is a very important role as PEFs are also called upon to attend to students during practice placements when busy clinical staff are unable to dedicate sufficient extra attention to students who are struggling or are failing to make progress with their practice placement competencies. For students on practice placements, PEFs frequently also organise dedicated group discussion sessions away from the practice setting for particular categories of students for reflection and peer support purposes.

However, there are small differences in the way in which the role and title are implemented in different health and social care professions. The College of Social Work (2012: 12) for example, defines a practice educator as one who:'… takes overall responsibility for the student's learning and assessment, utilising information from his/her own assessment and other sources', which suggests that the practice educator role in social work (as well as in other AHPs) is largely similar to the mentor role in nursing and midwifery.

As with the mentor preparation programme (NMC, 2008a), some AHPs are fast moving towards the title of 'accredited practice educator', educational preparation for which can be through the taught route based at a higher education institute (HEI), or an experiential learning route (Society and College of Radiographers, 2014). The Society and College of Radiographers keeps a 'Register of Practice Educators to the Society and College of Radiographers', but this is not a requirement by the HCPC at this point in time.

A study by Carlisle et al. (2009: 715) on the impact of the PEF role in Scotland revealed that the PEF role is 'accepted widely across Scotland and is seen as valuable to the development of quality clinical learning environments, providing support and guidance for mentors when dealing with "failing" students, and encouraging the identification of innovative learning opportunities'. However, McArthur and Burns (2008), amongst others, have evaluated the role of PEFs and found that whilst various staff think that PEFs should work with students, the PEFs themselves feel that their main role is in supporting mentors, as also noted by Sykes et al. (2014).

Personal tutor

Each pre-registration student is allocated to a nurse lecturer who acts as a personal tutor to the student. This role normally lasts for the duration of the three-year under-graduate course and involves:

- supporting, advising and monitoring students' progress throughout the educational programme
- accessing students' practice records for required information, within an ethos of confidentiality and professional accountability
- liaising with the mentor, link lecturer and student and, where concern is expressed, considering evidence and developing an action plan with the student.

Link lecturer

The link lecturer is usually a university lecturer whose responsibility is to assist clinicians in named practice settings. They assist mentors to interpret students' practice competencies and are available to support mentors when required. They might also assist in the development of the practice setting as a more effective learning environment for all learners. Students tend to receive a visit by the link lecturer early in the placement, especially first year students, to ascertain which learning objectives are realistically achievable. Further visits are arranged as required.

Some of the functions of the personal tutor and the link lecturer have increasingly become part of the PEF's remit but they continue to provide an essential complementary function.

Mentoring activities in allied health and social care professions

The role of practice educator in AHPs was examined briefly in the above paragraphs. Naturally, enabling students and learners to acquire skills for safe and effective practice prevail in all health and social care professions. In addition to knowledge gained from research and the planned activities of professionals to enable learning, professional and regulatory bodies provide informed guidance on how this can be achieved. For instance, several healthcare profession organisations publish separate profession-specific standards for mentors, such as the College of Operating Department Practitioners' (CODP) (2009) Standards, Recommendations and Guidance for Mentors and Practice Placements.

The HCPC's (2012a) *Standards of Education and Training Guidance* provides guidance on the design of pre-qualifying AHP education curricula, which is supported by specific standards of proficiency (SOP) for each of the 16 allied healthcare professions (HCPC, 2013) that it currently regulates, including chiropodists/podiatrists, clinical scientists, dietitians, radiographers, etc.

In addition to the role of the radiography practice educator that was referred to earlier in this chapter, the HCPC identifies the 'practice placement educator' as:

'A person who is responsible for a student's education during their period of clinical or practical experience' (HCPC, 2012a: 61). It indicates that 'Practice placement educators must have relevant knowledge, skills and experience' to support students and provide a safe environment for effective learning. The HCPC, however, does not currently set specific requirements about the qualifications and experience that practice placement educators must have to fulfil the role effectively. But some AHPs have formalised mentoring/clinical educator activities, as for example physiotherapy has done through the Accreditation of Clinical Educators (ACE) Scheme (CSP, 2014).

The titles 'practice placement educator' and 'practice placement coordinator' are also utilised in various AHP documents with reference to designated healthcare professionals who provide support and information to clinical educators (akin to the mentor role in nursing and midwifery), and also monitor the standards of practice placement being experienced by students (HCPC, 2012a).

Hinton (2009) reports on her experiences of mentoring Operating Department Practitioners' (ODP) students in which she indicates that it is an activity that is beneficial for students as well as for ODP mentors. In contrast, Mallik and McGowan (2007) completed a scoping exercise on the nature of practice education in five healthcare professions, namely dietetics, nursing, occupational therapy, physiotherapy and radiography, and concluded that although there are areas of good practice, 'these do so against the provision of well-supported, clearly supervised and adequately quality-assured practice education' (ibid.: 58). They recommend that such issues should be resolved by the various healthcare professions and need to be recognised and rewarded, and that collaborative work across the professions should be enhanced for achievement of more well-rounded practice education.

On the other hand, Lakasing and Francis (2005) argue that because a number of healthcare profession lecturers are not active clinicians, this tends to create a theory–practice gap that mentors have to redress during student practice placements, unlike medical academics who are also practising doctors. They indicate that mentors should therefore be provided with protected time and extra remuneration to enable them to fulfil this demanding role more effectively. Where extra funding is made available for mentoring activities, the money can be utilised to employ additional pro rata staff to allow the mentor protected time for more effective mentoring.

Lack of funding for mentorship in general medicine in the USA was also identified in a study by Luckhaupt et al. (2005). However, Barton (2006) reports on a study that explored the experiences of doctors mentoring students on nurse practitioner courses, and concludes that medical mentors (clinical educators) experience conflict in that as the students acquire new clinical skills and roles, this also amounts to the mentors feeling that their traditional medical authority is being challenged. This led to a renegotiation of professional boundaries between nurse practitioners and doctors.

In summarising this section on mentor and similar roles, it is clear that there are areas within these roles that overlap, and there are distinctions between them when current national policy and professional bodies' definitions are considered. However, as these roles evolve and different models of implementation are applied in different settings, endeavouring to disentangle the educational philosophy underlying these roles – such as differentiating between coaching and mentoring – is seen by Megginson et al. (2006: 5) as a 'sterile debate'.

Why Do Learners Need Mentors?

The mentor role is widely implemented and utilised and it may now appear to be an obvious facility afforded to learners. A more detailed examination of why we need mentors for mentoring students and learners reveals a number of reasons.

Activity 1.2   Why mentors?

The idea of this activity is to explore the variety of reasons why mentors are required in healthcare professional education, particularly in the context of the prevailing definition of the term. Therefore, consider and make notes on the question, Why do we need mentors (and preceptors) in: (a) nursing, midwifery and allied health professions; and (b) personal life? List as many reasons as you can think of.

When students on mentoring courses are asked to cite as many reasons as they can think of for requiring mentors, they tend to be able to identify several. The reasons given include the need to ensure safe practice by learners, to enable students to achieve their course practice competencies, and to listen and act as a sounding board for any worries or fears or the mentee's ideas on care delivery. Further reasons cited by students for mentoring learners in: (a) nursing, midwifery and allied health professions, and (b) personal life are listed in the box below.

Why we need mentors

In nursing and other health professions

- For guidance and support
- To structure working environment for learning
- For constructive and honest feedback
- For debriefing related to good/bad experience during placement
- As a link person with other areas
- As a role model
- To assess competence
- As a friend and counsellor
- For encouragement

- To provide the appropriate knowledge base for nursing interventions
- For questioning
- For protection from poor practice
- To build confidence
- For sharing learning, i.e. learning from each other
- It is an NMC requirement
- To keep your own skills and knowledge up to date
- For linking theory to practice
- For developing one's work skills in teaching and explaining
- To provide structured learning programmes during practice placements

In personal life

- For the development of one's self
- To share experiences
- For encouragement
- To build up confidence
- For honest opinions and views
- As a role model (may be a parent figure, etc.)
- For socialisation
- For support and guidance

One of the advantages of mentoring is that students who have been on placement in the particular practice setting might apply for a post in that setting after qualifying, i.e. they can have recruitment benefits. Furthermore, van Eps et al. (2006) explored the benefits of mentoring in a study that evaluated students' perceptions of mentorship and concluded that mentorship does enable the development of competent practice, especially if it is founded on supportive longer-term mentor–mentee relationships.

It could be argued that everyone could benefit from having a 'mentor' in their personal lives, at times referred to as a 'soulmate'. This privileged role is self-selected by both parties and could be fulfilled by a friend, partner, parent or senior peer. It is consistent with the definition of mentor in current medical mentoring, which suggests that the mentor is selected by the learner for support and guidance. In addition to the reasons for mentoring identified by student mentors and the above-mentioned benefits, there are also various research and policy reasons for the requirement for this role. The most significant ones for healthcare are now discussed.

First, mentoring has become an increasingly popular concept in a wide range of settings, for example:

- In schools and other educational institutions – for initial teacher training.
- In business – to support personal development of business skills, human resource strategies, and business development and self-employment. Further guidance on business mentoring in the UK is available from the Institute of Directors.

- In support of young people who are, or are at risk of becoming, disaffected or excluded from society – to raise achievement, self-confidence, personal and social skills.
- Medical mentoring – as for a doctor or medical student receiving guidance from an identified more senior or experienced colleague on a range of work-related matters.
- Management mentoring – incorporates coaching, and is discussed later in this chapter.

Thus, mentoring has already been implemented quite effectively in non-healthcare professions and social contexts. For instance, mentoring has worked successfully in initial teacher training (see, for example, Furlong and Maynard, 1995; Kerry and Mayes, 1995) for some time. The concept has developed continuously in this context since then, and international journals such as *Mentoring & Tutoring: Partnership in Learning* report on the latest developments and research on various aspects of the concept. Harrison et al. (2006: 1055), for instance, conducted an analysis of mentoring new teachers in secondary schools and found that: 'best practice for "developmental mentoring" involves elements of challenge and risk-taking within supportive school environments with clear induction systems in place and strong school ethos in relation to professional development'.

Furthermore, Barnett (2008: 3) notes that mentoring new teachers results in benefits for the mentor as well in terms of professional stimulation and collaboration, personal fulfilment, friendship and support, motivation to remain current in one's field and networking opportunities; and benefits to the institution include more satisfied staff and greater scholarly productivity.

As for medical mentoring, whilst in other countries, for example the USA, medical mentoring refers to mentoring medical students, in the UK the mentoring relationship is confidential between two qualified doctors, the mentor and the mentee (NHS England, 2014a; Viney and McKimm, 2010), and is more akin to clinical supervision in nursing, midwifery and AHPs, which was explained earlier in this chapter. For this, doctors adopt the Standing Committee on Postgraduate Medical and Dental Education's (SCOPME) definition of mentoring, which is:

> the process whereby an experienced, highly regarded, empathic individual [the mentor], by listening and talking in confidence, guides another individual [the mentee], often but not always working in the same organisation or field, in the development and re-examination of the mentee's own ideas, learning, personal and professional development. (McKimm et al., 2007: 15)

A second reason for the need for mentoring is the one identified when nurse education moved into the higher education sector en masse during the 1980s and 1990s with the restructured Project 2000 pre-registration curricula and a change in emphasis in certain aspects. The findings of various research studies on these novel programmes were eventually captured in the United Kingdom Central Council for Nursing,

Midwifery and Health Visiting's (UKCC) (1999) *Fitness for Practice* publication. This publication documented the strengths of these programmes, but one of the prominent findings of these studies was that at the point of registration students were not clinically as skilled as those who emerged from pre-Project 2000 programmes. This reinforced the need for wider availability of competent clinically based mentors to enable students to learn clinical skills so that they are 'fit for practice'.

The *Dearing Report* on learning in higher education, and other related national reports, also strongly advocates that higher education courses should enable students to become fit for practice, fit for purpose and fit for award (National Committee of Inquiry into Higher Education (NCIHE), 1997).

Third, the findings of Kramer's (1974) study mentioned earlier indicated the need for preceptors for newly qualified nurses. The notion was extrapolated to pre-registration students and is also a reason for the introduction of the term 'mentor' in the UK in the 1980s as a means of supporting student nurses with their learning during practice placements.

Fourth, the standards or codes of professional (or good) practice for nurses, doctors, social workers and AHPs usually indicate that qualified practitioners have a duty to facilitate students' learning during practice placements so that students develop their competence under supervision (for example, NMC, 2015: clause 9.4). Similar requirements feature in healthcare professionals' job descriptions, which are also guided by the *NHS KSF* (DH, 2004a).

Mentoring of course also provides registrants with an opportunity to teach, which in itself is a feature of their own professional development and can constitute a stepping stone in their own career trajectories.

Yet another reason for mentoring is the concept of work-based learning, which constitutes practice-based development of skills and (practical) knowledge. Its main features are reflected in the social learning theory that was constituted by Bandura (1986, 1997), and which centres on learning skills by observing skilled professionals perform them first. Social learning theory therefore also involves mentors being role models, and comprises four processes of learning (see Figure 1.1).

FIGURE 1.1 The four processes of learning

In more detail, the four processes of learning that the learner goes through are:

1 Observation of skilled performance

- The individual observes a skilled performance ('modelling stimulus').
- The observed behaviour is seen as useful and distinctive.
- Observer's level of arousal pertaining to the skill is raised.
- Observer is keen to learn the skill.
- Observer has previously felt positive reinforcement for learning skills.

2 Mental retention of the skill

- Step-by-step performance of the skill is mentally assimilated.
- Mental rehearsal of modelled behaviour.

3 Motor reproduction of the skill

- Observer carries out observed behaviour or skill, and self-evaluates it in terms of performance.

4 Reinforcement and adoption

- The behaviour is reinforced by external reward such as praise or through self-reinforcement, and is likely to be adopted.

According to Bandura (1986), we do not possess any inherent behaviour patterns at birth except reflexes, and therefore learning occurs by observing other people, which is the essence of social learning theory and which therefore includes learning from social situations. In healthcare, learners (mentees and preceptees) learn and acquire practical skills from mentors and other healthcare professionals through the four processes identified in Figure 1.1.

Bandura's (1986) social learning theory had previously been termed 'observational learning' or 'modelling', and was built on behaviourist learning theory (see Chapter 2). It is a component of work-based learning, a concept that is examined in some detail in Chapter 4 in the context of learning in practice settings.

Yet another reason for mentoring is that it can be effective in management mentoring, which is an activity wherein trainee managers are mentored by named highly experienced managers to enable those less experienced to develop their management skills (for example, Megginson et al., 2006). Waters et al. (2003), for instance, report on a very successful tailored mentoring programme for newly appointed nurse managers where mentees can choose their mentors.

Activity 1.3 Management mentoring

All nurses and the majority of healthcare professionals have a management and organisation of care role. Some healthcare professionals opt to develop their careers as clinical managers. Explore with a band 6 colleague how management mentoring is utilised informally, and possibly formally, to enable healthcare professionals to develop as clinical managers.

Brooke and Ham (2003) also report on a successful programme that enables managers to develop their leadership skills. A small number of healthcare professionals have had experience of management mentoring, which on occasion is referred to as 'management coaching'. This is a longer-term role than mentoring pre-registration students on practice placement. The management mentor role can initially take the form of a coach that advises the mentee to explore utilisation of particular management techniques, and takes a more directive approach. When the mentee has developed substantial management skills, the role can become more akin to a mentor's, i.e. less directive; and much later mentor–mentee activities become more akin to those of 'buddies', i.e. equals.

Mentoring and coaching

Other learning support roles that utilise aspects of mentoring have been identified by various agencies, some of which are still developing, and include *practice facilitator*, *buddy*, *coach* and *co-tutor*. The more developed terms 'coach' and 'coaching' tend to surface sporadically in nursing. Coaching itself is defined as 'the art of facilitating the performance, learning and development of another' (Downey, 2003: 21, cited in Byrne, 2007); and the Chartered Institute of Personnel and Development (CIPD) (2013: 1) indicates that:

> Coaching targets high performance and improvement at work and usually focuses on specific skills and goals, although it may also have an impact on an individual's personal attributes (such as social interaction or confidence). The process typically lasts for a relatively short period.

'Performance', 'specific skills' and 'goals' are key common words used in determining a common understanding of the term coaching, which in turn usually incorporates a more directive and prescriptive approach. This term and title, however, is more closely linked to sports, which involves training coachees using individually tailored programmes aimed at enhancing their physical performance so that they are able to take part in competitions in specific sports. Other prominent areas include life coaching (enabling the coachee to live a healthier and more fulfilled life); health coaching (enabling individuals with long-term conditions such as chronic obstructive pulmonary disease (COPD) to self-care; and business coaching (guiding someone who is starting their own business for the first time and helping them to succeed).

Reporting on the findings of an audit of a new role termed 'clinical coach', whereby an appointed academic coaches underachieving (referred to as 'marginal' or 'at risk') student nurses during practice placements, Kelton (2015) indicates that a systematic approach to clinical coaching can significantly enhance students' successful completion of the placement. Clinical coaching entails the appointed clinical coach providing additional support and guidance to the identified student. Another application of coaching in healthcare is management coaching, to guide more junior registrants to develop their management and organisation of care skills, whereupon the coaches are very experienced more senior healthcare managers enabling coachees to develop skills through one-to-one guidance and support that can enhance their management and leadership performance in the organisation (for example, Haidar, 2007; Coleman and Glover, 2010). It also applies to more senior managers such as he Executive Nurse receiving coaching from independent appropriate personnel.

Furthermore, there are endeavours to institute management and leadership coaching for healthcare students on their final practice placement at the end of their course when in addition to consolidating their patient or service user care skills, they also learn the practicalities of organising and managing care in the practice setting (for example, Eades et al., 2005), that is they begin to learn management skills. Management activities are identified by Gopee and Galloway (2014), some of which the third year student can learn, include:

- delegation of duties
- supervising care delivery
- organising transfers of patient care
- receiving/giving reports on patient/service users care needs and progress
- working with multidisciplinary team (MDT) members
- doing the off-duty/facilitating self-rostering
- managing space, i.e. extra beds/patients on trolleys
- ensuring the health and safety of staff/patients/visitors.

The competencies that student nurses or midwives have to learn have been identified by the NMC (2010a) for instance, and the GROW model (also referred to as: GROWing – which stands for Goal, Reality, Options, Will/Wrap up) is advocated (for example, Connor and Pokora, 2012) as a framework for effective coaching. There are several other books on coaching, and short courses and modules are available from various organisations.

Who Can Be a Mentor?

Despite all the reasons for mentoring discussed so far, it should not be taken for granted that all qualified healthcare professionals wish to undertake mentoring work, for all or even some of the time. Some healthcare professionals feel that continuous allocation of students to them all year round can be detrimental to their own effectiveness with their workloads, and they would like some space for reflection and to focus on their own professional development.

In the selection of mentors, it is important to ensure that they have the necessary skills and expertise for mentoring, which according to Neary (2000a) include coaching, counselling, facilitating, setting standards, assessing and giving feedback. Other writers and researchers identify similar lists of skills. Such lists initially appear simplistic but a whole range of expertise is required to undertake the mentorship role, and this can usually be developed through appropriate educational preparation.

In some professions, such as in medicine in the UK, the very definition of mentor suggests that students should be able to select their mentor. However, in reality, in healthcare professions, students on practice placement do not usually have the opportunity to select their mentors due to various factors such as RNs' increased workload. Nonetheless, there are situations when mentees are encouraged to or have the option to choose their mentor, such as if they go back to a particular practice setting for a second placement later in their course.

There are occasions when RNs may be able to select one individual to whom they can relate throughout an entire programme as a personal mentor or a 'buddy'. On the other hand, the NMC (2008a) also identifies the criteria for who can be mentors for nursing and midwifery students, which are as follows:

- Be registered in the same part or sub-part of the register as the student they are to assess and, for the nurses' part of the register, be in the same field of practice (adult, mental health, learning disability or children's nursing).
- Have developed their own knowledge, skills and competence beyond registration, and have been registered for at least one year.
- Have successfully completed an NMC-approved mentor preparation programme, or a similar previous programme.
- Have the ability to select, support and assess a range of learning opportunities in their area of practice for students undertaking NMC-approved programmes.
- Be able to support learning in an interprofessional environment – selecting and supporting a range of learning opportunities for students from other professions.
- Have the ability to contribute to the assessment of other professionals under the supervision of an experienced assessor from that profession.
- Be able to make judgements about [the] competence of NMC students on the same part of the register, and in the same field of practice, and be accountable for such decisions.
- Be able to support other nurses and midwives in meeting continuing professional development (CPD) needs in accordance with *The Code: Standards of Conduct, Performance and Ethics for Nurses and Midwives* (NMC, 2008b). [The NMC (2008b) Code has since been superseded by NMC (2015) *The Code: Professional Standards of Practice and Behaviour for Nurses and Midwives.*]

These criteria clearly imply that not all registrants are suitable for mentoring, at least not for all categories of learners. The competencies and outcomes for mentors are discussed next.

How to Mentor

In a systematic review of mentoring, Jokelainen et al. (2011) concluded that mentoring comprises two main themes. These are, first, facilitating student learning and, second, strengthening students' professionalism (professional attributes and identities). Four subthemes were deduced as well as a number of categories under each subtheme. Thus, the principles and methods of mentoring incorporate a number of factors that are essential for effective student learning. They include meeting NMC's (2008a) standards for mentors that are identified under eight domains, these being:

1 establishing effective working relationships
2 facilitation of learning
3 assessment and accountability
4 evaluation of learning
5 creating an environment for learning
6 context of practice
7 evidence-based practice
8 leadership.

The first domain, 'establishing effective working relationships', encompasses:

- how effective working relationships are developed and maintained
- effective mentor–mentee communication
- characteristics of the mentor
- actions by the mentor that support learning.

Each of the other domains is addressed separately in subsequent chapters as detailed in the introduction to this book.

Effective working relationships

In a study conducted by Johansson et al. (2010) to measure the quality of teaching and learning in practice settings, it emerged that the supervisory relationship between mentor and mentee is the most important factor contributing to effective clinical learning experiences. Eller et al.'s (2014) study of effective mentor–mentee relationship concluded that there are eight components to this, including open communication and accessibility, mutual respect and trust, and role modelling.

However, for two individuals who are usually initially unknown to each other, adopting the mentor–mentee roles presupposes that they are able to communicate with each other, develop a rapport and cultivate a 'working' relationship at the very least. The word *rapport* means 'a state of deep spiritual, emotional or mental connection between people', including understanding and empathy (Brown, 2002: 2465), and *relationship* refers to 'the state or fact of being related, an emotional association between two people' (Brown, 2002: 2520).

The requirement for effective working relationships is recognised by the NMC (2008a). But how are relationships formed between two designated parties? According to Rogers and Freiberg (1994), counsellors and helpers build a trusting and working relationship by ensuring first of all that certain key conditions prevail. These conditions are:

- *Acceptance (or unconditional positive regard)* – of the individual for who they are, that is, for their individual strengths and weaknesses; and mutual respect.
- *Genuineness* – as a person, honesty.
- *Empathic understanding* – being able and willing to view situations from the other person's perspective.

These key conditions are explored in some detail in the context of student-centred learning in Chapter 3. Rogers and Freiberg (1994) emphasise that 'trust' underpins these key conditions, which they suggest in reality permeate all mutually beneficial relationships. It is akin to a 'psychological contract' between the mentor and mentee, or between patient and carer, or colleagues and friends. The two parties also have to be willing to spend time together to maintain this relationship and to work towards the achievement of practice objectives, for instance. Although the mentee has to actively seek out relevant learning opportunities, the mentor also needs to take actions that support the mentee's learning, for example by familiarising themselves adequately with the mentee's educational programme.

Effective mentor–mentee communication

The skills and techniques of communication are some of the most important tools the practitioner undertaking the mentoring role has to utilise. The healthcare professional is normally already a skilled communicator in healthcare settings through initial educational preparation, and therefore it is important to establish which other communication techniques they need to develop in order to extend their skill base. Effective communication skills are essential within all teaching and learning situations.

Various modes of communication are available to the mentor to choose from, including:

- written, for example handwritten, typed, emailed, faxed, printed
- oral (spoken), for example face to face, one-to-one, in groups, by telephone
- non-verbal, for example body posture, eye contact, tone of voice.

Oral (spoken) communication is always accompanied by non-verbal messages, vocal and non-vocal. In fact, non-verbal hues are more powerful than verbal messages. Furthermore, Argyle (1994) suggests that non-verbal signals of a friendly attitude (as opposed to an unfriendly attitude) are:

- *proximity*: closer, leaning forward if seated
- *orientation*: more direct, but side to side for some situations
- *gaze*: more gaze for each other, and mutual gaze
- *facial expression*: more smiling
- *gestures*: head nods, lively movements
- *posture*: open arms stretched towards each other rather than arms on hips or folded
- *touch*: more touch in an appropriate manner
- *tone of voice*: higher pitch, upward contour, pure tone
- *verbal contents*: more self-disclosure.

After reflecting on a former framework for non-verbal communication referred to as SOLER (which stands for: 'sit squarely'; 'open posture'; 'lean towards the other'; 'eye contact'; 'relax'), Stickley (2011) suggests that the framework (or model) can be enhanced by using the acronym SURETY (which stands for 'sit at an angle'; 'uncross legs and arms'; 'relax'; 'eye contact'; 'touch'; 'your intuition'). This latter model incorporates the function of touch as a means of non-verbal communication, and intuition. Normal communication processes however are often presented as the information processing theory in the context of cognitive learning theory, which is dicussed in Chapter 2.

Generic and specialist communication skills

In addition to general communication skills, the mentor is likely to need to develop specialist communication skills to manage more complex mentee issues. Scammell (1990) suggests a communication continuum that spans generic communication at one end to specialist communication at the other, with the associated specific purposes and specific skills for each component on the continuum. These components and their associated purposes and skills are as follows:

Primary communications	*purpose*: initial contacts with others; brief encounters
	skill: simple interpersonal or social skills, e.g. ability to listen, etc.
Secondary communications	*purpose*: ongoing relationships – verbal, non-verbal, written; informal support groups
	skill: interpersonal or social skills, knowledge of how groups work, etc.
Advice giving	*purpose*: to offer factual information; to teach, instruct, supervise
	skill: when to give advice, ability to impart knowledge of subject area, etc.
Primary counselling	*purpose*: support for friend or work colleague
	skill: listen non-judgmentally, help with problem-solving, etc.
Secondary counselling	*purpose*: therapeutic counselling for specific mental health problems
	skill: advanced accurate empathy, self-disclosure, etc.

Primary and secondary communication occurs between mentor and mentee when exchanging information and establishing a working relationship. Beyond this level, the mentor may need to give direct advice to the student, especially when teaching, as well as when advice is requested. This, however, does not go as far as counselling, for which the individual requires more extensive training.

Primary counselling is a specialised communication skill that the mentor needs to develop to deal with difficult mentoring situations. Secondary counselling will be required for more intense psychological problems, which the mentor can deal with by directing the student to appropriate support services, or, if trained, by using a systematic approach such as Heron's (1989) six-category intervention analysis (see the box below).

The six-category intervention analysis as a
specialised communication skill

Authoritative intervention

- Prescriptive: giving advice
- Informative: imparting information
- Confrontational: directly challenging

Facilitative intervention

- Supportive: understanding and encouraging
- Cathartic: allowing the release of emotions
- Catalytic: encouraging deeper exploration

Heron's (1989) six-category intervention analysis therefore entails six possible actions that the counsellor can choose from. In difficult mentor–mentee situations, for every interaction, the mentor may decide which of the six categories is most appropriate. For instance, for a student who frequently claims to be feeling unwell, physically or psychologically, the mentor might use the prescriptive category of helping, and advise the mentee to consult the occupational health department. They might also give further information about where the department is, and the likely outcomes of this situation. In other situations, the mentor might use another one of the categories, for example cathartic, to enable the mentee to elaborate in detail how they feel about a patient whom they have looked after but who has passed away rather suddenly, for instance.

Ways in which the mentor can usefully apply Heron's model of intervention towards their mentees are discussed in Chapter 7.

Mentors' characteristics and roles that support learning

In addition to effective communication skills and the ability to form effective mentor–mentee relationships, various researchers have examined the characteristics and roles of mentors that play crucial parts in enabling the mentee's learning during practice placements.

Characteristics of mentors

Activity 1.4   Characteristics of an effective mentor

Make a list of what you consider to be the characteristics of a registrant who is effective in their mentoring role for either undergraduate or postgraduate students. Consider their characteristics from such perspectives as personal qualities, approach/actions and skills.

Responding to Activity 1.4 must have been straightforward as all healthcare professionals who have undertaken preparatory educational programmes that include practice placement will have encountered mentors. Some mentors may have been excellent, while there might have been reservations about others. Most of the characteristics identified by groups of student mentors are listed in the box below.

Characteristics of the person who is an effective mentor

- Patient
- Open-minded
- Approachable
- Has a good knowledge base
- Knowledge and competence is up to date
- Has good communication skills, including listening skills
- Provides encouragement
- Is self-motivated
- Shows concern, compassion, empathy
- Has teaching skills
- Provides psychological support
- Counsellor

- Tactful
- Diplomatic, fun and fair
- Willing to be a mentor
- Versatile, adaptable, flexible
- Allows time and commits self to it
- Confident
- Enthusiastic
- Advisor
- Is honest and trustworthy
- Trusting
- A role model
- Non-judgemental
- Resource facilitator
- Able to build working relationship

Drawing on their study of students' perspectives on the qualities of the effective mentor, Gray and Smith (2000) list several characteristics, many of which are also identified in the box above. In another study of the personal characteristics of mentors, Huybrecht et al. (2010) concluded that the perceived characteristics of mentors include:

- ability to give feedback
- make time available for mentee
- positive attitude
- transferring of enthusiasm onto students in spite of workload, lack of time, etc.
- closer follow-up of new developments
- teaching ability
- sharing of experiences.

From their concept analysis of mentoring, Hodgson and Scanlan (2013) identified the characteristics of effective mentors as: approachable, knowledgeable, honest, friendly, patient, experienced, enthusiastic, willing to spend time with the mentee, have a strong belief in the mentee's capability, they challenge, support and encourage a mentee, but also expect the mentee to be willing to learn, be career committed, competent, and have strong self-identity and initiative.

Roles of mentors and enabling functions

In addition to personal characteristics of mentors, other researchers explore the 'roles' of mentors. The roles of mentors refer to what mentors do to enable or facilitate mentees' learning. Deducing from an earlier substantial study on various aspects of mentoring, Darling (1984) identified fourteen roles of mentors that enable learning. These roles are being a(n):

- role model
- energiser
- envisioner
- investor
- supporter
- standard prodder
- teacher–coach

- feedback giver
- eye-opener
- door-opener
- ideas bouncer
- problem solver
- career counsellor
- challenger.

Taking a broader perspective, Hall et al. (2008) explored mentors' perceptions of their role in teacher training in the USA and found that it comprises nine roles and responsibilities for supporting learning of individuals engaged in teacher training. These roles are:

- parent figure
- trouble shooter
- scaffolder
- counsellor
- supporter
- instructional model
- coach or guide
- source of advice
- a sounding board for concerns about teaching.

Activity 1.5 Ascertaining mentorship potential

Consider Hall et al.'s (2008) or Darling's (1984) roles of the mentor, and identify situations from the past when you needed to be in these mentoring roles, or will be in forthcoming mentoring opportunities.

1 For each role, do a self-rating of yourself as a mentor using the numbers 1 to 4, with 1 indicating development or learning need and 4 indicating skilled.
2 Next, focus on one or two of the roles on which you rate yourself as low, and consider why this is (e.g. lack of opportunity), and how you can develop your competence in that role.

The above exercise based on roles of the mentor is also referred to as 'measuring mentorship potential' (MMP) (Darling, 1984). Of course, the teacher mentor has to be a role model in teaching in the first place, and in healthcare the mentor has to be a role model as a healthcare professional, i.e. as a clinician, as well. Alternatively, with reference to research mentors in medicine, Tobin (2004) identified seven roles of the physician-researcher: as teacher, sponsor, advisor, agent, role model, coach and confidante.

Each of these mentor roles can be explored in detail as a concept in its own right, and to illustrate this, the next section explores the features of being a 'role model' and then of 'challenger and supporter' that were identified by Darling.

The mentor as the role model

Various research studies indicate that mentors should be role models for their mentees (for example, Tobin, 2004; Billay and Yonge, 2004; Darling, 1984).

<table>
<tr><td rowspan="2">Reflection Point 1.1</td><td>

A role model

Consider the terms 'model' and 'modelling'. Next, consider what a role model is. Consider also why healthcare professionals need to be role models, who else for, and what it is about a person that makes him or her a role model.
</td></tr>
</table>

In response to Reflection Point 1.1, you might have felt that a mentor who is a role model is someone who fulfils NMC's (2008a) standards for mentors, as identified earlier in this chapter. Although the mentor would be a role model predominantly for clinical skills, they should also be a role model as an organiser of care, a researcher and a teacher within the parameters of their post.

As with most nascent and tentative concepts, a concept analysis or a STEP (social, technical, economic and political) analysis can enable further clarification of the concept, and a systematic understanding of various facets and components of the concept. Alternatively, a SWOT (strengths, weaknesses, opportunities and threats) analysis can be undertaken. Such an analysis can help the individual decide whether any problem-solving, avoidance or developmental actions need to be taken.

Activity 1.6   STEP analysis of role model

Using the headings 'social', 'technical', 'economic' and 'political', conduct a STEP analysis of 'the mentor as a role model'.

Being a role model is a feature of Bandura's (1997) social learning theory, which stipulates that substantial learning occurs as a result of observation of appropriate professionals. Bahn (2001) suggests that role modelling is consistent with social learning theory, as substantial socialisation occurs in clinical learning environments. It is also a significant component of 'work-based learning', which is discussed in Chapter 4.

There can also be bad role models, that is, how not to come over as a healthcare professional. Bad role models can therefore not be seen as a model at all, considering what the word 'model' means. A role model is 'an exemplary person, a perfect exemplar of excellence' (Brown, 2002: 1806), that is, someone whose practice standards, attitudes and beliefs can be emulated by the observer. Individuals choose their role models, such as someone who is good at time management, at self-organisation or at how they interact with colleagues.

Donaldson and Carter (2005) report on an evaluation of the perceptions of undergraduate students on role modelling within the clinical learning environment. They indicate that students stressed the importance of good role models whose competence they could observe and practise. Constructive feedback was needed on their practice from their role models to develop their competence and build up their confidence, and to convert observed behaviour into their own behaviour and skill set.

Faugier (2005a) suggests that role models are those whom we look up to, emulate and admire as professionals, but in society in general, she suggests, people base their character identities, values and lifestyles on celebrities and characters in television programmes. All teachers in the practice setting (for example, mentors) should therefore be aware of their impact as role models on students' learning of skills and professional attitudes.

Thomas (2005) reports that there are mixed views about nurses being role models of healthy habits when off duty, and therefore a certain level of self-awareness of one's public behaviour is necessary to keep their credibility as role models intact.

The mentor as a challenger and supporter

During their practice placements students are likely to encounter patient or service user situations that they find challenging, and being a 'challenger' is one of the roles of the mentor identified in Darling's (1984) research, and other situations that they will find much less challenging especially in the latter part of their pre-registration programme as they acquire various clinical skills. How much support (also a mentor role according to Darling) should the mentor provide to the student when the latter encounters very challenging situations?

Mentoring support and challenge

Consider the mentor's roles as 'supporter' and 'challenger', and think of patient or service user care situations (or clinical interventions) in your workplace that, say, a second year student will find highly challenging, and others that will be much less challenging. Often mentors have to comment on the level of initiative that their

(Continued)

Reflection
Point 1.2

(Continued)

mentees show. So think for yourself (or discuss with a peer) if the mentee encounters highly challenging patient or service user care situations, what level of support you would provide your mentee.

What is the result if the student consistently encounters situations that are of 'low challenge' to them?

Of course, students have to be supervised all the time, either directly or from a distance. There are various examples of situations that present high or low challenges for learners in practice settings, and the level of support required. Asking a third year student nurse consistently to perform clinical skills for which they have already been signed as competent would provide a lesser challenge to them, and lesser support might be required. But if the same student has not yet learnt how to provide care in epidural pain control, for instance, then this would present a higher challenge and the student is likely to need a high level of support.

Daloz (1989) explored these two mentor roles further and concluded that high challenge and high support can lead to growth and achievement of aspirations (or vision), while low support and low challenge can result in stasis and apathy. However, high challenge and low support, according to Daloz leads to 'retreat and burnout' (see Figure 1.2).

Mentor actions to support learning

The roles and responsibilities of the effective mentor are regularly researched to ascertain the more contemporary nature and perceptions of this function. For example, Carnwell et al. (2007) explored NHS and HEI managers' perceptions of

FIGURE 1.2   The effects of support and challenge on the mentee's development

learning support roles. They found that the mentors' primary role is in clinical practice, their primary skills constituting clinical expertise, teaching clinical skills and
student support, and their primary focus is the individual student, that is student
supervision and the assessment of students' clinical skills. However, they also identified potential for role conflict, particularly if the mentor is relatively recently qualified and therefore still developing their own repertoire of clinical skills.

> ### Activity 1.7   Actions that support learning
>
> In addition to having the characteristics of an effective mentor, think of and make
> a list of a number of actions that can be taken by mentors that support learning.

No doubt a range of components that support learning can be identified. One of the
key functions of the mentor is to help the student integrate into the practice setting,
which entails managing the practice placement, receiving the student and conducting
initial, mid-placement and final interviews, and preferably using learning contracts.
'Acceptance' of the mentee (Rogers and Freiberg, 1994) signifies that the mentor
accepts the student for their current levels of knowledge and competence, which may
be extensive or minimal.

As for managing the placement, the designated mentor would have been nomi-
nated before the student starts on the placement, and would need self-preparation
time beforehand. Time would also have been set aside for receiving the student and
introducing them to the team, and associate mentors may have been identified.

Seeing the practice placement from a student's viewpoint suggests that they
might be experiencing different feelings in anticipation of the placement. They are
likely to appreciate any prior information sent to them, which might include any
preparatory reading that the student can do. On the first day, they tend to appreciate an introduction to the clinical area, making them feel comfortable about learning, a professional but friendly environment, student involvement and continuity
of mentorship. These perspectives are consistent with 'empathic understanding'
identified as a key condition of effective working relationships by Rogers and
Freiberg (1994).

Furthermore, the NMC (2008a) indicates that to enable effective learning, at least
40 per cent of the student's placement time must be spent working with the mentor.
Similar rules apply to the practice teacher role. Moreover, the NMC (for example,
2008a) has identified the need for 'protected time' for mentoring, as has the
Department of Health (1999).

Adverse Effects of Poor Mentoring

A common experience in nursing in the twenty-first century is that nurses working in
many practice settings feel that they are managing their workload with ongoing staffing

constraints. Indeed, Phillips et al. (2000) noted that mentors fulfil their mentoring role as one of several other roles they have during any span of duty. Despite 'protected time' for mentoring having been advocated for over a decade (DH, 1999), the implementation of this mechanism remains slow for many mentors due to the demands on their time. When working within these constraints, knowingly or unknowingly, the mentor may be taking (or omitting) actions that discourage learning.

Activity 1.8   How the mentor might discourage learning

Think of, and make notes on, a range of actions on the part of mentors that, deliberately or not, may be seen as discouraging or disabling learning.

The following case study presents an example of poor mentoring.

Case Study

Poor mentoring

Mel Alexis is a second year student nurse on a rehabilitation ward. One day, she finished her shift early, having told the staff nurse in charge that she had a terrible headache, while in fact she was extremely upset regarding her placement.

That morning she had felt that the staff nurse had spoken to her in a very unprofessional manner, as she does to patients as well. This is what bothered Mel the most. She also challenged the staff nurse over her drug administration that morning. A patient was left her morning medication in a pot on the table, but was unable to swallow it as she needed assistance due to her having a weak side and problems with her other hand. As Mel walked past the patient's room, the patient called her and indicated that she had not taken her tablets yet. As Mel was not the nurse who administered the drugs, she called the nurse to the room for her to administer the drugs. The nurse said that she did not have time to do this but the tablets were correct for the patient.

Mel agreed to assist in giving the medication but noticed three tablets lying on the table beside the pot. Mel asked the nurse what these tablets were and she was advised they were morning medications as well. Mel doubted this as they were not in the medicine pot and asked the nurse why they were not in the pot, but the latter did not give an answer and instead picked them up and put them into the pot. The nurse then told Mel to assist with the medications and Mel made it clear that she did not feel that the medications were correct, as there seemed to be more tablets than the patient usually took in the morning. The nurse told Mel not to question her drug administration, so Mel felt that she had no choice but to assist the patient in taking the drugs.

This event highlighted Mel's unhappiness with this ward. She had started feeling like this on day one when she was not introduced to any staff members or shown around.

She had had to find things out for herself during her time on this ward and if she asked where something was, the staff said it would be quicker for them to get the item themselves rather than show Mel. As a second year nurse, she was expecting to do many nursing activities but instead she felt that she was being treated like a support worker. Although Mel loves providing basic nursing care to patients, she expected a lot more out of this placement than she was actually achieving. Mel appreciates that on a rehabilitation ward nursing takes on a different role but she feels that she has yet to see what this role is.

Mel says she has always wanted to be a nurse and really loves the job, but this ward has now made her question this and it makes her very sad to feel like this.

In response to Activity 1.8, you may have felt that one of the problems that students experience is the lack of opportunities to work with their named mentor. Other actions on the part of mentors that you might have thought of that can discourage learning are:

- lack of interest in students and in their learning needs
- lack of knowledge about the student's course
- lack of evidence-based practice or research utilisation
- hierarchical, and a lack of team approach
- not acknowledging student's previous experience
- negative attitudes
- reluctant to change practice.

There is a possibility that you have yourself witnessed poor mentoring, directly or indirectly. Other problems with mentoring remain prevalent. Earlier research into mentoring and assessing had identified personality characteristics that discourage learning. For instance, Darling's (1985) qualitative study revealed what she termed the characteristics of the 'galaxy of toxic mentors' (see box).

The 'galaxy of toxic mentors'

Types	Features
Avoiders	Mentors who are not available or accessible, also referred to as 'ignorers' or 'non-responders'.
Dumpers	Throw people into new roles or situations and let them flounder, or let them 'sink or swim', often deliberately.

(Continued)

(Continued)

Types	Features
Blockers	Actively avoid meeting the mentee's needs by refusing requests, by controlling through withholding information, or by blocking the mentee's development by over-supervising.
Destroyers/ Criticisers	Set out to destroy the mentee by subtle attacks to undermine confidence, and open and public verbal attacks and arguments, questioning the mentee's abilities, and deliberately destroying confidence.

Source: Darling (1985)

Based on extensive experience in management and decision-making, Heirs and Farrell (1986) explored the mindsets of individual employees who enable an organisation to progress with its aims, and those of people who block such development. While the focus is on looking for, and developing, 'talents' in junior employees, in reality the mindset of some employees can stifle development of juniors and mentees. The researchers grouped the problematic or disabling traits of those who block development as 'three mental poisons', in terms of the functioning of rigid minds, ego minds and Machiavellian minds (see box). Such ways of thinking are not always obvious, nor easily detected, but do affect learning adversely.

The functioning of rigid minds, ego minds and Machiavellian minds

The rigid mind:

- Personal values are set or stereotyped
- Unable to see the positiveness in others' thoughts if they conflict with their own thinking
- Continually blocks the openness of more creative thinking
- Loyal to traditional thinking and rejects novelty
- Appears to lack imagination or creativity
- Stifles use of originality and encourages complacency

The ego mind:

- Sees elements of a problem only in terms of self-interest and self-importance
- Fairly ambitious and has a high opinion of own abilities
- Looks after number one to the exclusion of other considerations

- Pays little attention to what others think and say
- Unsociable and does not contribute to collective thinking
- Will betray colleagues and even the organisation if it serves his or her ends

The Machiavellian mind:

- Quickly sees the range of likely outcomes of any decision
- Manipulates the feelings and ambitions of others to deceive
- Devious and calculating
- Intimidates and engages in politicking
- Perpetuates worry in the organisation and perpetually currying favour with superiors
- Scheming, cunning and suspicious of subordinates

Source: Heirs and Farrell (1986)

Mentoring was formalised with increased emphasis with the introduction of diploma in higher education programmes in Nursing (Project 2000) (UKCC, 1999). In this context, Gray and Smith (2000) conducted a study to explore students' experiences of mentoring, and found that whilst effective and good mentoring did prevail, the majority of students also experienced poor mentoring, as some mentors:

- break promises
- lack knowledge and expertise
- have poor teaching skills
- have no structure to their teaching
- 'chop and change their minds'
- allow students to observe only (i.e., not participate)
- are unclear about their students' capabilities
- throw students in at the deep end
- delegate unwanted jobs to students
- dislike their job and/or students
- may be disliked by other members of the team
- are distant, less friendly, unapproachable
- intimidate the students
- have unrealistic expectations.

Activity 1.9 Mentors who disable learning

Discuss with a peer or in a small group why any mentor would behave in the negative ways described by Darling or Gray and Smith. Discuss also if and how such behaviours can be changed.

Darling (1985) makes a number of suggestions on how to deal with 'toxic' mentors. For instance, if the particular mentor–mentee allocation is unavoidable, then the mentee can try and keep the relationship balanced by building a support network with other students or registrants within the team, and drawing on his or her own personal strengths (for instance, problem-solving skills). Heirs and Farrell (1986) suggest that it is the responsibility of the organisation's managers to identify employees who block development and learning. 'Poisonous' thinking endures, but can be changed gradually through formal and informal meetings. Decisions about delegation of responsibilities and roles need to be applied selectively and overseen with appropriate intensity or leniency.

At times, mentors are ineffective because of a lack of detailed knowledge of their mentee's educational programme (or course), regarding which the PEF should be able to advise. Other actions that can be taken if ineffective mentoring is detected is to implement co-mentoring, which involves two mentors jointly mentoring the student. Temporary non-allocation of a student to the ineffective mentor is another alternative that might work. Managers can formally or informally ask the mentor how well they feel they are fulfilling their mentoring role. The line manager may be able to confront the ineffective mentor if poor mentoring has been observed, or a complaint received. There can be other alternative strategies, but they will be dependent on local circumstances. Ethical aspects of poor mentoring are discussed in Chapter 7.

Approaches and Models of Effective Mentoring

Despite the multiplicity of likely mentor behaviours that could inhibit learning, mentoring remains a necessary role for supporting learning in healthcare professions. A mentor in personal life is also advocated. Due to the humane, personal and suffering-prevention nature of healthcare provision, professional education programmes need to be appropriately structured and carefully monitored. Mentoring students must also be a structured or planned exercise, as discussed earlier in this chapter. An appropriate combination of directive and facilitative approaches may be adopted, depending on the knowledge and competence that the student displays.

The underlying principles on which each mentor bases their mentoring vary according to the personal beliefs and approaches of the mentor towards this role. The underpinning beliefs of the mentor about student learning therefore determine their approach to mentoring, and the model or framework of mentoring they use.

The differences between the terms *approach*, *model* and *framework* are as follows. 'Approach' to mentoring is personal to the mentor and is based on his or her own life and professional experiences, and personal views and beliefs. In mentoring, it would depend on the mentor's beliefs about nursing, undergraduate course design, student and learner populations and their styles of learning.

A 'model', however, can be defined as a research-deduced, and therefore informed, set of interrelated components that enable the activity to be addressed comprehensively. A 'framework' takes this further, whereupon the components of the model are utilised as sections or headings for planning and implementing the activity, and may even have been empirically tested.

All three perspectives indicate a planned and systematic approach to the mentee's placement experience to make it more effective. Few frameworks for mentoring in healthcare are currently available. Darling's (1984) roles of the mentor constitute such a model, the NMC's (2008a) eight domain standards for mentoring are another. Despite the pragmatic nature of frameworks, it is important to examine other approaches and models of mentoring that are available, such as those identified in the box.

Approaches, models and frameworks for mentoring

Approaches to mentoring

Classical mentoring	Also known as informal or primary mentoring. A natural, mutual and self-chosen relationship that can usually be terminated by mutual decision.
Reflective practitioner	Based on learning theories, e.g. andragogy, styles of learning and student-centred approaches, the mentor is a critical friend and co-enquirer.

Models or frameworks of mentoring

Apprenticeship model	The mentor as skilled crafts person, and the mentee learns by re-enacting their actions.
Competence-based model	The mentor enables the mentee to learn specific practice objectives, and assesses their competence in them.
Team mentoring model	A team of mentors mentor one or more students jointly, as recommended by Phillips et al. (2000), for instance. Is akin to team supervision for doctorate students.
Contract mentoring	Formal mentoring that is time- or objectives-restricted, e.g. when on practice placement at another institution.
Pseudo-mentoring	Also known as quasi- or partial mentoring, may be in appearance only and for a specific task, e.g. dissertation supervision.

A model is of course useful if it can be used as a framework for action. Kerry and Mayes (1995) tend to use the terms 'strategies', 'approaches' and 'models' interchangeably. They suggest four models of mentoring, namely the:

- *colleagual model* – similar to team mentoring or the use of associate mentors
- *counselling model* – refers to facilitation of learning using humanistic theories (discussed in Chapter 2)
- *professional model* – similar to the contract model, for example for a student on a practice placement, or in dissertation supervision (i.e., for a specific task)
- *process model* – also referring to facilitation of learning but enabling the mentee eventually to become an independent practitioner.

Activity 1.10   Application of models of mentoring

In your own experience of mentorship, which of these approaches, models or frameworks apply to learning professional skills in your own practice setting, and why? Which ones suit you most? Make some notes.

It could be argued that often the apprenticeship model applies more to the training of support workers in that an apprentice normally learns skills and crafts at the level of task performance, along with associated practical knowledge, unlike the holistic psychobiosocial approach taken by nurses and midwives. The competence model might apply to nursing but the reader needs to be aware of varying definitions of the term 'competence'. Some definitions see competence as the ability to perform a skill in accordance with agreed procedures and incorporate practical knowledge, while others see it as including theoretical knowledge as well.

The reflective practitioner approach is one that is frequently favoured within health profession circles, and advocates the mentor taking a less directive approach to their practice-based teaching. Consider the following reflective recording in the portfolio of a student social worker called Sheila.

Case Study

Sheila's portfolio

I visited Mr J while his care coordinator, who is also my practice supervisor, was on annual leave. At this time Mr J expressed concern about his care coordinator and questioned her supportive abilities. My initial reaction was to explain that different practitioners would use different approaches, and advised him to raise the issue with the care coordinator. In a further conversation by telephone, Mr J reiterated the issue but in a more agitated manner and asked me to speak to the care coordinator. His care coordinator suggested that we visit Mr J to question him about what he actually wanted from the service and what type of support he felt she should offer. She felt Mr J didn't always engage with services (he frequently missed appointments), and that his drug-addiction problem was the issue he most needed to address, but which she did not specialise in. Mr J was receiving services from the drug team but, again, he didn't always attend his appointments. However, it was clear Mr J felt he needed more support. As a result we discussed a referral to an agency which provided outreach support specifically for people with a history of offending and drug/alcohol abuse problems. Mr J was keen to accept this support.

....

Reflective recordings from clinical situations provide an essential learning vehicle for mentees. The approaches and models presented in the box above titled 'Approaches, models and frameworks for mentoring' may not all be seen as frameworks, although they can be systematic and comprehensive. Most of the approaches are relatively recent concepts that await further empirical exploration or testing. Other frameworks and models of good practice are identified as specific sets of actions for specific professions, such as in business mentoring (Institute of Directors, 2014). The Royal College of Nursing (RCN) (2002) presents them as the 'responsibilities' of mentors.

Further dimensions of mentoring

To enable healthcare professionals to fulfil their mentor role effectively, especially towards students on pre-qualifying education programmes, they are required to undergo specified educational preparation. They thus have to attend and successfully complete an NMC-approved mentor course. One requirement for such courses is that they address the theory and practice related to the mentor outcomes under the eight NMC (2008a) domains referred to earlier in this chapter.

Fulton et al. (2007) explored the international literature for the content of mentor programmes and concluded that although the NMC domains (they were originally published in 2006) provide an acceptable framework for mentoring, it is reasonable to expect each country to be able to adapt the framework according to their own national and local needs.

The NMC (2008a) indicates that educational preparation for mentors needs to be at a minimum academic level 5 (Quality Assurance Agency for Higher Education (QAA), 2008), although most of these programmes are at degree and postgraduate levels (levels 6 and 7, respectively). They tend to be equivalent to 200 to 300 hours of student learning and are normally completed within four months. Mentor courses may be available with accredited CATS points or without, but in both cases the NMC's (2008a) standards are met and the level of critical analysis that student mentors engage in has to be at minimum level 5. Continuing learning for mentors subsequent to successful completion of a mentor preparation programme is discussed in Chapter 8.

Furthermore, as noted earlier in this chapter, mentoring is now an activity that is widely applied in various healthcare and non-healthcare fields and can take different forms. Previously, mentoring in nursing, and currently in medicine (NHS England, 2014a), comprised mentors and mentees being mutually selected for their respective roles by the two healthcare professionals for facilitation, guidance, assistance and support with student learning. The notion that students can select their mentor has currency in some situations, such as if the named mentor's job changes at short notice.

Gilmour et al. (2007) report on a highly successful peer-mentoring programme in which second year student nurses mentor first year students as they embark on their pre-registration university courses. Furthermore, a small-scale study by van Eps et al. (2006) suggests that year-long mentorship programmes yield more beneficial outcomes for students in terms of the variety of skills that they acquire through the longer-term relationship than the usual shorter-term ones.

Long-arm mentoring is another activity that tends to prevail primarily in certain areas of primary and social care where the mentor is not generally based at the same healthcare site as the mentee, and yet all criteria and activities comprising effective mentoring are fulfilled. Electronic or e-mentoring can also be implemented successfully, as demonstrated by Stewart and Carpenter (2009), whereupon the mentor and the mentee communicate entirely through their computers.

Moreover, increasingly, as interprofessional working and interprofessional learning is being systematically operationalised, the concept of interprofessional mentoring is also gaining in popularity and credibility. Lait et al. (2011), for instance, document the findings of evaluative research on the concept of interprofessional mentoring, indicating that:

- students learned about the roles of other professions and how to work together to provide patient-centred care
- interprofessional mentoring can be 'threaded' through all clinical placements rather than being offered only once on the three year pre-registration programme, or once a year.

Lait et al. (2011: 213) also point out that the activities that students engaged in varied in complexity and that 'provider commitment' is important. Furthermore, Lloyd-Jones et al. (2007) report on the successful implementation of interprofessional learning (IPL) across the whole curriculum of healthcare profession courses, on campus and in practice settings, and also that it figures in assessment strategies.

However, in a study of students' experiences and staff perceptions of the implementation of placement development teams, Williamson (2009) reports that students indicate a need for more direct, personal and organisational support, and better communication between university and placement areas. Furthermore, research also suggests that the effectiveness of the mentor role also depends on the level of the mentor's interest in mentoring (for example, Hallin and Danielson, 2009).

Chapter Summary

This chapter has focused on mentoring as a concept and professional role, and has therefore addressed:

- Current and recent perspectives on the concept of mentoring; and definitions of and distinctions between the mentor's and various other learning facilitation roles, such as preceptors, clinical educators, assessors and supervisors, practice education facilitators, link lecturers and personal tutors. All these roles are established so as to facilitate healthcare learners to acquire clinical skills, knowledge and appropriate attitudes.

- A number of reasons for requiring mentors to support learning for healthcare students on preparatory education programmes during practice placements, and the criteria for who can be a mentor.
- Effective mentoring, which encompasses effective working relationships; relevant mentor–mentee communication, which includes generic and specialist communication skills; the characteristics of mentors; and ascertaining own mentorship potential.
- Research findings on detrimental effects of poor, inefficient or adverse mentoring, and ways of addressing this issue when it occurs.
- The use of different models or approaches that identify mentors' perceptions of their mentoring role.

📖 Further Optional Reading

1 For an exploration of research on mentoring and coaching in a wide range of settings in the UK and abroad and discussion on a range of perspectives and issues, see:

- Garvey, B., Stokes, P. and Megginson, D. (2014) *Coaching and Mentoring: Theory and Practice*, 2nd edn. London: SAGE.

2 For details of the successful implementation of preceptorship, see:

- Scottish Government (2014) *Flying Start NHS*. Available at: http://www.flyingstart.scot.nhs.uk (accessed 21 April 2014).

3 For an easy-to-follow and yet extensive and well-informed exploration of the concept and practice of supervision, including the qualities needed to be a good supervisor, see:

- Hawkins, P. and Shohet, R. (2012) *Supervision in the Helping Professions*, 4th edn. Milton Keynes: Open University Press.

4 Having examined a range of components of the mentor role in this chapter, whilst also addressing the NMC's mentor outcomes under the domain Establishing effective working relationships, if you are a student mentor, you should now be in a position to identify a selection of evidence that you can provide to demonstrate your competence on the mentor outcomes under this domain. Please see the companion website where a number of items of evidence are identified under each NMC domain.

To access further resources related to this chapter, visit the companion website at https://study.sagepub.com/gopee

2
How Learners Learn

Introduction

Chapter Outcomes

On completion of this chapter, you should be able to:

1 Identify the specific knowledge and competencies that healthcare students learn during their pre-registration education programmes, including different types of knowledge and professional skills.
2 Identify various reasons for learning by different individuals, and the nature of professional competence.
3 Analyse prevailing major views and perspectives on learning, teaching and education.
4 Understand and critically analyse key theories of learning and indicate how they can be applied to learning in practice settings.
5 Comprehend the different styles and approaches to learning and ways in which mentors can adapt their approaches to teaching to match mentees' individual learning styles and approaches.

As patient or service user care interventions are the main part of healthcare professionals' work, an appropriate proportion of their pre-registration education courses are dedicated to developing students' clinical and psychosocial care skills. In the nursing pre-registration course, for instance, which amounts to a total of 4600 hours of learning in three years, the NMC (2010a) requires a minimum of 50 per cent of this learning time to be utilised in learning patient or service user care skills in practice settings (of which a small number of hours of practice learning can be facilitated by 'simulation' in skills laboratories). Learning in practice settings therefore occupies a pivotal role in pre-registration education. Indeed, learning is an ongoing requirement for all healthcare professionals throughout their careers.

Consequently, this chapter and Chapter 3 are based on 'facilitation of learning', which is also one of the eight domains in the NMC's (2008a: 51) standards for supporting learning, and under this domain the NMC indicates that mentors must 'facilitate learning for a range of students, within a particular area of practice where appropriate, encouraging self-management of learning opportunities and providing support to maximise individual potential'. The outcomes for mentors under this domain are:

- use knowledge of the student's stage of learning to select appropriate learning opportunities to meet individual needs
- facilitate the selection of appropriate learning strategies to integrate learning from practice and academic experiences
- support students in critically reflecting upon their learning experiences in order to enhance future learning.

Chapter 2 draws on multiple theories of learning and focuses on ways in which healthcare learners learn the competence and knowledge required for patient or service user care delivery that is safe and effective. Ways in which the mentor facilitates learning are examined in Chapter 3, and how practice settings can also be effective learning environments in Chapter 4.

What Do Healthcare Learners Learn, and Why?

The first section of this chapter begins by identifying the specific knowledge and competencies that learners in healthcare professions learn, in particular during their initial preparatory programmes.

Healthcare competencies

For nurse education programmes, in *Standards for Pre-Registration Nursing Education*, the NMC (2010a) identifies the knowledge and skills that students have to acquire in order to gain the Registered Nurse (RN) qualification. These standards have been implemented since 2011, and are the latest update on sets of standards and competencies that have been developed over a number of years by nursing regulatory bodies. The preceding one was published in 2004.

The NMC (2010a) standards comprise those that all HEIs currently offering pre-registration nurse education programmes have to incorporate in their pre-registration nursing courses. In its 'competency framework', the NMC (2010a) identifies: first, 'generic competencies' that student nurses in all four 'fields' of practice (previously referred to as 'branches') must achieve during their education programme. The four fields are: (1) adult nursing; (2) mental health nursing; (3) learning disabilities nursing; and (4) children's nursing.

Second, the standards identify a set of field-specific competencies. Both generic and field-specific competencies are grouped under the following four domains:

- professional values
- communication and interpersonal skills
- nursing practice and decision-making
- leadership, management and teamworking.

As can be expected, the NMC provides comprehensive details of all areas of competence that students must achieve to be able to have their name entered into the NMC's register as a 'registrant' in the particular field of practice. Under the domain 'Nursing practice and decision-making', for instance, it identifies the generic competencies as well as ten field-specific competencies – a few examples of field competencies under this domain for 'adult nurses' are reproduced in the box.

Field standard of competence for adult nurses under the domain 'Nursing practice and decision-making'

1 All nurses must use up-to-date knowledge and evidence to assess, plan, deliver and evaluate care, communicate findings, influence change and promote health and best practice. They must make person-centred, evidence-based judgements and decisions, in partnership with others involved in the care process, to ensure high quality care. They must be able to recognise when the complexity of clinical decisions requires specialist knowledge and expertise, and consult or refer accordingly.

   1.1 **Adult nurses** must be able to recognise and respond to the needs of all people who come into their care including babies, children and young people, pregnant and postnatal women, people with mental health problems, people with physical disabilities, people with learning disabilities, older people, and people with long term problems such as cognitive impairment.

2 All nurses must possess a broad knowledge of the structure and functions of the human body, and other relevant knowledge from the life, behavioural and social sciences as applied to health, ill health, disability, ageing and death. They must have an in-depth knowledge of common physical and mental health problems and treatments in their own field of practice, including co-morbidity and physiological and psychological vulnerability.

3 All nurses must carry out comprehensive, systematic nursing assessments that take account of relevant physical, social, cultural, psychological, spiritual, genetic and environmental factors, in partnership with service users and others through interaction, observation and measurement.

   3.1 **Adult nurses** must safely use a range of diagnostic skills, employing appropriate technology, to assess the needs of service users.

> 4 All nurses must ascertain and respond to the physical, social and psychological needs of people, groups and communities. They must then plan, deliver and evaluate safe, competent, person-centred care in partnership …
>
> *Source*: NMC (2010a: 17–18)

As can be seen in in the box, there are also sub-competencies identified under some of the competencies. These standards of competence and sub-competencies are then translated into specific practice competencies locally that students will need to achieve during practice placements. No doubt it should prove useful for all mentors to have a hard copy or PDF copy of the whole *Standards for Pre-registration Nursing Education* (NMC, 2010a) document handy to refer to as and when required.

In *Standards for Pre-registration Midwifery Education*, the NMC (2009a) identifies the competencies that midwifery students have to achieve to register with the NMC as 'Registered Midwife' (RM). These standards documents are available free from the NMC. 'Standards of proficiency' for the preparation programmes of the AHPs managed by the HCPC have also been identified in appropriate HCPC publications for each allied health and social care profession that it regulates. The General Medical Council (GMC) and other healthcare regulators publish their own corresponding standards.

In addition to the regulatory bodies' standards, each healthcare profession's professional body, for example the Royal College of Nursing and the British Medical Association, tend to publish further guidance to facilitate implementation of the regulatory body's standards in professional preparation programmes. So other healthcare professions – such as clinical perfusion scientists, dance movement therapists, sports therapists and complementary therapists, who are not yet regulated by the HCPC and generally already have their own separate professional bodies – can join the HCPC at some point through a formal process of application and approval, and thereafter their standards of proficiencies can be identified.

Every two to three years, one or more major organisational inquiry on nurse education publishes its findings and makes recommendations. Because of recent reports of poor nursing care, mainly in the media, the RCN commissioned one such inquiry with the remit to explore the nature of 'excellent preregistration nursing education in the UK' and how it should be delivered. The recommendations of the inquiry, known as the Willis Report (Royal College of Nursing, 2012: 6) includes:

Nursing education should foster professionalism which includes embedding patient safety as its top priority, and respects the dignity and values of service users and their carers.

Patients' safety and dignity are key concepts in this recommendation, and clearly such recommendations directly indicate elements that pre-registration education should cover and that student nurses must learn – see also the section in Chapter 8 under the heading 'Students raising concerns'. The DH's (2013a) *Education Outcomes Framework*

(Gov.uk, 2013) is another prominent publication that is being instituted to influence the content of pre-registration programmes. The framework is a parallel document to the *NHS Outcomes Framework* (Gov.uk, 2014) that was developed as a component of the Health and Social Care Act 2012 (DH, 2012a).

The Act comprised a radical change in the management of healthcare delivery in England ever since its implementation in April 2013. In relation to the education and training of healthcare workforce in England, the Act includes the establishment of Health Education England (HEE) (Gov.uk, 2013) and Local Education and Training Boards (LETB) for overseeing and operationalisation of funding, respectively. The Act also included other policy changes, such as the establishment of clinical commissioning groups (CCG) for commissioning care and treatment and the strengthening of public health activities through instituting *Public Health England*.

Essential skills clusters, care and compassion

The NMC undertakes a number of public and professional consultations to arrive at the content of the pre-registration nurse education programme, and following one of these consultations it was decided to include 'essential skills clusters' (ESCs) within these programmes. These skills are now fully integrated into both nursing and midwifery pre-registration programmes. The NMC Circular 07/2007 (NMC, 2007c: 1) indicates that 'essential skills clusters' are 'UK-wide generic skills statements set out under broad headings that identify skills to support the achievement of the existing NMC outcomes for entry to the branch, and the proficiencies for entry to the register'.

For nursing, there are 42 areas of essential skills that pre-registration students must learn in practice and be assessed on, some by the end of the first year of the programme (first 'progression point'), some by the end of second year, others by the end of third year. The skills are grouped into five clusters, for nursing these being:

1 care and compassion, communication
2 organisational aspects of care
3 infection prevention and control
4 nutrition and fluid management
5 medicines management.

For midwifery programmes, the cluster headings are:

1 communication
2 initial consultation between the woman and the midwife
3 normal labour and birth
4 initiation and continuance of breastfeeding
5 medical products management.

These skills are incorporated into the respective pre-registration programmes. They do not comprise all practice skills that students have to learn to register with the NMC as an RN or RM, but instead they can support the achievement of the set practice competencies for each placement.

ESCs apply to midwifery and to all fields of nursing, and therefore both generic and field-specific ESC skills should be addressed within the context of each of the four fields of practice, which students have to demonstrate competence in by specific progression points.

Care and compassion, which is the first cluster for nursing identified above, is further strengthened by more recent guidance jointly issued by the Chief Nursing Officer for England (CNO) and the Director of Nursing at the Department of Health as they identify the 6 Cs of Nursing (NHS England, 2014c). The 6 Cs stand for: care, compassion, competence, communication, courage and commitment. These concepts therefore also form part of pre-registration curricula, and of practice competencies that mentors enable students to achieve during practice placements. 'Compassion' is examined in some detail in Chapter 5.

The student's learning needs: knowledge and competence

In addition to the placement competencies that students are required to learn, they are likely to have their own aims and thoughts on specific healthcare knowledge and competence that they would wish to acquire during particular practice placements, as adult learners (Knowles et al., 2011). This should be encouraged and explicitly supported, as appropriate.

Students acquire knowledge in, say, human physiology, pharmacology and treatment methods, which is consistent with the generic and field competencies under the four domains identified by the NMC (2010a). The terms *competence* and *competency* are often used in relation to the skills that healthcare students learn. Different types of knowledge are discussed shortly but, first, what do the terms 'competence' and 'competency' mean?

Defining 'competence'

There are conflicting definitions of the terms 'competence' and 'competency' in the literature.

Being competent

Focusing on your own experience of working with colleagues in your healthcare profession, and of students approaching the end of their pre-registration courses, consider what being competent means. For example, which pay band or what amount of experience makes a healthcare professional 'competent'?

Reflection Point 2.1

Although the term *competence* is used rather glibly, it is a term that has several definitions, as identified by Bradshaw (1997) for instance. Benner (2001) sees being competent as being at the midway point in the 'novice to expert' stages of skill acquisition.

This is the point when the learner is deemed able to perform the skill safely and effectively unsupervised, but further learning is required to become 'proficient' or 'expert'.

Benner (2001) suggests that competence is an interpretively defined area of skilled performance identified and described by its intent, function and meanings (as in competency statement). Policy and research documents therefore indicate that the terms *competence* and *competent* apply to the person, that is, the professional's overall knowledge, skills and attitudes and their 'fitness to practise'. The term *competency*, however, applies to specific clinical skills, which in nursing also include the associated knowledge and attitude components.

The NMC (2005a) identifies competence as relating to the student demonstrating their 'capability' in particular skill areas to a required standard at a particular point in time, and that competencies are component skills that contribute to being competent. A widely accepted definition of competence is 'a term used to describe the skills and ability to practise safely and effectively without the need for direct supervision' (UKCC, 1999: 35). The NMC (2010a: 11) defines it as 'the combination of the skills, knowledge, attitudes, values and technical abilities that underpin safe and effective nursing practice and interventions'. Thus, the concept 'competence' is fundamental to the autonomy and accountability of healthcare professionals and therefore also to their codes of practice (for example, NMC, 2015).

The NMC (2004a) sees a competent nurse as one who consistently demonstrates fitness for practice. Essentially, it can be argued that competence implies being able to perform the clinical intervention safely, confidently and effectively according to the approved procedure or clinical guideline and without the need for direct supervision. Others argue that competence refers to ability or capability as well as the associated practical knowledge, and yet others feel that competence signifies manifesting theoretical knowledge as well. As a term that is also used in NVQ and in medical education, its profession-specific definition should be accepted, in that in the former the remit for NVQ courses signifies the ability to perform the relevant skill and having the associated practical knowledge. In medical and non-medical professions, competence signifies having the ability, together with the practical and theoretical knowledge.

Nevertheless, a 'lack of competence' is seen as 'a lack of knowledge, skill or judgement of such a nature that the registrant is unfit to practise safely and effectively in any field in which the registrant claims to be qualified, or seeks to practise' (NMC, 2004a: 3). Peers, managers and employers as well as the general public are expected to report lack of competence through the appropriate channels.

Types of knowledge associated with professional skills

The knowledge required for clinical competence can be grouped or classified in different ways. Schon (1995) notes that healthcare professionals have an accumulated repertoire of knowledge, with mastery over its manipulation, production and application. Benner (2001) identifies practical knowledge and theoretical knowledge, as well as tacit knowledge. She suggests that novices – that is, healthcare professionals who are new to healthcare – are more inclined to use rules and guidelines, such as practical knowledge, while 'expert' healthcare practitioners tend to use intuition more.

Different types of knowledge bases that professionals use can also be viewed from Carper's (1978) 'patterns of knowing' perspective. They are:

- *empirical knowledge*: knowledge derived from research and scientific experiments, which therefore can be measured, tested and corroborated
- *ethical knowledge*: knowledge based on morals and philosophy, but which is usually difficult to test
- *aesthetic knowledge*: knowledge based on sensitivity or intuition, such as in the 'art of nursing'
- *personal knowledge*: knowledge of one's self and how it influences one's professional practice.

Each of these 'patterns' is seen as equally important for healthcare practice and for developing further knowledge. Therefore, in relation to physiotherapy and knowledge regarding hip replacement, for instance, empirical knowledge relates to the research evidence for hip replacement operations, the patient experiencing less chronic pain and a better quality of life afterwards. Ethical knowledge could refer to whether, say, an 80-year-old widow consents to such an operation, and whether it is right to subject her to such a potentially traumatic experience. Aesthetic knowledge refers to the expertise and extensive experience of the physiotherapist to enable the patient to mobilise fully after the operation. Personal knowledge refers to the physiotherapist knowing himself or herself as a person, their preferences and values, and the effect that these might have on their professional practice.

The mentor's role towards the physiotherapy student would be to enable the mentee to acquire skills and practical knowledge, but includes having a good insight into the mentee's level of scientific, ethical and personal knowledge.

In a study exploring whether nurses use knowledge from research findings to inform decision-making, Thompson et al. (2002) found that although colleagues are the more immediate source of information on which to base decisions, they are also a source of research (or data-based empirical) knowledge and useful networks. However, although various decisions made by clinical managers are based on empirical knowledge, other decisions are often influenced by previous experience and intuition.

Major Views and Perspectives on Learning, Teaching and Education

What is learning?

How individuals learn has been researched and defined over a number of years. So what is learning? How do you define 'learning'? Generally, dictionaries provide a broad explanation of the term. For instance, to learn is to 'acquire knowledge (of a subject) or skill as a result of study, experience or instruction; to acquire or develop the ability to do' (Brown, 2002: 1562). More specific definitions have come from philosophers and educational psychologists. The latter generally agree that learning is a process that leads to modification in behaviour or the acquisition of new abilities or responses, and which is additional to natural development, growth or maturation.

Accordingly, Gagné (1983) defined learning as a change in human disposition or capability, which persists over a period of time and that is not simply ascribable to the process of growth. Curzon and Tummons (2013: 11) define learning as 'the apparent modification of a person's behaviour through his activities and experiences, so that his knowledge, skills and attitudes, including modes of adjustment, towards her or his environment, are changed, more or less permanently'.

These definitions tend to concur that:

- learning is reflected in changes in behaviour, physicality and attitudes
- learning occurs in day-to-day life experiences, in addition to planned formal education
- learning a psychomotor skill is permanent in nature in that the individual subsequently has the capacity to perform the skilled act at a future point in time.

Specialist skills may 'decay' mainly due to environmental factors such as changes in medical devices, social values and so on. Learning in healthcare professions is about learning competence and knowledge, the nature of which was discussed earlier. In healthcare professions, learning is a lifelong process of skill and knowledge acquisition and updating them through planned participation in focused reading and structured programmes of study.

Perspectives on learning

Learning experiences are influenced by where the learner 'is coming from', as each person perceives new experiences in a different way, depending on how the new experience relates to the individual's past. However, two opposing views about formal learning are suggested by Ramsden (2003), who identifies learning as either: (a) a quantitative accretion of knowledge, i.e. facts and procedures; or (b) a change in the way in which people interpret and understand the world around them.

However, according to Socrates (2000 years ago), education is not merely transferring knowledge of facts and procedures from 'teacher' to 'pupil'. Rather, it is 'an adventure, an activity of the mind, a pursuit demanding reflection, analysis and investigation, a social activity undertaken by equals freely associated to engage in dialogue' (Jeffs, 2003: 28).

Radical distinctions are also made by Freire (1996), who argues that there are two contrasting perspectives on education and learning, which he identifies as the 'banking' concept of education versus 'problem posing'. On the one hand, the banking concept is the traditional mode of learning and involves the teacher helping a student fill their minds with knowledge, which is later 'cashed out' relatively unchanged, for example in

examinations. On the other hand, the problem-posing approach to education is education through dialogue, in which the facilitator and students meet and exchange ideas
and experiences through critical discussions and debate. Neither the facilitator nor the
students necessarily have the 'right' answer as there is room for 'multiple realities'.

Another perspective is provided by Peters (1966, 1973) regarding the differentia-
tion between training and education. What distinctions would you draw between
education and training, between nurse education and nurse training? Peters (1966)
notes that training means knowledge and skill development devised to bring about
some specific end. However, the aims of education, he notes, are that:

- something of value is being passed on and learned
- the individual comes to care about the learning involved, to develop understanding, and to achieve
- what is being learned must have a place in a coherent pattern of life, that is, relevance among other things in life.

Therefore, education 'implies that something worthwhile is being, or has been, intentionally transmitted in a morally acceptable manner … The educated person is one
whose life has been transformed by the deepening and widening of his understanding
and sensitivity. To be educated is not to arrive at a destination; it is to travel with a
different view' (Peters, 1973: 122).

These perspectives on learning correspond with the concepts of teacher-centred
learning and student-centred learning, which are discussed in Chapter 3. So how do
the definitions and these views on learning and education apply to, or compare with,
approaches taken in healthcare profession education curricula?

Activity 2.1   Different perspectives on nurse education

Discuss with a course or work-based peer your thoughts on how far Ramsden's
(2003), Freire's (1996) and Peters' (1966, 1973) perspectives on learning apply to
nursing, midwifery or to AHP professional education.

In nurse education, the difference between education and training is that the word
'training' is usually associated with developing the ability to take an approved set of
actions to perform a certain clinical task. This is thought of as a convergent process of
learning to complete a task competently. Education, however, is seen as a divergent
process that in addition to initially learning the step-by-step actions, the healthcare
professional is constantly reflecting on each action in the context of their deep knowl-
edge-base background, principles, values, ethics and effect on the recipient individual.

Education does not stop at a predetermined point of attainment, but progress further in development of critical ability and, consequently, the individual remains open
to new impressions, principles and perspectives. Education facilitators should therefore

provide an environment where students feel sufficiently supported to decide on areas and depth of learning, as long as the core curriculum aims are achieved.

Where do healthcare learners learn?

Naturally, learning does not occur only in university classrooms through lectures, workshops and books, but it also occurs in work-based settings, during patient or service user contact. Learning also occurs in skill laboratories and in the ward, teaching room or office. Furthermore, learning occurs in the trust's postgraduate or in-service training departments. In the practice setting, learning can take the form of informal and structured teaching sessions.

Additionally, learning occurs in the student common room, in informal social meetings and even 'in car parks, in corridors, over tea as well as through unnoticed patterns of behaviour and interaction in the classroom itself' (Field, 1999: 12). This notion that learning can occur from friends and peers and in a whole range of settings is referred to as 'social capital' (Gopee, 2002a). A corresponding notion is 'human capital', which refers to self-investment of time and effort by individuals through learning at university or in public libraries, as well as at home and in the non-traditional places suggested by Field (1999). Learning occurs everywhere, including, for example, in therapeutics or propaganda practices. Learning contributes to progress, and notions such as 'learning society' and 'learning organisation' (in that most companies have training and customer services departments) have evolved.

Lately, other effective ways of 'social' learning have been recognised, such as 'communities of practice' and 'action learning sets', the first is more informal and the latter more formal, but both are equally effective. Communities of practice refer to groups of people sharing a passion for something of interest, which they want to know more and more about or do, and learn by interacting regularly, as identified by Lave and Wenger (1998). The learning that ensues is not necessarily intentional, but is achieved by sharing information with each other, and building relationships that enable them to learn from each other.

Students studying for a specific subject have an overall common interest, but smaller groups of students may develop a 'passion' for specific sub-topics and meet informally to learn more and more about it. The same may apply to health and social care professionals in relation to their specialist area. Action learning sets are more formal classroom- or meeting-room-based discussions on pre-identified curricular topics, which is based on research by, for example, McGill and Beatty (1998) and Currie et al. (2012).

Theories Underpinning Learning

There are a number of theories of learning that can underpin professional education programmes. Exploration of these theories has taken place over several decades. It has swung between theories of learning, models of learning, principles of learning and styles of learning, with theories and styles of learning being the more popular concepts in the twenty-first century.

There are at least ten schools of thought, theories or models of learning, which have all created different definitions and incorporate a variety of concepts, but most of them have evolved from the three more robust learning theories, namely:

- behaviourist learning theories
- cognitive learning theories
- humanistic learning theories.

Behaviourist learning theories

Most learning theories belong to the field of psychology, which in the earlier part of the twentieth century used to be about introspection, that is, how mental processes are structured. However, gradually there was a move away from this paradigm (see, for example, Watson, 1978) and it was suggested that psychology should be a science, and psychological theories should be based on observable and quantifiable data, that is, those manifested in changes in behaviour. Initially, psychologists worked with animals to observe behaviour changes, and later worked with people.

Behaviourist learning theories refer to learning through response to particular stimuli, resulting in classical conditioning or operant conditioning. Classical conditioning refers to changes in behaviour through stimulus–response, whereby desirable responses to particular stimuli, that is, newly learned behaviours are rewarded. Operant conditioning is a subsequent development by Skinner (1971) and others, whereby approximations of desired behaviour are rewarded and thereby the target behaviour develops gradually. Being rewarded for new learning is also known as 'positive reinforcement', and can be external, in the form of verbal affirmations from the teacher (or close relatives) such as 'well done', or material rewards, or they can be internal through self-satisfaction.

Behaviourist learning theory can be applied in healthcare professionals' education programmes. For instance, operant conditioning can be effectively applied when students with weak academic backgrounds could achieve high levels in academia if earlier attempts are positively reinforced. Overall, healthcare learners are positively reinforced both by feeling a sense of achievement on being able to perform new healthcare skills, and by their mentors/supervisors acknowledging or recognising their newly developed competence.

Another example is that gaining praise for becoming competent at a particular clinical skill, or part-skills towards the desired competent performance, can positively motivate the student and make them want to learn new skills. Thus, praiseworthy performance or approximations of competent practice or of part-skills by healthcare learners are rewarded or positively reinforced.

Social learning theory builds on these early behaviourist theories whereby the individual observes competent behaviour or skill performance by professionals, learns and reproduces it, and if the attempt is positively reinforced then that behaviour or skill is likely to be adopted. It refers to behaviour, attitudes and values of teachers or other role models that may be copied by learners (Bandura, 1986, 1997) and thus learned in social situations, as discussed in Chapter 1.

Cognitive learning theories

As just indicated, behaviourist learning theories initially constituted an attempt to make psychology more scientific and empirical. More recently, various education sectors, including nurse education, have incorporated aspects of behaviourist theories and social learning theory into professional education programmes (for example through systematic feedback to students on their knowledge and competence, and through active role-modelling).

Subsequent work by Piaget (1962), Ausubel et al. (1978) and others led to the evolution of cognitive learning theories, which take the view that learning is an internal purposive action involving thinking, perception, information processing and memory. Cognitive learning theories include:

- gestalt theory of learning – entailing insightful learning, the 'aha' phenomenon
- Ausubel et al.'s assimilation theory – which incorporates information processing
- experiential learning – learning through engaging in practical activities, followed by reflection.

Cognitive learning theories were initially based on animal experiments by Kohler (1925), but all three above-mentioned theories can be applied to healthcare professional education programmes. They include learning by insight (or insightful learning) – which overlaps with gestalt learning theory, which in turn refers to seeing the whole picture, and insight is gained through the 'aha' phenomenon and the sudden realisation of a solution to a problem, or how various parts fit into a pattern, for instance the 'penny dropping' experience.

Gestalt theory of learning can be applied to professional education programmes by structuring learning so that learners are given problem situations to resolve (usually referred to as problem-based learning), and through group discussions, analysing ideas and trial and error, whereby particular insights are gained. Thus, group discussions as well as project work, self-directed learning and peer learning can enable this process. Implementation of problem situations that can be used in teaching include, for instance, asking a small group of students to resolve a snapshot of a clinical situation such as helping a patient with partial paralysis move from a bed to a chair.

To a notable extent, Bruner's (1960) discovery learning theory refers to insightful learning. It involves situations that are devised in such a way that the learner can discover principles and underlying techniques for themselves. It also involves the use of past experience and existing knowledge to form new insights. For instance, a student who witnesses a patient with asthma gain relief from distressed breathing by using their inhaler can gain further insight into the specific functions of bronchioles and alveoli in oxygen transfer previously encountered in books or lectures.

Ausubel et al.'s (1978) assimilation theory is based on the view that most meaningful cognitive learning takes place as a result of interaction between the knowledge (cognitive structures) that the individual already possesses, and new information that the individual encounters. Thus, the single most important factor influencing learning is what the learner already knows. This forms the basis for the transfer of learning, in that, for instance, once the learner comprehends the principles of asepsis in hospital settings, the knowledge can be adapted in community care settings.

Ausubel et al.'s (1978) assimilation theory refers to activating the relevant knowledge the student already has so as to assimilate new knowledge into their existing mental structures. This also increases retention, and is therefore also relevant for adult learners, as they already have substantial knowledge prior to starting on an academic course.

For new information to be 'received and assimilated' or subsumed into an anchoring structure or schema, Ausubel and his colleagues suggest giving the learner prior reading or the opportunity to engage in particular activities in preparation for the teaching session (referred to as 'advanced organisers', and more recently as 'flipping'). The advanced organiser creates an anchoring structure for the new knowledge, like a scaffolding of ideas on which to build what the student needs to know. For instance, prior to a practice placement with a physiotherapist, the learner could be advised to revise or learn about the microstructure of muscles, in readiness for learning how they are strengthened through exercises by a patient who has had a broken leg operated on.

Cognitive learning theory therefore involves learning by participation and continually taking into consideration the person's previous knowledge and competence, such as clinical skills already learnt by the student on previous placements, and university skills laboratories.

Experiential learning refers to learning by doing, rather than by merely being informed by others about a particular topic. It is achieved by building simulation activities in teaching–learning sessions, for instance, as advocated by Kolb (1984), among others. Experiential learning is therefore a component of reflective learning.

Learning from experience

Consider the question: Do we learn from all experiences we come across in our day-to-day activities?

Reflection Point 2.2

In his study of experiences that individuals encounter as they go about their normal day-to-day business and how much they learn from them, Jarvis (1995) deduced a typology of learning that identifies three categories and nine types of potential learning experiences as follows:

- Non-learning

  ○ presumption
  ○ non-consideration
  ○ rejection

- Non-reflective learning

    ○ preconscious learning
    ○ skills learning
    ○ memorisation

- Reflective learning

    ○ contemplation
    ○ reflective skills learning
    ○ experimental learning.

The typology also acknowledges the reality that there are particular situations that do not lend themselves to much learning for particular individuals, that is, non-learning experiences. The second category in the typology is non-reflective learning, which includes rote learning and memorising, for example temporary or one-off use of telephone numbers.

However, the third category is reflective learning, which focuses on the important part that experience plays in the learning process. Contemplation refers to thinking about life situations, and hopefully learning from them; and 'experimental learning' refers to learning from findings of well-designed research. Reflective learning refers to the learning that occurs as a result of systematic reflection on situations encountered.

Kolb (1984), for instance, suggests that learning can be conceived of as a four-stage learning cycle that involves identifying the immediate concrete experience or an incident as the basis for observation and reflection. Out of this arise new concepts for hypothesis and theory building. Implications of these are considered in new situations and then theory is confirmed, adjusted or advanced.

This form of learning is widely used in general and professional education programmes. Individuals are encouraged to learn from situations or 'critical incidents' that they encounter, to analyse them in the context of published literature and to record them systematically in their portfolios. These can comprise assessed work components of their programme of study.

The rationale for reflective practice in healthcare is that it is also a means of constructing or generating knowledge from particular incidents. The origins of reflection on incidents go back to times when, for instance, techniques for dealing with aggressive behaviour in mental health nursing were minimal. When clinical staff met after such incidents to discuss the situation, they started realising that if cues and signs of potential violence were identified in the individual patient before the disruptive incident actually occurred, they can take certain actions to prevent it from happening in the first place. This was formalised and seen as a therapeutic means that could be used, step by step, to prevent the disruptive incident. This also constituted constructing knowledge from clinical practice. The lack of knowledge and theory development from day-to-day experiences in practice settings was a weakness identified by Phillips et al.'s (2000) study of mentoring practices.

Similar 'concrete experiences' have led to changes in clinical practice, such as use of the triage system in Accident and Emergency departments and ensuring that normal saline solution is at room temperature or above prior to using it for wound cleansing. Several of these examples are noted in Chapter 5.

Kolb's (1984) learning cycle comprises four stages in the learning process, from the initial concrete experience or incident, through to exploring the experience retrospectively so that it leads to new learning, generalising from the new learning, to applying new learning to similar new situations. The original Kolb's cycle is presented as a closed circle with the fourth stage (applying new learning) leading to the first (the initial concrete experience). However, it is likely that the new learning may not be fully effective when applied to new situations that are similar, or even identical, to the initial concrete experience or incident, and therefore it becomes another new experience or incident to learn from. Consequently, the experiential learning cycle can be presented more meaningfully as a spiral that shows that applying new learning to similar situations must be undertaken with an open mind, as further learning might ensue in the light of new evidence and evolving social changes, as well as possibly research (see Figure 2.1).

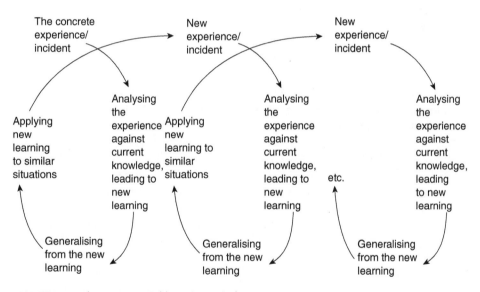

FIGURE 2.1   The experiential learning spiral

Adapting (i.e. making small changes) to published models and frameworks in one's teaching and learning is not uncommon, and can in fact be recommended as they are applied to specific groups of people or activities. This is also because Kolb's model of learning has its critics. For example, Bergsteiner et al. (2010) thoroughly examined Kolb's learning cycle and argue that the graphics of the model are flawed and suggest changes. Rogers and Horrocks (2010) argue that since learning from new experiences requires 'critical reflection', all learning cycles need to be adapted in the search for new principles before new conclusions are reached.

Nonetheless, teachers and students can alternatively utilise other models of reflection, such as the one by Boud et al. (1985), Gibbs (1988) or others that are generally available in the literature. Boud et al.'s model of reflective practice involves identifying the concrete experience, observation and reflections, attending to feelings, re-evaluating the experience and new learning.

For instance, when the student encounters a new experience during the practice placement, they observe the experience as a critical incident and later they recall the incident, and describe it, reflect on it and explore it in the context of existing knowledge within professional and other relevant literature. As a result of this, they develop and generate further insight by identifying and redefining the problem in a climate of mutual support (at university reflection-on-action workshops, for instance). They can share their newfound knowledge in as much detail as appropriate, even make a presentation, as it might have teaching implications for future practice. However, to benefit from this concept, the scheduling of the learning process should ensure that time is made available following practice placements for reflection, consolidation and evaluation.

Constructivism

Also gaining in popularity is a further development from the three groups of cognitive learning theories, one that is referred to as 'constructivism'. As a concept that was earlier pioneered by Berger and Luckmann (1967) as the social construction of reality, constructivism previously signified how individuals construct new thoughts, images, concepts and theories from structured and incidental experiences, that is 'scaffolded' onto the individual's existing current and past knowledge. An evolving ensuing term is 'constructionism', which refers to specific instances of creation of knowledge from life experiences and encounters with learning situations.

Currently, as a learning theory, constructivism is founded on the premise that, by reflecting on our experiences, each one of us constructs our own unique understanding of learning encounters, and in the quest for meaning we construct our own images and models of reality. Thereby the student does not accept verbatim all knowledge presented to them, but assimilates it in the context of their prior knowledge and their current social surroundings. More recent research findings on constructivism as a basis for effective learning include those of a study by Duane and Satre (2014) that supports the uses of this theory.

Humanistic learning theories

A third group of theories that have been developed with regard to how learning occurs are humanistic learning theories, which include:

- Alan Rogers' characteristics of adult education and andragogy
- Carl Rogers' student-centred approach to learning
- Maslow's learning as self-actualisation.

Humanistic learning theorists claim that preceding theories omit aspects of human existence such as feelings, attitudes and values, and thereby overlook the more holistic perspective that incorporates attitudinal components of learning. They suggest that learning should be concerned with personal human growth. Students can therefore learn concepts, theories, models and propositions (i.e., 'propositional knowledge') from books and other learning resources, and spend more classroom time on experiential learning activities, which include thinking processes that also incorporate exploration of values, attitudes and feelings.

Adults as students on healthcare profession courses

In the context of the more holistic and humanistic approaches to learning, adult learning is another concept in its own right.

Adult learners

Consider the question: Should ways of teaching adults be different from ways of teaching school children or college students? That is, what is different about adult students in contrast to school or college pupils? Think of reasons for your answer.

Reflection Point 2.3

Knowles et al. (2011), Rogers and Horrocks (2010) and Tennant (2005) suggest various ways in which teaching adults, or adult education, is different from teaching children. A prominent underpinning assumption about the preferred way of learning by adult learners is that they are competent at self-directed learning. Teaching adults includes teaching university students on generic or professional courses. Some of the differences suggested by nurses on post–registration courses are identified in Table 2.1.

TABLE 2.1 Differences in the ways in which adults and children learn

How children learn	How adults learn
• Children have a shorter attention span, and therefore a variety of learning activities is needed, including starter activities. • Teaching children is pedagogy, e.g. telling them. • Children are more open to new ideas. • There is a need to reinforce information over time.	• Adults are (usually) self-motivated to learn. • Adults may have relevant (or faulty) professional and life experiences. • Open discussion is more feasible in adult groups. • Lesson content can be adjusted based on ongoing evaluation of learning needs.

Source: Gopee (2000)

However, in both instances, the learner–teacher relationship is important and needs to be based on mutual trust. Different teachers may have their own repertoire of different teaching styles and techniques when teaching adult students. Rogers and Horrocks (2010) conclude by identifying the characteristics of adult students or learners as individuals who:

- define themselves and have a self-image as adult students
- are in the middle of a process of growth, not at the start of the process
- bring with them a package of experience and values
- come to learning with intentions
- bring with them expectations about the learning process
- have competing interests
- already have their own set of patterns of learning.

Reflection Point 2.4

Adult education in healthcare courses

How far is the adult learning approach relevant or applicable to nursing and other AHP education?

Rogers and Horrocks' characteristics of adult learners suggest that adult students' learning can be facilitated more effectively within an ethos of self-directed learning. Mentors can build self-directed learning into practice placement programmes for learners by allocating time for exploring further relevant clinical experiences or consulting relevant learning resources.

Andragogy and self-directed learning

Andragogy is an approach to teaching and learning aimed at enabling individuals to become aware that they should be the originators of their own thinking. Accordingly, although substantial knowledge and skill acquisition begin on qualifying (for example, becoming a registered nurse), it is up to the individual professional to determine the necessary areas of learning for themselves. This learning could be instigated by ward-based experiences and the self-direction developed should become career-long.

In a qualitative study of lecturers' and students' perceptions of self-directed learning and factors that facilitate or impede them, Lunyk-Child et al. (2001) found that students who engage in self-directed learning undergo a transformation that begins with negative feelings (i.e. confusion, frustration and dissatisfaction), but ends with confidence and skills for lifelong learning.

However, another side to self-directed learning is highlighted by Hughes (1999), who indicates that this approach is not necessarily 'emancipatory' as it can be a 'repressive instrument' in that it can marginalise the benefits of collective and cooperative learning, that is, learning in groups in classrooms. Hughes suggests that governments can use self-directed learning to argue that less central funding would be required to educate self-directed students. Furthermore, Knowles et al. (2011) suggest that the teacher needs to develop specific competencies to accommodate effective self-directed learning. In light of these issues and reservations related to andragogy and the benefits as well as Rogers and Horrocks' (2010) general characteristics of adult learners, it can be concluded that in healthcare:

- Adult education constitutes collaborative activities between teachers and learners.
- Teaching should build on learners' professional experiences.
- Learners should participate in identifying learning needs, setting objectives and evaluating learning.
- The level of effective application of theory to clinical practice must always be identified.
- The role of the teacher is that of a facilitator.
- The outcome of the teaching and learning encounter should be to enable the individual to develop into a responsible autonomous practitioner.

Student-centred teaching

Carl Rogers (1983) is well known for suggesting that teaching may be an overrated activity, as it is learning that should be in focus. For this to happen, he advocated the use of empathic understanding, genuineness and being non-judgemental in learning situations. These activities are helping skills that Rogers successfully transferred from therapeutic counselling situations to student-learning situations (Rogers and Freiberg, 1994). The teacher thus becomes the facilitator of student-centred learning, as is also advocated by Freire (1996) and Knowles et al. (2011). The facilitator achieves this by creating the appropriate environment for learning and identifying resources, and therefore empowering students to become responsible, to develop self-awareness and to think of alternatives. Student-centred teaching is discussed in some detail in Chapter 3.

Learning and self-actualisation

Maslow's (1987) theory of a hierarchy of human needs suggests that our highest-level need, which is also lower priority, is our need for self-actualisation. Our physiological needs are highest priority, followed by safety needs, the need for belongingness and love, our self-esteem needs and finally the need for self-actualisation. It could be argued that the goal of education is to assist individuals to achieve self-actualisation, to help the person to become the best that they are able to become with the resources that are accessible. Maslow observed that there are a number of characteristics of self-actualising individuals, which include:

- demonstrate acceptance of self and others
- are problem-centred
- demonstrate democratic character

- have a philosophical, non–hostile sense of humour
- show creativeness
- seem to transcend any culture.

Teachers might argue that they apply the above-mentioned theories of learning as appropriate, with particular groups or with individual learners. However, from adult educators' professional perspectives, andragogy also requires consideration of whether the adult student is merely biologically adult or merely of legally adult age or is also being a psychologically and socially responsible adult.

Furthermore, Race (2010: viii) reviewed the main prevailing theories of learning, and observed that most theories are worded in academic technical language used by educational psychologists that the majority of readers find cumbersome and not easy to comprehend. He therefore constituted his theory of learning using much simpler words, which he termed 'ripples on a pond' model of learning, which in turn identifies fundamental factors underpinning successful learning, namely:

- wanting to learn
- taking ownership of the need to learn
- learning by doing
- learning through feedback
- making sense of what is being learned
- explaining or teaching or coaching
- making informed judgements – assessing.

The ripples model of learning is a more recent further development of experiential learning and is therefore rooted in 'learning by doing'. Race argues that the seven factors underpinning learning occur in sequence, with each stage interacting with those next to it, much like a pebble falling into a pond and creating ripples with each stage moving in backward and forward directions. It is presented as concentric circles. It is interesting to note that the first three 'ripples' tend to represent learners' motivation and the actions that they take to learn, both being components that have featured for decades as crucial for effective learning.

Race's ripples model of learning can be implemented in educating healthcare profession students by ensuring that each factor is achieved, such as enabling students to become motivated to learn, creating the medium for 'learning by doing', by giving feedback and creating opportunities for students to teach others.

How Else Do We Learn Healthcare Skills?

In addition to different theories of learning, learning is also influenced by the different styles and approaches to learning adopted by individuals. The distinctions between theories and styles can be explained as follows.

A theory tends to imply cause and effect, that is, if we do x, then y will happen. For instance, if the Smiths send their child to an independent school, then they will have a better chance of securing a student place in a reputable university. According to the dictionary (Brown, 2002: 3236), a theory is 'a systematic statement of rules or principles to be followed; a system of ideas or statement explaining something, especially one based on general principles, independent of the thing to be explained'. Alternatively, Lindberg et al. (1998: 62) define a theory as 'a group of concepts, definitions, and statements that presents an organised view of phenomena ... with the intent of describing, explaining, or controlling these phenomena'. A learning theory, the humanistic theory for instance, comprises an organised view of a group of concepts that should result in much more effective learning.

In contrast to a learning theory, a learning style refers to the unique way in which the particular individual tends to respond to learning situations so that they acquire the targeted skill or knowledge. For example, do they accept new learning instantly, or do they prefer to reflect on it before accepting it fully? Do they question first whether the learning has practical applications or do they first accept new concepts at theoretical levels? Alternatively, approaches to learning tend to depend on the level of individual commitment to particular episodes of learning, as discussed shortly in this chapter.

Major learning styles

The foregoing discussion on learning styles was largely related to learning theories and concepts, and partly to learning clinical skills.

How do you prefer to learn? What is your learning style?

We are all unique as learners. How does each of us prefer to learn? What is your preferred learning style, for learning in practice settings and for learning in classroom settings? Which style does not suit you?

Reflection Point 2.5

Learning styles have been researched over a number of years, and Honey and Mumford's (2000) classification of styles of learning is one that has been most widely published. You might have responded to Reflection Point 2.5 by identifying that you prefer to learn by attending a course or lecture, that is, in formal teaching situations. Others may prefer to learn by:

- watching others and seeing the end-product first
- trial and error, generally through experience
- reading and other forms of personal study such as distance learning
- discussion with others.

Another well-accepted proponent of learning styles is Kolb (1984), who identifies four styles of learning manifested by students, namely the converger, the diverger, the assimilator and the accommodator. Honey and Mumford (2000) suggest that individual learners vary between whether they are activists, reflectors, theorists or pragmatists. Jarvis and Gibson (1997) add other learning styles such as focusers, scanners, impulsivity and reflectivity. The main learning styles are summarised in the box.

Popular learning styles

Converger vs Diverger	Convergers are individuals who tend to use abstract thinking, progress to active experimentation and generate a single correct solution; divergers tend to start from concrete experiences, generate ideas then speculate on broader perspectives.
Impulsivity vs Reflectivity (similar to Accommodator vs Assimilator)	Using the 'impulsive' style means the individual tends to respond first, at times spontaneously (is accommodating) and reflect later; those who use reflectivity tend to reflect first (assimilate) and respond subsequently.
Activists vs Reflectors	Individuals who are activists tend to involve themselves fully in new experiences; reflectors ponder on experiences from different perspectives, thoroughly analysing them before participating in the experience in practice.
Theorists vs Pragmatists	Theorists are individuals who start from observations and develop or synthesise them into theories; pragmatists tend to consider the practical application of novel encounters first and theorise afterwards.
Focuser vs Scanner	Focusers are individuals who examine the whole problem and develop solutions from them; scanners tend to solve one aspect of the problem at a time and assume that it is the correct one unless it is disproved.
Holistic vs Serialistic	Individuals using the holistic approach tend to prefer to see a phenomenon as a whole; while serialists prefer to identify its components and their roles as part of the whole phenomenon.

Styles of learning are explained in full detail in the relevant literature. For instance, the style 'Impulsivity vs Reflectivity' implies that some individuals respond to new learning stimuli first and reflect later, while other individuals reflect first and respond afterwards. Although the latter might be intellectually sounder, the former has its uses in certain situations, especially by those who are in a position to use intuitive knowledge.

To enable utilisation of styles of learning, Honey and Mumford (2000) designed a Learning Style Questionnaire (LSQ) that is widely used. The LSQ constitutes a self-assessment tool that indicates which style is generally utilised by the individual completing it, and the main uses of knowledge derived from the LSQ are:

* increased awareness of learning activities that are congruent with the individual's learning style
* a better choice of activities leading to more effective and economical learning
* identification of areas in which an individual's less effective learning processes can be improved
* development of ways in which specific learning skills can be improved, for example reflective learning.

A number of questionnaires and inventories on learning styles are available in education literature and through the Internet, but research on learning styles almost always indicates that students do not choose and use only one style of learning as they use different styles or a combination of styles. James et al. (2011), for instance, explored the learning styles of first year nursing and midwifery students utilising the VARK (visual, aural, read–write and kinaesthetic) questionnaire, and found that the majority of students were 'multi-modal', that is they use all four modes of learning identified in VARK. Fleming et al.'s (2011) longitudinal study also concluded that student nurses do not use one 'dominant learning style', although they do recognise that educators should be aware of students' learning styles and endeavour to maximise students' learning potential by utilising a range of teaching and learning methods.

Adapting to students' styles of learning

As implied in Reflection Point 2.5, the individual's learning can also vary, depending on whether the individual has to learn clinical skills or professional theories and concepts. Despite different research findings, it is arguable that, where feasible, the mentor should endeavour to be aware of their mentee's learning style and approach to see if they can adapt to them in order to make their teaching more effective. This could make the achievement of practice objectives easier and more efficient.

An example of the adaptation of the 'Theorists vs Pragmatists' style of learning is as follows. For instance, if the mentor finds that a particular student has leanings towards the pragmatist style for any particular component of learning – that is, they immediately want to know how the learning applies to actual patient or service user care situations – then the mentor can first focus on the practical application of the learning and subsequently move on to underpinning theories. The practical knowledge can follow immediately afterwards and the theoretical knowledge later. Another student may wish to acquire all necessary theoretical knowledge before engaging in its practical application.

Applying the 'pragmatist style' to learning drug calculation

Another example of the application of learning styles can be with regard to students acquiring drug calculation skills. Competent drug calculation is naturally a crucial nursing or midwifery skill, as too much or too little medication can either harm the patient or delay their recovery (which the 'theorist' would need to know before learning the skill). But some students struggle to become competent at drug calculation, which is a problem that has been highlighted for over a decade. A literature search in just one journal (*Nurse Education Today*) presented over 100 articles on the topic area, and recently there has been a proliferation of books (and even e-learning packages) on drug calculation. Many universities also have a mathematics support department to help students who need to refresh their calculation skills.

Coincidentally, mentors are in a suitable position to help their mentees learn these skills, as instead of being a classroom-based potentially dry topic, during practice placements drug calculation directly applies to the individual patients or service users in their care. During drug administration, the mentor could seize the opportunity to ascertain his or her mentee's drug calculation skills. Subsequently, if appropriate, for the learner who is more of a pragmatist than a theorist (or leans towards the 'visual' style), the mentor can show the learner step by step how patient X's medication dose is calculated, preferably long before they learn to administer the medication. It is a competency that simply has to be mastered (NMC, 2009a, 2010a).

To conclude this examination of learning styles, there are also individuals who do not adhere to a specific learning style, as noted by Fleming et al. (2011) for instance, and the individual may even consciously change their learning style according to the situation. Learners could develop their ability in all styles of learning and change or adapt them as new knowledge and skills are encountered, which might depend on how novel the new experience is to the individual. Style may also change through new experiences and at different stages of maturation. Additionally, mentors can make their facilitation of learning even more efficient by the use of learning contracts.

Using learning contracts

Learning contracts are very much a feature of adult education (or andragogy) as discussed earlier in this chapter, and involve negotiated learning between teacher and student. As the word *contract* implies, a learning contract is a written and signed agreement between teacher (mentor in this case) and learner resulting in the latter's active involvement in decisions over practice objectives and other components of learning. Therefore, it is often a feature of practice placement learning, whereby the mentor and student agree on specific practice objectives and on each party's responsibility in the achievement of the objectives.

The use of learning contracts is advocated by Knowles et al. (2011) in the context of adult learners needing to exercise more self-direction in their learning. The agreed set of objectives in the learning contract includes those of the course curriculum for practice learning, and those of the student and the mentor. Therefore, the learning contract affords the student some control and responsibility over their learning, motivates them to engage with the placement experience and to learn. It is also a medium for identifying the student's pace of learning, to explore the means of theory and practice integration, and can be supported by ascertaining the student's preferred learning style.

However, the requirements and objectives set by the course curriculum have to be met. A learning contract section or template may already have been included in the student's placement competencies booklet. Basically, the mentor and student discuss and agree on specific practice learning objectives for the student, how the learning will take place and precisely how they will know that the objectives have been achieved. These are usually written down by the student and, when agreed, both mentor and student sign and date the contract. Learning pathways based on patient journeys can be incorporated as a strategy for achieving particular objectives. An example of a learning contract is presented in Template 2.1.

TEMPLATE 2.1   A learning contract

Name of student:			Cohort:	
Placement:			Mentor's name:	
Learning needs	Objectives	Resource and strategies	Target date	Evidence
What do I want to learn? – Topic area	What do I want to have achieved at the end of this learning? – Specific objectives	How will I learn, and who will support me? – Learning strategies	Date of achieving the objectives	How will I know I have achieved my intended learning?
1. Assessment of a new patient	Able to assess the health and social care needs of newly admitted/ referred patient/service user	Mentor, social worker	30–11– 2014	Mentor reviews and agrees with my assessment and care plan

(Continued)

(Continued)

2. Teach patients	Able to teach a type 2 diabetic patient how to control their dietary intake	Mentor, dietician. Consult diet sheets, guidelines. Read up on type 2 diabetes	30–11–2014	Mentor observes my teaching and signs me as competent in this skill
3.	...			

Pre-contract

Signature of student:	Date:
Mentor's signature:	Date:
Name of link lecturer/practice education facilitator:	Name of personal tutor:

Comments on achievement of contract objectives

Signature of student:	Date:
Mentor's signature:	Date:

Crucial components of the learning contract are also the specific resources (human and material) that are required to enable the student to achieve the agreed objectives and also the specific dates by which each objective will have been achieved. An alternative to a learning contract is a 'learning agreement' (Open University, 2001; RCN, 2002), which has similar features but might not include the signatures of those involved nor rigid 'achieve-by' dates.

Reflection Point 2.6

The learning contract

What would logically happen after both parties have signed the learning contract? Do you feel that it should be constantly reviewed to monitor the student's progress with its content, or only reviewed on the 'target date'?

Learning contracts may be seen by some as a chore. Others may prefer to write something, treating it as a mere formality. But the benefits of learning contracts have been reported by Ghazi and Henshaw (1998), for instance, who found that learning contracts help to improve student performance in assessments and student attendance at lectures. Timmins (2002) and others reported similar benefits.

An important step involved in constructing a learning contract is the mentor facilitating self-assessment of clinical skills and knowledge by the student and identifying pre-requisite learning. Naturally, when a contract has been drawn up, then on the 'achieve-by' date there will be a need to ascertain whether the activities identified in the contract were undertaken and the objectives achieved. The review time will of course have been determined at the beginning when the content was being discussed and documented.

The mentor will have developed knowledge and understanding of the use of learning contracts as part of the mentor preparation programme, along with how they can deliver these functions in the context of other roles that they have to fulfil.

Rogers and Freiberg (1994) indicate that learning contracts endow the student with some freedom to learn aspects that they wish to learn and pursue areas that they find particularly interesting. A learning contract is also a medium for resolving any doubt that there may be about specific purposes of the learning experience. It clarifies the activities that the student would engage in and provides motivation and reinforcement through the achievement of objectives.

For learning contracts to be effective, they need to be skilfully constructed. Guidelines for constructing them are provided by educational researchers Knowles et al. (2011), as well as by Bailey and Tuohy (2009), and an example of a well-constructed learning contract is presented in Template 2.1 above.

Students with special education needs (SEN)

In addition to theories and individual styles of learning, facilitators of learning should also heed the special education needs (SEN) of individual students. The number of students disclosing that they have a disability is increasing, including those who are students on healthcare profession courses. Universities have an obligation to comply with legal requirements, such as those of the Disability Discrimination Act (DDA) (Office of Public Sector Information (OPSI), 2005), and the Special Educational Needs and Disability Act (OPSI, 2001), which are now incorporated into the Equality Act 2010 (Equality Challenge Unit, 2012). As it is mandatory for students to acquire professional skills in practice settings for a specified number of hours during the course (for example, NMC, 2010a), mentors have to be aware of their obligations towards students with disabilities as well under these Acts.

The QAA (2010: 7) prefers to refer to the student with SEN as a 'disabled student' but retains the DDA's (OPSI, 2005) definition of disability. The Equality Act defines disability very similarly as: 'a physical or mental impairment, which has a substantial and long term adverse effect on his or her ability to carry out normal day to day activities'.

The above-mentioned Acts also identify a list of different impairments that constitute a disability, including dyslexia, visual or hearing impairment and mental health conditions. In addition to disabilities, the Equality Act, which came into force on 1 October 2010, encompasses other human characteristics that employers could willingly or inadvertently discriminate against. It identifies nine such 'protected characteristics', namely:

- age
- disability
- gender assignment
- marriage and civil partnership
- pregnancy and maternity
- race
- religion or belief (including lack of belief)
- sex
- sexual orientation.

Furthermore, the above Acts indicate that institutions must provide 'reasonable adjustment' facilities to support SEN students with their learning and with their course assignments. Almost all organisations concerned with the education of healthcare profession students, including the RCN (2007) and the QAA (2010), prepare their own written statement on how they make 'reasonable adjustments' for SEN. The RCN's (2007: 19–20) guidance on how reasonable adjustments can be made in the practice setting for students with dyslexia is as follows:

- the use of coloured overlays to assist in reading text on white paper
- the use of coloured paper
- additional training and support
- giving verbal rather than written instructions
- allowing plenty of time to read and complete the task
- giving instructions one at a time, slowly and clearly, in a quiet location
- reminding the person of important deadlines and reviewing priorities regularly
- using a wall planner, and creating a 'to do' list
- the use of modified/specialised equipment
- provision of a quiet area to write up notes, or for when specific tasks require intense concentration
- flexible working hours/frequent breaks.

For advice and support on how to make adjustments for students with SEN, mentors can consult various named individuals and departments such as the local university's lecturer(s) who specialises in this topic area, Occupational Health services and students' unions.

Research on the extent to which the needs of students with SEN are met include those by White (2007) and Tee et al. (2010). White, for instance, conducted a qualitative study to explore how far the education needs of students with dyslexia are met during their prequalifying programme. She found that students experienced particular problems during practice placements, but none of the mentors in the study felt adequately educationally prepared to help students with disabilities. Students with SEN do develop their own coping strategies, and the study recommends that a more concerted effort should be made to support both students and their mentors to make the necessary 'reasonable adjustments'.

Griffiths et al. (2010) provide a six-phase framework for supporting disabled students systematically for more effective learning during practice placements. However, other than in the context of policies related to disabilities, there is also an abundance of literature and research on the topic area. Scullion (2010), for instance, identifies the two most prominent perspectives on disability: the medical model and the social model. As the term implies, the medical model endeavours to enable people with disabilities to function to their maximum by rectifying the problem as far as they can at the pathophysiological level.

The social model tends to view those with disabilities as those who should not be stereotyped and stigmatised, but adjustments should be made to their social environment to enable them to function to their maximum. Scullion indicates that, as a strategy to challenge discrimination, healthcare professionals should promote and enhance the social model of disability through 'social advocacy'.

However, a literature review of 'reasonable adjustments in nursing and midwifery' conducted on behalf of the NMC by Kane and Gooding (2009) revealed that there are still various issues related to this, including the resources required for reasonable adjustments to be made and non-disclosure of a disability for fear of social discrimination. Furthermore, Tee et al. (2010) found that disabled students require 20 per cent more contact time with lecturers than non-disabled peers, and they therefore recommend the appointment of a 'student practice learning advisor' whose primary role will be to support disabled students by ensuring that opportunities to succeed are maximised by operationalising recommended adjustments in practice.

....

Students with Disabilities

Student nurse Vicky informed the pre-registration Course Director by the end of the first week of the start of the course that she has been told previously when she was at college that she might have dyslexia. The Course Director advised the student to attend the Student Welfare Department of the university for an assessment of

(Continued)

Case Study

(Continued)

her particular difficulties, and to determine the adjustments that should enable her to undertake her course activities with more ease. Consequently Vicky was issued with the following facilities and advice, some of which should help in academic settings, others in the practice setting:

- Provision of notes from the lecturer on coloured paper if possible, or use of coloured overlays
- Use of coloured overlays for reading text on white paper
- A spell checker, or a specialised computer with built in spellchecker, etc
- Permission to have a person take notes for Vicky at lectures or to use a tape recorder to audio record lectures
- Visual diagrams to explain things
- Allowing additional time when taking written examinations
- Allowing extra time to complete nursing tasks in the practice setting
- Giving instructions one at a time, and allowing to ask for clarification, or double checking on instructions
- Use of pocket books to write words or instructions to remember during a clinical shift
- Use of check lists
- Allocating a quiet uninterrupted area and additional time to write up nursing patients progress notes

Vicky was understandably apprehensive about how quickly she was going to be able to adapt to activities in the practice setting during practice placements, and on the other hand although her mentor has attended lectures on 'students with special education needs' both during the mentor course and at a mentor update session some months ago, she hadn't actually anticipated that one of her own mentees would be dyslexic. At the initial individual interview with the student, when the student mentioned her disability, and also indicated that she has been able to use certain contraptions to cope with university lectures and simulation activities, the mentor remembered that in the course her normal duties, she has to adjust to people with various individual differences, and did not pursue this aspect of the conversation too far at that point in time.

However, by the end of the second shift with the student, the mentor had investigated various ways in which students with special needs can be supported in practice settings, including in a Royal College of Nursing (2007) document, and noted continuing use of the term 'reasonable adjustments'. Giving the student extra time with clinical activities and extra support were deemed essential, as well as asking Vicky how she normally manages her particular dyslexia problems. By the end of the practice placement, the student had achieved all her practice objectives and passed her first placement.

Reference: Royal College of Nursing (2007) *Guidance for Mentors of Nursing Students and Midwives: An RCN Toolkit.* London: RCN.

See also: Child, J. and Langford, E. (2011) Exploring the learning experiences of nursing students with dyslexia. *Nursing Standard*, 25 (40): 39–46.

Approaches to learning

Evolving from different theories and styles, research has also identified different approaches to learning. Marton et al.'s (1997) research on approaches to learning identified individuals who take a deep approach to learning, those who take a surface approach and those who take the strategic approach. Students tend to use one of these three approaches. The defining features of each approach are presented in the box.

Deep, surface and strategic approaches to learning

Deep approach	• Relates ideas to previous knowledge and experience • Looks for patterns and underlying principles • Checks evidence and relates it to conclusions • Examines logic and argument cautiously and critically • Engages with full interest with the course content
Surface approach	• Studies without reflecting on purpose and strategy • Treats the course as unrelated bits of knowledge (discrete elements) • Memorises facts and procedures in relation to assessments • Finds difficulty in making sense of new ideas presented • Feels undue pressure and worry about coursework
Strategic approach	• Puts consistent effort into studying • Ensures conditions and materials for studying are appropriate • Manages or organises time and effort to greatest effect • Is alert to assessment requirements and criteria, and pays attention to cues about marking schemes • Gears work to the perceived preferences of lecturers

---

Whether a student takes the deep or surface approach to learning (Marton et al., 1997) might also depend on the stage of development of the subject area. Social sciences and arts may warrant a deep approach, while parts of science subjects such as biology and law might only require surface approaches, at least at earlier stages because they often constitute factual, single-answer knowledge. Newer and less factual subjects might also warrant a deep approach.

Approaches to learning also relate to the quality of the learning undertaken. Ramsden (2003) reports that if someone treated learning as an external imposition and concentrated on memorising facts, then that person was taking a surface approach to learning, and this would result in poor knowledge and understanding of the subject. Alternatively, 'if they intended to understand, and interacted vigorously with the content of the text (a deep approach), they stood a better chance of getting the author's message and being able to remember the supporting facts' (ibid.: 2003: 19). As for adapting to the student's approach to learning, the mentor would prefer the student to take a deep approach but, during very busy times, strategic and surface approaches might temporarily be relevant.

Principles of learning

Based on the views, theories, styles and approaches to learning discussed in this chapter, there are certain generally agreed principles of learning that can be concluded from them, which can make learning more effective from the standpoint of both facilitators and learners. Mostly derived from Gagné (1983) and Knowles et al. (2011), these are:

- Whatever a student learns, they must actively learn it themselves – no one can learn it for them.
- Each student learns at their own chosen pace, as this varies depending on their particular circumstances, mental abilities and various other factors.
- A student learns more when each step is immediately reinforced or corrected.
- Full, rather than partial, mastery of each step makes the total more meaningful.
- When given responsibility for their own learning, the student can become more highly motivated and likely to learn and retain more.
- The teacher as manager of learning should assume that McGregor's (1987) theory Y prevails, that is, learners are self-motivated to learn, and they seek out learning opportunities for themselves (theory X implies learners have to be directed or coerced to learn).
- Students who come to education expecting to be passively fed information and knowledge should be eased into andragogical principles of learning and teaching soon after.

Chapter Summary

This chapter has focused predominantly on the 'what' and 'how' of learning professional knowledge and competence, and has therefore explored:

- What healthcare learners learn, and why, in the context of the student's learning needs and the different types of knowledge associated with professional skills.
- The definitions of competence and healthcare competencies, and issues related to them.
- Major views and perspectives on learning, teaching and education, which include what learning is, and where and how individual healthcare learners learn.
- Theories underpinning learning, in particular behaviourist learning theories (including Bandura's social learning theory), cognitive learning theories and humanistic learning theories, such as andragogy and self-directed learning, student-centred approach to learning and learning as self-actualisation.

- How learners learn healthcare skills, which included an examination of major styles of learning, and approaches to learning, such as deep, surface and strategic learning, and how the mentor can adapt their mentoring activities to students' individual styles and approaches; use of learning contracts; and strategies for facilitating learning for students with SEN.

📖 Further Optional Reading

1 For full details on all the NMC's requirements for effective and quality-assured pre-registration nurse education in the UK, see:

- Nursing and Midwifery Council (2010a) *Standards for Pre-registration Nursing Education*. Available at: http://standards.nmc-uk.org/PreRegNursing/Pages/Introduction.aspx (accessed 15 April 2014).

2 For a detailed discussion on 'vicarious learning' in relation to social learning theory, see:

- Roberts, D. (2010) 'Vicarious learning: a review of the literature', *Nurse Education in Practice*, 10 (1): 13–16.

3 For updates on the current provision for students with SEN and detailed guidance on how to support learning for students with disabilities, see:

- Quality Assurance Agency for Higher Education (QAA) (2010) *Code of Practice for the Assurance of Academic Quality and Standards in Higher Education Section 3: Disabled students*. Available at: http://www.qaa.ac.uk/Publications/Information AndGuidance/Pages/Code-of-practice-Section-3.aspx (accessed 4 January 2014).

To access further resources related to this chapter, visit the companion website at https://study.sagepub.com/gopee

3

Facilitating Learning

Introduction

Chapter Outcomes

On completion of this chapter, you should be able to:

1 Identify a wide range of students and learners whose learning qualified health-care professionals facilitate.
2 Differentiate between teaching and facilitation of learning, and the different contemporary perceptions of, and approaches to, teaching and learning.
3 Evaluate a number of ways in which mentors can enable healthcare students to acquire health and social care skills, the steps involved in effective planning for skills teaching, along with the underpinning knowledge base.
4 Demonstrate knowledge of structured and systematic methods of teaching that can be implemented by mentors to enable students and learners to acquire health profession skills and knowledge.
5 Evaluate various methods of teaching and presentation aids that can be selected for effective teaching, and also ways of managing some of the likely problems with them.

Having explored in Chapter 1 what mentoring, preceptoring and similar roles signify, the reasons for the mentor role and how it can be performed effectively, and then in Chapter 2 the different major perspectives on learning, along with learning theories, styles and approaches, this chapter focuses on the teaching and facilitation of learning roles of the mentor. Over the years, both the UKCC and the NMC have identified the mentor as the main 'teacher' in practice settings. This chapter therefore considers the various professional groups of learners whose learning healthcare professionals facilitate; whether to teach or facilitate learning; systematic ways of facilitating learners' acquisition of practice skills and knowledge; as well as some of the main issues related to facilitation of learning in practice settings. The mentor's competence under the 'facilitation of learning' domain and the related outcomes identified by the NMC (2008a) were noted in the introductory section of Chapter 2.

Whose Learning Do Healthcare Professionals Facilitate, and Why?

Activity 3.1   Whom do healthcare professionals teach?

To start exploring facilitation of learning, first make a list of all the groups of people whom nurses and other healthcare professionals teach. Having done this, add the exact healthcare topic areas that they are likely to teach to the different groups of individuals.

The healthcare professional's role includes a substantial teaching component and you might therefore have felt that Activity 3.1 was rather simplistic. However, it does reflect the reality of the extent of teaching that RNs and RMs do, and in response to the activity you might have mentioned:

- Nurses teach student nurses (first, second and third year), healthcare assistants on national vocational qualification courses, patients/service users, patient's relatives, and junior doctors.
- Midwives teach women/service users, for example new mothers and fathers, how to look after a new baby.
- The practice nurse teaches primary (and secondary) level ill-health prevention, for example how to quit smoking, lose weight, expectant mothers regarding their diet and relaxation for those with high blood pressure.
- SCPHNs teach mothers with different needs, such as single teenage mothers or those in different age groups.

Why Do Healthcare Professionals Need to Know How to Facilitate Learning?

On a day-to-day basis, the healthcare professional's role focuses largely on attending to patients' and service users' health problems. Teaching activities generally tend to be more transient and are engaged in at opportune moments. Nevertheless, there are several reasons why healthcare professionals teach and facilitate learning. First, in addition to teaching colleagues and juniors being a job requirement for most health-care professionals by virtue of their contract of employment, it also constitutes one of the four essential components of nursing and midwifery, as identified by Wright (1990), the Scottish Government (2014) and in DH policy documents – the other components being clinical practice, care organisation and involvement in research. Correspondingly, the *NHS KSF* (DH, 2004a: 57) notes under 'personal and people development' that healthcare professionals have to contribute to 'the development of others during ongoing work activities [by] structured approaches ... informal and ad hoc methods' and demonstrate and share skills and knowledge.

Similarly, teaching usually forms part of healthcare professionals' codes of practice, which stipulate that they must be willing to share skills and experience. For instance, the NMC's (2015: clause 9) code of practice specifies that the RNs and RMs 'must' share their skills, knowledge and experience for the benefit of their colleagues and people receiving their care, and also support their students' learning. This form of teaching includes teaching new skills to colleagues (RNs/RMs), for example the use of new medical devices such as a new glucometer, how to conduct a patient assessment, the Doppler technique and teaching healthcare profession students.

Teaching is also an integral component of healthcare professionals' pre-registration education programmes as identified by the NMC (2010a), under the domain 'Communication and interpersonal skills', for instance, indicating that nurses must educate patients and service users 'to encourage health promoting behaviour' (ibid.: 2010a: 16); and under 'Leadership, management and team-working', 'All nurses must facilitate nursing students and others to develop their competence using a range of professional and personal development skills' (ibid.: 2010a: 20).

Furthermore, specialist RNs and other healthcare professionals are at times required, or invited, to do small-group teaching on specific aspects of their specialist areas within the healthcare trust or classroom teaching on specialist university-based courses.

Additionally, healthcare professionals might also engage in teaching merely to advance the teaching or presentation skills that they have previously acquired to varying degrees. They could thereby also start to develop public speaking skills. For more experienced mentors, teaching provides them with an opportunity to apply the principles of teaching and learning, and experiment with new teaching techniques. Furthermore, mentors have to teach because of variable levels of success in joint education–trust roles such as lecturer–practitioners and the clinical teaching role of nurse lecturers.

Facilitating Learning or Teaching?

At times we hear the statement, 'John (or Jane) is an excellent (or a born) teacher,' but, as with most skills, teaching can be regarded as an 'art' and a 'science'. This means that although someone may appear to have a natural knack for teaching, it is also a skill that can be learned, using scientifically deduced theories. Short or long teaching courses such as the City and Guilds 7307 'Certificate in Teaching Adult Learners' and the 'Postgraduate Certificate in Education' courses are specifically designed for this purpose.

After several years of teaching experience, eventually the skill becomes so well developed and refined that it appears akin to an artistic talent. However, thinking about some of the concepts discussed in Chapter 2, such as self-directed learning and reflective learning, consider the question: Should mentors teach mentees and juniors, or facilitate their learning? Both concepts are suggested for contemporary mentoring activities.

Approaches to teaching and learning

Dictionaries tend to define teaching as 'to tell or show, to give instruction or lessons in' or 'to enable (a person) to do something by instruction and training'. Such definitions tend to signify teaching as one-way traffic, that is, the teacher controls the content, direction and flow of the session's content. It also reflects one of the earlier approaches to teaching. However, various other approaches to teaching and learning have evolved over the years, so much so that Joyce et al. (2009) indicate that there are more than 22 models of teaching, some of which are well researched whilst others still need rigorous testing.

An underlying trend that figures clearly in all these approaches and models of teaching is the transition from the rather derogatory term 'teacher-centred' teaching to 'student-centred' teaching. Three stages of evolution of approaches to teaching can be identified, which are as follows:

1 In the earlier stage, teaching was seen as the teacher imparting selected and predetermined knowledge and skills to students as he or she is the expert in that subject area. In such approaches, students in turn are passive recipients of the instruction, but this results in students feeling inhibited from exploring alternative views.

2 In a gradual change in attitude towards teaching and learning, teaching was viewed as enabling active learning, an approach in which teachers structure learning activities for students so that the latter actively engage with the subject matter and explore specific topic areas in the curriculum or syllabus. Thus, the teacher leads students to conclusions by enquiry and questioning.

3 In the third and current stage, teaching is viewed as 'facilitating learning', whereby teachers work in partnership with students and jointly determine their learning needs in the overall context of the curriculum and the means by which those learning needs will be met. The teacher creates the conditions for learning and does not control all learning outcomes, thus allowing the student a substantial degree of choice in what to learn.

These three stages of development in ways of teaching therefore reflect an evolving trend from the earlier one implying a teacher-centred approach to the latter being much more student-centred, and therefore progressing from teaching to facilitation of learning. The approach chosen of course depends on several factors such as the particular student group's motivation to learn, the teacher's own beliefs about teaching and learning, and the subject matter, or a deliberate combination of these as the teacher feels appropriate.

The three teaching approaches can also be categorised as didactic, Socratic or facilitative, respectively. Contemporarily, Ramsden (2003) refers to these approaches as theories 1, 2 and 3. However, Biggs and Tang (2011: 16–20) interpret these three approaches at three 'levels of thinking about teaching' and note that at stage (or level) one, if the student does not 'absorb' the knowledge and skills imparted to them, because they either have not got the ability or the motivation to do so, then the teaching is unlikely to be effective.

In the level (or stage) two approach, in addition to the ability to impart knowledge and skills, the teacher needs additional skills such as that required to structure learning activities and to negotiate student learning so as to ensure the curriculum's learning outcomes are met. Yet further skills are required at the third and current level of thinking about teaching, which is facilitation of learning as this is based on the student's own learning needs and is about enabling students to engage with their learning more actively. The earlier approaches were also reflected in the method of assessment used by educators, which had negative effects on students' learning and achievement.

The trend in moving away from teacher-centred approaches to student-centred approaches was suggested several years ago by Bruner (1960), for instance, who advocated 'discovery learning' theory, indicating that this approach can make learning more effective as it is an active process that is stimulated through student curiosity. The teacher therefore devises situations, poses problems or questions, and creates the medium for the student to discover the structures and principles underlying the situation or topic area. This approach feeds into the currently advocated methods such as problem-based learning, which is an instructional method in which students work in small groups or individually to gain knowledge from simulated problem situations and acquire problem-solving skills at the same time.

Mentors can use these approaches in their learning facilitation roles. Problem-based learning can be implemented in the form of self-directed learning in clinical practice, in, for example, management of a staff conflict situation, management of a new illness or syndrome and the use of limited learning resources. The teacher, however, must ensure that the learning is directly linked to achieving learning outcomes or competencies identified in the module or the course.

Current definitions of teaching take these evolving learning philosophies into account. For example, according to Curzon and Tummons (2013: 20), teaching is 'a system of activities intended to allow learning to happen, comprising the deliberate and methodical creation and control of those conditions in which learning does occur'. The definition thus does not reflect teacher-centred one-way information giving.

Teacher-centred or learner-centred approaches

Teacher-centred teaching approaches clearly imply that the teacher directs the content of the teaching session. This may have advantages in being economical, in that with their deep knowledge of the subject the teacher can maximise the allocated time by selecting and focusing on the most significant areas of the topic.

Drawing on the theories underlying patient or service user-centred therapy for people with psychological problems, Rogers (1983) formulated the student-centred approach to learning, which formed a major landmark in approaches to teaching and learning. Rogers suggested that:

- Human beings have a natural potentiality for learning.
- Much significant learning is acquired through doing.
- Learning is facilitated when the student participates responsibly in the learning process.
- The most socially useful learning in the modern world is the learning of the process of learning, a continuing openness to experience and incorporation into oneself of the process of change.

Activity 3.2   Teacher-centred or student-centred teaching

To follow up on the aforementioned approaches to teaching, identify a number of factors that you consider to be the strengths and weaknesses of teacher-centred and student-centred teaching methods in healthcare professional education programmes.

Jarvis (1995) notes that using teacher-centred methods of teaching reinforces hierarchical social relationships between teachers and learners (or mentor and student), and thereby replicates models of authority in which the teacher might be seeking to control and mould individuals to fit into social systems. Rogers (1983) suggested earlier that such approaches cause learners to become dependent on teachers and thereby obstruct growth and development. The possible weaknesses of teacher-centred methods or strategies include the following:

- They assume that students usually lack discipline and are irresponsible.
- They disregard experience as a resource for learning.
- The orientation to learning is subject-centred rather than building on the individual student's existing knowledge.
- The motivation to learn is external, for example by passing coursework.
- They can suppress the individual's creative powers.
- Student's opinions and questions tend to be largely overlooked.

Rogers sees the teacher as a facilitator of learning, a provider of resources for learning and someone who shares feelings as well as knowledge with learners. Furthermore, he indicates that crucial to effective facilitation of learning is the relationship between individual learners and the facilitator. The prerequisites for being an effective facilitator of learning are awareness of self and being oneself in the teaching situation, through (as mentioned in Chapter 1 in relation to building an effective working relationship):

- *Genuineness* – The facilitator portrays full honesty and willingness to declare their strengths and the areas in which they are lacking, where appropriate. They remain a real person and are not sucked into the image of a distant and authority-vested teacher.
- *Trust and acceptance* – The facilitator must be able to gain and retain the student's trust, and vice versa, and overtly accept any limitations that students might have.
- *Empathic understanding* – The facilitator consistently endeavours to see situations from the learner's viewpoint.

Rogers contrasts the kind of learning that is concerned solely with cognitive functioning, for example acquiring knowledge, with that involving the whole person. The learning naturally needs to be guided by the approved curriculum for the course the student is on to be able to obtain the relevant award (i.e., qualification). Rogers suggests that it is possible for the teacher to build into a programme this freedom to learn. This can be done by using students' own experiences and problems so that relevance is more obvious, and by identifying relevant resources both material and human for their students. The goal of education is therefore to enable the student to become a fully functioning person as a whole (Rogers and Freiberg, 1994).

In healthcare learning, the student-centred approach is reflected in andragogy, but the latter needs to be tailored to the individual student's responses to it. Facilitation of learning is also consistent with the andragogical approach to teaching and learning, as advocated by Knowles et al. (2011) (and discussed in Chapter 2) and with 'learning by insight', that is 'a perception of a whole group of relationships … a suddenly occurring re-organisation' (Curzon and Tummons, 2013: 62). A concept analysis of facilitation of learning by Cross (1996) revealed that the:

- prerequisites of being a facilitator are the facilitator's qualities of realness, that is, caring and empathy, access to learning situations and the motivation of students and social influences
- defining attributes of facilitation are a process of enabling change, a climate of learning which includes mutual trust, acceptance and respect, and the nature of interaction being student centred, negotiated and collaborative
- consequences of facilitation are reciprocal change and feedback, and increased independence.

Case Study

Mentoring Jane

Consider the following case study. Jane is a 34-year-old ex-schoolteacher who is now a first year midwifery student. Jane is a graduate, who, after initial teacher training, soon found the job easy but had no wish to take on management responsibilities. The job was soon becoming too routine when she realised that in fact she had always wanted to be a midwife instead. Jane is also raising her own family and has remained an active member of the Parents and Teachers Association.

Consider the ways in which Jane's mentor, Julie, can take a learner-centred approach to learning facilitation during the practice placement. Make some notes taking into account Jane's previous vocation.

Mentors can consider ascertaining and adapting their facilitation of learning role to mentees' previous knowledge of health and their preferred styles and approaches to learning, as noted in Chapter 2. Jane's age, responsibility and discipline as a qualified teacher and a mother can be taken into account when taking a learner-centred approach to placement learning. A self-directed approach to learning in consultation with Jane can be warranted.

Despite these benefits of the student-centred approach to teaching, there could also be drawbacks, some of which are identified in the box.

Arguments for, and criticisms of, the learner-centred or person-centred approach to teaching

Arguments for:

- Motivates, as aims and objectives are clear and relevant.
- Learning is meaningful.
- Encourages divergent and critical thinking through dialogue.
- Allows autonomy and creativity.

Criticisms:

- Can be time consuming if emphasis is on how much ground is covered, rather than the nature of learning that occurs. Rogers (1983) was aware of this, and suggested that there should be freedom within a system of constraints.
- Structure and guidelines may suffer.
- Timetables and deadlines might not get adhered to.
- Assumption that everyone engages in self-directed learning.

Despite likely weaknesses, the student-centred approach to facilitation of learning is preferred as it entails more active involvement in learning. This is also consistent with old sayings such as, 'What we do we understand, what we see we remember, what we hear we forget' (Neary, 2000a: 93); and in relation to the senses and remembering, in that we remember 90 per cent of all we do, 50 per cent of all we see, but only 10 per cent of all we hear.

In experiential learning, as a way of adapting learning theories to methods of teaching, students need to be given opportunities for 'doing', that is, applying or using the knowledge or skill. For example, most healthcare courses include the topic 'moving and handling patients'. This is an apt example that lends itself to experiential learning, in that having been exposed to the knowledge base (for example, principles of moving and handling), students can then learn by doing. This can occur in university skills laboratories under close supervision of the facilitator. Students can be given problem situations to solve, which could enable them to make the topic their own and internalise it.

A concluding suggestion on facilitation of learning is that, in the context of the current-day vehement push towards efficiency, mentors and mentees need to seize learning opportunities as they arise, which is also referred to as opportunistic learning or teachable moments.

Facilitating Learners to Acquire Clinical Skills

Healthcare professions are skill-based vocations, which means that pre-registration education leads to becoming competent at performing specific clinical interventions to improve patients' or service users' health. Competence was defined and discussed in Chapter 2. According to Curzon and Tummons (2013), a skill signifies having expertise in an activity that has been developed as the result of training and/or experience, enabling the individual to perform the particular task with effectiveness and flexibility. It requires effective mind and muscle coordination, resulting in the production of appropriate, swift and meaningful patterns of movement. These are the distinguishing features of a 'skilled activity', which also include dexterity, the ability to respond quickly, spatial ability and the capacity to share attention among a number of more or less simultaneous demands (Curzon and Tummons, 2013). These defining features of skills also apply to healthcare clinical skills and competencies.

Learning motor skills

Progression with learning and mastering clinical skills can be identified along a continuum that identifies early attempts at learning a skill to becoming proficient. A widely used framework for identifying levels of psychomotor skill development and testing in healthcare courses is that suggested by Steinaker and Bell (1979) in a taxonomy of experiential learning. The term *taxonomy* broadly refers here to levels of learning, that is, learning from lower levels to higher levels. In Steinaker and Bell's model, skill development progresses from the lower-level exposure, through participation, identification and internalisation to dissemination.

Experiential learning refers to learning that involves going through the experience of actually doing or engaging in the skill. Competency or skill development through the different levels occurs over the three-year course. The five levels and the likely interpretation (or criteria) related to a clinical skill are presented in the box.

Taxonomy levels and criteria

Levels	Criteria
Exposure	Have some knowledge of concepts, terms and methods used in clinical practice Show willingness to participate
Participation	Interact well with patients/service users Carry out activities under supervision Explain activities when questioned
Identification	Apply theory to practice Demonstrate awareness of situations Interpret information correctly Act on one's own without having to be prompted
Internalisation	Consistently apply theory to practice in a range of settings Compare and contrast different approaches to practices Determine implications of practices Solve problems by analysis and evaluation Show willingness to share experiences
Dissemination	Use opportunities to teach service users and families Share experiences with peers and others Accurately write and verbalise information about teaching and management issues

Consider a mental health student who has to demonstrate a certain level of proficiency in helping or counselling skills by the end of their third year of professional education:

1 *Exposure* – refers to the student observing the mentor helping or counselling appropriate service users and becoming aware of the pre-conditions and specific helping skills being used by the mentor.
2 *Participation* – refers to when, under mentor supervision, the student attempts to use selected helping skills, e.g. low-level self-disclosure.
3 *Identification* – is when the student starts to feel competent at some of the helping skills and this is acknowledged by their mentor.
4 *Internalisation* – can be difficult to achieve within the constraints of the pre-registration course, as this implies that the learner is so proficient at these skills that they see them as part of themselves as a person.
5 *Dissemination* – refers to being so knowledgeable and competent in a skill that the person can have specific and valid opinions about the skill, can explain them and even teach them, which is difficult to achieve in a pre-registration course.

To teach competencies at the appropriate level entails careful planning that determines the teacher's approach, student behaviour and assessment techniques. Another well-established model of learning a clinical skill is Benner's (2001) stages of skill acquisition, which is based on a framework initially deduced from how trainee pilots learn their vocations and eventually become experts in flying aeroplanes. These stages are novice, advanced beginner, competent, proficient and expert, in this sequence, and they relate to longer-term activities on expertise development as they progress from initial cruder attempts to more refined performance with a substantial associated knowledge base.

Fitts and Posner (1973) earlier suggested that there are three phases of learning a skill – the cognitive phase, associative phase and autonomous phase:

1 *Cognitive phase* – concerned with the learning of the procedure, but the more complex the skill, the longer the learning will take.
2 *Associative phase* – engaging in skilled performance of part-skills or in whole practical skills, and interfering responses are eliminated.
3 *Autonomous phase* – in the long-term, the skill becomes automatic and can be performed without the student thinking much about it.

The three phases are not completely distinct as they overlap, with one phase leading to the next.

Teaching psychomotor skills

A major component of the mentor's role is to teach clinical skills. Various aspects need to be considered in relation to this.

Activity 3.3   Skill acquisition and maintenance

Think of, and list, all factors that the mentor as a teacher needs to consider, and all preparations that they need to make to teach a particular clinical skill in the practice setting. Then list all the factors that the mentor might affect enabling efficient acquisition of the psychomotor skill in the practice setting. Finally, list all the factors that might affect maintenance and performance of the clinical skill at the same or higher standard in practice settings.

There are several factors that need to be considered when preparing to teach a clinical skill. Those required for teaching blood glucose monitoring, for instance, include:

- which patient?
- condition requiring it
- equipment needed
- approved procedure for taking a blood sample
- gain patient's consent
- factors affecting reading of results
- ensuring there's enough blood on the test strip

- safety aspects
- own knowledge
- the student's knowledge base – practical and theoretical
- reading result – up/down/normal
- record the result, and take any necessary action
- opportunities to practise
- frequency of measurement
- testing the equipment and cleaning it after use
- evaluate, observe, supervise
- what if?!!
- time allocated
- record learner's competence.

A list of factors that need to be considered for a particular clinical activity like the one above is rarely fully prescriptive as there are other variables that need to be taken into account in relation to the individual patient's health problems or needs, and the equipment and other resources that are available.

Teaching a clinical skill requires first of all a skills analysis. Generally, the trust's procedure for the clinical action constitutes a very good basis for structuring a lesson plan for the skill. The mentor can also consider how the task is performed or executed, step by step, by those who are recognised as competent at the particular clinical action. These are discussed shortly. Such a detailed analysis of the clinical skill constitutes its performance or assessment criteria, which is discussed in Chapter 6. In the box below a set of principles of teaching a skill or competency is presented that stands the test of time (adapted from Curzon and Tummons, 2013). These are generally fully used when teaching a skill in the HEI's skills laboratory, but can be easily adapted by the mentor when teaching in the practice setting.

Principles of teaching a skill or competency

1 *Initially demonstrate the skill in its entirety as a fully integrated set and cycle of operations.* The demonstration needs to be accompanied by a clear step-by-step commentary, and it must be a demonstration of mastery of the skill. The correct movements that go to make up the skill must be in evidence from the outset.

2 *Break the skill down into its component and subordinate activities.* Each action must be demonstrated, explained and analysed. The relation of separate activities to one another and their integration into a hierarchy of sequences that make up the skill must be stressed.

3 *Skill acquisition lessons require supervised, reinforced and carefully spaced practice by students.* It is only by experiencing and repeating the essential movements that the learner can discover the kinaesthetic cues of successful performance.

(Continued)

(Continued)

4 *Continuous, swift and accurate feedback must be provided for the learner.* Delayed feedback on performance makes the feedback less effective.

5 *Assess part-skills or the whole skill regularly and in work-related realistic conditions.* Evidence should also be sought on the ability of the student to transfer the acquired skill to related situations.

Source: Adapted from Curzon and Tummons (2013)

The principles presented in the box constitute a firm foundation for developing a skill-teaching session. Achievement of competence at one level ought to be accepted as a necessary preparation for moving to higher level of skill. The learner should be able to progress from competent performance to proficient, etc. Drawing on this, and on healthcare professionals' perceptions of factors that need to be considered when preparing to teach a psychomotor skill, the teacher should also consider taking the following actions before the actual skill-teaching session:

- Practise the skill yourself, using the relevant procedures and equipment.
- Ensure that, as the teacher, your practice is up to date and evidence-based.
- Have all equipment and materials ready.
- Arrange for your learner(s) to hear and see the skill demonstration.
- State the aim of the session.
- Show the finished product if possible.
- Ask the student/patient to verbalise the action.
- Arrange for the student/patient to practise the skill.

Domains of learning and levels of skill acquisition

Precisely which areas of knowledge and competence do healthcare students learn on their pre-registration courses? Well, students learn a comprehensive range of knowledge base and competence that are required for healthcare interventions. Each intervention comprises three domains of activity: psychomotor (skill), cognitive (knowledge) and affective (attitude) (for example, Bloom, 1956; NMC, 2010a). The psychomotor domain refers to motor, muscular and coordination skills; the cognitive domain refers to the use of knowledge and information; and the affective domain refers to attitudes, emotions and values. The three domains equating broadly with skills, knowledge and attitudes, also equate largely with doing, thinking and feeling, respectively. The three domains are integrated essential components of each competency and not necessarily distinct and separate activities. All healthcare interventions incorporate these three domains and therefore learning the clinical skill must also incorporate all three components.

Psychomotor, cognitive and affective domains of competencies

Consider any two clinical interventions (e.g. blood pressure taking, counselling, ward management) to ascertain whether each of them contains all three components: skill, knowledge and attitude.

The sequence of events that both teacher and learner should engage in during skill acquisition is summarised in Table 3.1. It captures the principles of teaching and facilitation of learning of a psychomotor skill or competency that incorporates the cognitive and affective domains. The five components of the affective domain to be achieved by the learner are: *receiving, responding, valuing, organising* and *characterising* (Krathwohl et al., 1999).

After practising the skill on several occasions, a summative assessment of competence will be performed by the mentor and, if the learner is deemed competent, he or she is usually permitted to practise the skill without direct supervision. One of the key purposes of Table 3.1 is to highlight how the cognitive and affective domains of learning are integral components of learning any clinical intervention.

As a general guide, 25 per cent of the lesson time should be used to demonstrate the skill, 15 per cent in verbal explanation and 60 per cent for guided practice. So, for effective acquisition of the skill or competency, it is important to consider the requirements for effective teaching. Other factors that affect effective and efficient acquisition of the skill include:

- the complexity of the skill
- individual differences in speed of learning, or background
- its transferability to real-life settings
- teaching situation – environment, light, space, room temperature
- the quality of instruction
- knowledge of progress
- availability of practice opportunities
- availability of necessary equipment – checking them beforehand, describing them
- getting feedback on skill performance
- a positive approach
- a running commentary if appropriate
- a true-to-life setting
- allowing time for discussion
- time for practice – with positive reinforcement.

The types of knowledge associated with skills teaching is practical knowledge (i.e., 'knowing how') and theoretical knowledge (i.e., more in-depth 'knowing that'). Healthcare courses involve acquisition of both types of knowledge, and students

TABLE 3.1   Skills teaching sequence

Psychomotor domain	Cognitive domain	Affective domain
Awareness that learner lacks the skill or is deficient in it ↓	Establish learner's existing knowledge base underpinning the skill	Receiving – i.e., ensuring learner realises that it will be beneficial to learn the skill
Ensure the learner is motivated to learn the skill ↓	Permit learner to be active in seeking related knowledge	Responding – learner is willing, and takes action to learn the skill
Analysis of the step-by-step procedure/components of the skill ↓	Having clear objectives in learning the skill, and seeking out possible sources of learning	Responding – learner appreciates the step-by-step procedure and the materials required at every step
Prepare equipment, etc. to teach the skill ↓	Assembling appropriate equipment/devices and materials	
Demonstrate the skill at normal speed ↓	Enable learner to observe and assimilate all details of the procedure	
Discuss each step just performed; re-demonstrate part skills as required ↓	State rationale for each action; emphasise important points; discuss safety points; encourage learner to ask questions	Valuing – the rationales for each step taken; learner is willing to participate in performing the skill or part skill
Allow learner to perform whole skill/part-skills ↓	Select components to work on, and actually 'doing' the skill, i.e. experiencing it	Organising – mental rehearsal of each skill component, with rationales; asking questions when unsure
Allow learner to perform the skill under supervision ↓	Observe in silence, and with confidence in the learner	
Praise and review ↓	Give feedback on performance. Reward progress. Correct any mistake.	Organising – reinforcement and sense of achievement, confidence
Allow to apply/repeat the skill under supervision	Using the learning in real situations. Assess progress and knowledge of rationales	Characterising – accepting the procedure is the correct way of performing the skill

are assessed on them at different academic levels, as detailed shortly in this chapter. Also see this book's Companion Website for an example of a lesson plan for teaching a clinical skill.

Facilitating Knowledge Acquisition

Despite the current paradigm shift away from teaching to facilitation of learning, formal teaching also has its place in professional preparatory programmes. Many clinical skills and knowledge components are best imparted to learners through teaching. There will be times when the mentor will have to conduct short structured teaching sessions, probably in a room in the practice setting that can be used for this purpose. These sessions can be quite short or last an hour or more, delivered to a small group of learners or colleagues. Therefore a good insight into how to structure and deliver a teaching session is a useful component of the mentor's armoury of capabilities.

Effective teaching requires careful and thorough planning. The lesson needs to be fully structured, with flexibility built in, depending on whether it is being delivered to a large group or to smaller group workshops.

Planning a structured teaching session

Logical sequencing of a structured teaching session constitutes lesson planning, an example of which is presented in the box.

Steps in lesson planning

1 Identify the topic of the lesson.
2 Research the subject.
3 Consider the students in relation to their previous knowledge.
4 Write down the aims and objectives.
5 Jot down as many points as possible in keeping with the objectives; then select, prune, sequence and structure these points.
6 Select the appropriate teaching methods.
7 Screen the activities against the objectives.
8 Write the lesson (include teaching aids).
9 Prepare aids, equipment and classroom.
10 Give the lesson.
11 Evaluate the lesson.

Each step presented in the box requires specific attention in its own right. For instance, the third step requires the teacher to consider the students in relation to the knowledge they already have, as well as any prior reading that was required or suggested before the teaching session. This accords with the use of appropriate learning theories such as Ausubel et al.'s (1978) assimilation theory (discussed in Chapter 2). It is also consistent with Bruner's (1960) notion of linking new learning to previous knowledge.

As to the sequencing of lesson content (step 5 in the box above), the Herbartian rule (Hughes and Quinn, 2013: 171) of sequence (or 'sequence procedures') for lesson presentation has stood the test of time and is also referred to as 'traditional rule'. It involves proceeding from:

1   *The known to the unknown* – link new concepts to what is already known by the learner (e.g. water to blood, water pipes to blood vessels).
2   *The simple to the complex* – simple explanations to more complex areas; increasing level of complexity (e.g. diffusion in a jar to movement of oxygen and CO_2 between alveoli and alveolar capillaries; intra- and extra-cellular movement of potassium).
3   *The concrete to the abstract* – demonstrate a link between visible components and invisible concepts (e.g. aspirates or infusion to acidity vs alkalinity).
4   *The particular to the general* – use specific examples to illustrate general theories (e.g. giving information reduces anxiety, people generally have a need to know what is happening).
5   *Observation to reasoning* – from how things are done to why.
6   *The whole view, to the parts, then return to the whole view* – the subject matter as an entity, analysis of component parts, return to the overall view.

Step 6 in the box above suggests selecting the appropriate teaching methods. A range of teaching methods is available to the teacher (see the box below). The teaching method(s) selected for the session must be based on principles of teaching and on learning theories. The appropriateness of the method depends on the teacher's level of knowledge of theories and principles and their values, research and verbal skills, facilitative skills and on the aims of the lesson, for instance.

Most frequently used teaching methods

- Lectures
- Buzz groups/work in subgroups
- Seminars
- Skills demonstration
- Guided study and open learning
- Role plays
- Problem-solving games/ exercises/workshops
- Case study/patient-centred discussions

- Video recording a teaching session
- Tutorial – individual/small group
- Ideas free flow exercises (previously known as brainstorming), e.g. concept-mapping
- Questions and answers
- Formal lessons
- E-learning and distance learning
- Group discussion
- Team teaching

Each of these methods has its advantages and disadvantages that are examined later in this chapter. The eighth step in box above titled 'Steps in lesson planning' is to 'write the lesson', and includes identifying the teaching aids to be used. An example of a lesson plan is presented in Template 3.1.

TEMPLATE 3.1   A lesson or session plan

Date: .... Cohort: .... No. of students: ....

Title of the course/module: ....

Subject of lesson: ....

Lesson aims:

Objectives:

Duration of lesson: .... (e.g. 1 hour)   Classroom: ....

Time	Lesson content	Method	Teaching aids
5 mins	Ascertain previous learning	Q & A*	–
2 mins	State and explain lesson objective	Verbal exposition	PowerPoint slides
10 mins	Concept I	Verbal exposition; Q & A	Whiteboard/flipchart
15 mins	Concept II	Verbal exposition; discussion	Whiteboard/flipchart
20 mins	Concept III	Students complete gapped handout; discussion	Gapped handout
3 mins	Recapitulation, and recommend further reading	Verbal exposition	PowerPoint slides
4 mins	Test and evaluation	Q & A	PowerPoint slides
1 min	Announce title of next lesson + pre-reading	Verbal exposition	PowerPoint slides Written guidance on pre-reading
*Q & A = Questions and answers			

In relation to steps 8 and 9 in the box titled 'Steps in lesson planning', or the use of an appropriate range of teaching aids such as whiteboard/flipchart or PowerPoint slides, some of these will be explained briefly and their advantages and disadvantages will also be explored later in this chapter.

In planning the lesson, the teacher needs to consider likely constraints such as class size (for instance, is it 10 students or 200 students?), the number of pages of handouts if any are given and the availability of articles to be recommended as further reading. The teacher's aim in a lesson is to motivate, stimulate and communicate, to hold the class's attention and to achieve the defined objectives (Curzon and Tummons, 2013), and therefore further essential considerations to be taken by the presenter are that:

1 The lesson must be appropriately pitched.
2 The teaching objectives must be realistic and clear.
3 Exposition must be ordered, simple and clear.
4 Development must be logical and sequential (flows coherently).
5 Presentation must be based on the essential 'social character' of the lesson (e.g. laboratory work or lecture).
6 Presentation must involve a variety of media.
7 Presentation must be carefully adjusted in the light of fluctuations in class attention.
8 Appropriate body language should be used.

Furthermore, a well-constituted presentation requires a clearly defined structure, the elements of which will normally include:

- an introduction, main part and conclusion
- a logical sequence within each of the three parts
- regular sign-posting – this is what we have covered so far, this is what we will explore next, and these are what we will address afterwards
- key learning points or main headings
- built-in monitoring and review – checking that the main learning points are being understood.

Appropriate communication and delivery skills are crucial. The presenter's role is also to engage with the audience, to challenge, to enthuse, to support, to motivate and to clarify. The next step is to give the lesson based on the lesson plan, and to evaluate it at the end of the lesson. The evaluation of the lesson can include use of an evaluation form, or the students can be asked to write three things that they liked or found most useful about the session, aspects that can be seen as weaknesses, and suggestions for improvement (see Chapter 8 for more on evaluation).

Levels of theory acquisition

The objective of many a teaching session is to impart knowledge and understanding of the designated topic area and, depending on various factors, it can cover application, analysis and synthesis. These concepts are largely enshrined in the cognitive domain of Bloom's (1956) taxonomy of learning, which follows six hierarchical levels. The first or lower level of learning is the acquisition of knowledge, followed by the higher levels – comprehension, application, analysis, synthesis and evaluation, as illustrated here:

1 *Knowledge* – refers to knowledge of topic area and content.
2 *Comprehension* – refers to knowledge, and comprehension or understanding of why things work the way they do.
3 *Application* – refers to knowledge and comprehension, and application of knowledge and understanding to general and specific settings.
4 *Analysis* – refers to knowledge, comprehension, application, and analysis of all components of knowledge and application; and alternative perspectives.
5 *Synthesis* – refers to knowledge, comprehension, application, analysis, and synthesis of components to arrive at solutions to problems.
6 *Evaluation* – refers to knowledge, comprehension, application, analysis, synthesis and evaluation (research, etc. on the topic).

Knowledge is the most basic level of learning, in which the student shows recall of specific facts, classifications, categories and sequences or methods in the topic area. It is a significant component of student assessment, as when the student has to demonstrate knowledge of human biology or of research methods. *Comprehension* refers to understanding and interpretation of the topic area, and can be shown by the student explaining theories and reasoning in their own words. It answers the question 'why' certain things happen or certain actions are taken, and the possible implications and consequences of these. *Application* occurs when the student applies knowledge and understanding to 'real-life' situations such as patient care.

Analysis entails the ability to break down theories and concepts into their component parts, and explain the relationships between elements and the whole. It considers strengths and weaknesses, and separates the important aspects of information from the less important ones. *Synthesis* requires the individual to recombine various components of the topic area into a newly reconstructed whole. The student thereby utilises creativity in producing something unique, for example a plan, a design or a proposal. *Evaluation* implies the ability to make judgements regarding the value of material learned.

A simple and brief example of levels of learning related to 'the heart and blood pressure' is presented here to illustrate how cognitive levels of learning (Bloom, 1956) apply to learning in healthcare:

* *Knowledge* – knowing the anatomy and physiology of the heart and that pressure is exerted on the blood vessels each time the heart pumps a certain volume of blood through them.
* *Comprehension* – understanding that the reason for the heart beating rhythmically at approximately 60 beats every minute, generating a blood pressure (BP) of approximately 110/70 mm Hg is to ensure that essential ingredients such as glucose and oxygen are transferred to every tissue in the human body, and continuously.

- *Application* – awareness that the above BP reading can change for a variety of reasons, which might include diseased organs, and its significance for patient care.
- *Analysis* – when a person is seen to have high BP, the nurse needs to consider the whole range of reasons for this.
- *Synthesis* – designing, and advising the individual on, a set of actions to take to reduce their BP, and explaining the effects of unstable or high BP based on their own unique aetiology and perceptions of high BP.
- *Evaluation* – ascertaining the value of the above set of actions, the skills and compliance of the patient in relation to them, and any research evidence on which actions are based.

The analysis of the cognitive domain of learning is essential as it involves critical analysis, which as already noted above entails breaking down information, exploring relationships between elements, or organisation and structure of information. Critical analysis involves the use of critical thinking, whereby we:

- examine all the component parts of a situation
- identify what existing knowledge or information we have, related to the situation
- distinguish relevant information from irrelevant
- challenge generalisations, assumptions and rituals
- imagine and explore alternatives and choose appropriate options.

Gopee (2002b) and Gopee and Deane (2013) discuss effective ways in which students can demonstrate critical analysis in their written assignments. Furthermore, Krathwohl (2002) has suggested a refinement of Bloom's (1956) level of knowledge acquisition by suggesting that the sequence be represented as follows:

1 Remember → 2 Understand → 3 Apply → 4 Analyse → 5 Evaluate → 6 Create

Krathwohl reverses the fifth and sixth levels, and this revised taxonomy is also a useful tool for identifying educational objectives but, as with any new framework, it requires further work in its applicability to education programmes for healthcare professions.

Teaching Methods and Teaching Aids

As discussed in the preceding section, skill demonstration is an effective way of teaching how to perform a professional skill. For structured lessons, effective teaching requires choosing and applying the appropriate teaching methods and aids, which are selected based on such factors as class size, aims of session, the students' existing knowledge levels and so on. The most frequently used teaching methods were identified in the box presented earlier titled 'Most frequently used teaching methods'.

Teaching methods – their advantages and disadvantages

Lectures remain an efficient teaching method for imparting knowledge and comprehension of a selected section of a subject area. A lecture is economical in that the knowledge can be imparted to hundreds of students by one lecturer during a particular teaching session. In fact, the lecture can be televised live to other lecture theatres in the same or other universities, even in other countries.

However, only a limited level of application and analysis can be achieved, as in very large groups it is difficult to cite examples of application to each student's field of interest. Moreover, it is easier for students to let their minds wander off the subject, which they generally cannot do in smaller groups. Discussions, workshops and group work to explore application, analysis and synthesis of components of the lecture should therefore always follow lectures. Similarly, the advantages and disadvantages of other teaching methods also need to be appreciated.

Optional activity – teaching methods: advantages and disadvantages

Taking an analytical approach, the strengths and weaknesses of each of the examples of different teaching methods listed in the box titled 'Most frequently used teaching methods' can be identified. Consider these different teaching methods, and feel free to add others of your own, and identify as many advantages and disadvantages as you can for each of these methods.

You should have been able to identify one or two advantages and disadvantages of each of the aforementioned teaching methods. With *skill demonstration*, for instance, the advantages include visual display of the skill being performed. It reinforces previously acquired knowledge of the skill, activates many senses, enables procedure-directed practice, correlates theory and practice and is economical on time. The disadvantages could be that the learner might be left-/right-handed related to positioning of equipment, the skill might involve movements that are too complex and too much information might be given. As learning and mastering a skill take time, there is also a danger that the learner might be expected to perform the demonstrated skill at similar speed to the skilled demonstrator too soon.

The advantages of using *case studies* or *patient-centred discussions* as a teaching method are that there is active participation by students, that they are useful in the application of theory to practice and that they present an opportunity for structured problem-solving. This increases understanding of the situation, diagnosing the problem, creating alternative solutions and predicting outcomes or implications. The disadvantages include insufficient patient data and extent of relevance for each student.

Presentation and teaching aids

There are several types of presentation aids that the teacher can utilise to vary the session and thereby to retain the audience's attention or to add emphasis to aspects of the session. These aids include:

- flipchart and pens
- whiteboard
- PowerPoint slides
- showing video-cassette or DVD recordings
- plastic models of body parts/objects
- gapped handouts
- simulated materials or liquids
- visualisers.

The purpose of teaching aids is therefore to introduce variety into the teaching process, to extend sensory perception, to extend visual perception, to give meaning to abstractions and to assist in conceptualisation of complicated issues. The choice of visual aids involves consideration of appropriateness to the context or message, its cost-effectiveness, its availability and its suitability for your style of presentation. Each teaching aid requires a good understanding of how it works.

> ### Activity 3.4   Strengths and weaknesses of different teaching aids
>
> Consider the strengths and weaknesses of the different teaching aids listed earlier, add other ones that you know of, and discuss with someone who has had some experience of classroom teaching what might be the strengths and weaknesses of each of these aids.

The *PowerPoint presentation* is a highly favoured method of presenting the knowledge base of a topic area to small or large audiences. The advantage is that it is prepared in advance and can be made very lively and colourful with pictures, cartoons and short films for more impact. The likely disadvantage might be that too many words are inserted in each slide, or if the slides are presented at a high speed which may not allow time for the audience to take the content in properly, or the equipment (for example, computers) may fail.

Issues with Facilitation of Learning in the Practice Setting

The mentor's role includes teaching mentees on a one-to-one basis, and at times in small groups in the practice setting. In both situations, the mentor needs to have a clear view of various components of the session, for example the content and sequence of the presentation, in order to ensure that the learner gains an orderly, systematic understanding of the topic or clinical skill. However, the problematic situations that might arise when facilitating student learning may present challenges to the mentor.

For a variety of reasons, in practice settings, it cannot be guaranteed that a planned teaching session will go ahead although most do go to plan. Urgent need to cover for sickness, emergencies such as cardiac arrest, patient not consenting to student involvement, are some of the reasons. However, many care provider settings now have dedicated teaching areas, which can help focus attention on teaching sessions.

Furthermore, there can be confusion in the interpretation of students' 'supernumerary status' during placements, in that the student may claim that they are there only to observe clinical activity, while the mentor believes that they should observe as well as participate. Supernumerary status can be manipulated by some students to the extent that they take excessive time off practice settings as study time, to the detriment of learning hands-on care and clinical skills, as many mentors claim that healthcare delivery is learned by doing, not by merely knowing about it.

In opportunistic learning, negotiating access to opportunities is a skill in its own right.

Chapter Summary

This chapter has focused on the mentor's role in the facilitation of learning, both formal and incidental, and has therefore examined:

- Whose learning healthcare professionals facilitate, and why; the various reasons for teaching; and the definitions and different perceptions of teaching, along with why healthcare professionals need to know how to facilitate learning.
- General perspectives on learning, indicating a move away from teaching to the notion of facilitating learning, with teacher-centred methods and student-centred approaches to teaching and learning, with the latter comprising a shift away from formal teaching to much more learner-centred facilitation of learning.
- Facilitating learning of clinical skills, teaching a psychomotor skill, the domains of learning, levels of psychomotor skills and stages of skill acquisition.
- Facilitating knowledge acquisition, include undertaking planned and structured short teaching sessions, either on a one-to-one level or in small groups of learners or peers.
- The types of knowledge associated with skills such as practical knowledge and theoretical knowledge, along with levels of theory acquisition, and levels and stages of skill acquisition (taxonomy levels).
- Step-by-step planning of teaching sessions, including utilisation of different methods of teaching and teaching aids, and an analysis of how they can be used effectively.
- Some of the issues that might surface in the facilitation of learning in practice settings.

Further Optional Reading 📖

1 For an excellent textbook on how to teach, see:

- Curzon, L.B. and Tummons, J. (2013) *Teaching in Further Education: An Outline of Principles and Practice*, 7th edn. London: Bloomsbury Academic.

2 For a concept analysis of the concept facilitation in the context of facilitating the implementation of new evidence into practice, see:

- Harvey, G., Loftus-Hills, A., Rycroft-Malone, J., Titchen, A., Kitson, A., McCormack, B. and Seers, K. (2002) 'Getting evidence into practice: the role and function of facilitation', *Journal of Advanced Nursing*, 37 (6): 577–88.

To access further resources related to this chapter, visit the companion website at https://study.sagepub.com/gopee

4

The Practice Setting as an Effective Learning Environment

Chapter Outcomes

On completion of this chapter, you should be able to:

1 Clearly identify the various reasons for healthcare students being required to undertake practice placements.
2 Recognise the reasons for ascertaining students' previous clinical experiences before identifying their learning needs, and identify their hopes and expectations with regard to the placement.
3 Identify how a functional learning ethos can be created and maintained in the practice setting, which includes interprofessional learning, implementation of research findings and conducting annual education audits of practice placement settings.
4 Analyse the benefits of, and issues related to, work-based learning and identify ways in which the utilisation of learning pathways can enhance the student's learning.
5 Identify guidelines, policies and standards for clinical learning environments, and how practice settings can become learning organisations.
6 Recognise the likely problematic aspects of practice placements, such as with integration of theory and practice, and with supernumerary status, and the likely solutions to these.

Having explored the concept of mentorship in Chapter 1, perspectives, theories and styles of learning in Chapter 2, and facilitation of learning in Chapter 3, this chapter focuses on the factors that make healthcare settings effective learning environments for healthcare profession students, as well as for qualified staff. Ensuring that the practice setting has an effective learning environment is a key role of the mentor according to research (for example, Darling, 1984; Phillips et al., 2000), and under the domain 'Create an environment for learning', the NMC (2008a: 55) indicates that the mentor should be competent in creating 'an environment for learning, where practice is valued and developed, that provides appropriate professional and inter-professional learning opportunities and support for learning to maximise achievement for individuals'.

This chapter therefore examines the nature of effective learning environments in practice settings, ways in which healthcare professionals can be involved in creating, maintaining and monitoring such environments, educational policies, along with the issues related to student practice placements. Other aspects related to learning environments are identified under the domain 'Context of practice' and managing change, which are analysed in Chapter 5.

Students on Practice Placements

This section of the chapter explores why practice placements are required, and students' perspectives, hopes and expectations in relation to practice objectives and clinical experiences during placements.

The requirement for practice placements

The key reasons for practice settings having to be learning environments for student practice placements are as follows. First, healthcare professions comprise skill- or competency-based activities, and these skills are acquired predominantly in practice settings. Several hundred student nurses, numerous AHP and medical students start their pre-registration or pre-service courses each year, and each student requires practice placements in practice settings to learn patients or service users skills directly, or to consolidate and extend their learning from university skills laboratories. Most suitable practice settings in the local trusts and the independent sector are used for placements, and the placement of all these students is arranged by the education institution's placement department.

Each practice setting is advised in advance of which students are starting on placement with them and when. Students arrive on placement with a document containing practice competencies that the student must achieve during the placement, which takes into account the specific clinical skills and knowledge that the particular setting can offer.

Pre-service education requirements include those identified in the *EU Directive [2005/36/EC Annex V.2 (5.2.1)]* (NMC, 2010b: 1; NMC, 2013a) for healthcare profession qualifications, which states that the duration of learning in practice settings must comprise at least one half of the minimum duration of the training (i.e. half of a total of 4600 hours of the total education programme).

With regard to mentoring during practice placements, the requirement by the NMC (2010a) (similar to other health and social care professions) in *Standards for Pre-registration Nursing Education* under 'Standards for Education' is that:

- Programme providers must ensure that students are allocated to an identified mentor, practice teacher or supervisor during practice learning (clause R4.2).
- Practice learning providers must ensure that students are supervised directly or indirectly at all times during practice learning by a mentor, practice teacher or other suitably prepared registered professional (clause R4.2.2).

These standards are in concordance with the NMC's (2008a) competence for mentors under 'creating an environment for learning':

- Support students to identify both learning needs and experiences that are appropriate to their level of learning.
- Use a range of learning experiences, involving patients, clients, carers and the professional team, to meet defined learning needs.
- Identify aspects of the learning environment which could be enhanced, negotiating with others to make appropriate changes.
- Act as a resource to facilitate personal and professional development of others.

Another reason for practice settings needing to be learning environments is the increasingly popular concept of work-based learning (discussed later in this chapter), which clearly recognises the wide occurrence and value of learning in practice settings. However, various research studies have in the past revealed weaknesses of practice settings as learning environments. Consequently, for learning to occur, the practice setting must embody an ethos that nurtures and supports learning, and does not deter it. Poor clinical learning environments as a major factor in student attrition emerged from a study by Crombie et al. (2013) who explored the factors that enhance rates of course completion by student nurses.

Students' perspectives, hopes and expectations

A number of practice settings have an established welcome and orientation programme for students starting practice placement with them, and an induction pack with specific clinical objectives for newly qualified healthcare professionals. A named mentor is allocated to each student prior to the start of the placement, along with associate mentors. Both the mentor and the mentee have certain hopes and expectations of each other. So what does the student anticipate encountering at the start of the placement?

Activity 4.1   Student expectations from the placement

Your work base clearly has a wide range of specific knowledge and competence to offer students during practice placements. From your experience of having students on placement, make some notes on what you feel are the expectations that students might have on starting placement in your practice setting.

On exploring students' expectations of mentorship, a study by Foster et al. (2015) at one UK university concluded that students value teaching, explaining, support and encouragement as some of the key features of a successful practice placement. In addition to students' expectations, the staff in the practice setting naturally also have certain expectations of students. They hope that the student will be punctual, make every effort to integrate with the team and be open-minded about the ways in which care is delivered in the particular practice setting. The mentor might expect the student to seek out learning experiences and opportunities, and ask questions about aspects that they do not understand. The box below lists some of the characteristics of 'good' learners that were identified by student mentors.

Significant characteristics of healthcare learners
for effective learning

- Keen, enthusiastic and motivated to learn
- Open-minded
- Identifies own learning needs
- Open to feedback and constructive comments
- Is punctual
- Reflects on experiences
- Knows own limitations

- Able to adapt to different practice settings
- Does not have negative thoughts prior to start of placement
- Utilises learning opportunities
- Communicates effectively
- Wants to self-improve
- Reads round the subject area

Advanced preparation of learners

Universities strongly advise students to contact practice placement settings prior to the placement start date, mainly to introduce themselves, but also to enquire about practicalities such as what time shifts start, a room for changing into uniforms, possibly travel or car parking facilities, as well as any other information that can be given (for example, named mentor's name). Initiating contact can be pivotal for a smooth and successful placement as according to Webb and Shakespeare's (2008: 563) research, good learning support depends to a good extent on students themselves initiating and building a relationship with their mentors.

However, students find it useful if, prior to the practice placement, they receive a welcome letter from the practice setting, and even invites the student to come over for an informal pre-placement visit. It is useful if the student can also be advised of any recommended preparatory reading related to the clinical specialism. This action is in line with Ausubel et al.'s (1978) concept of 'advanced organiser', which suggests that learning is likely to occur more effectively if new experiences are linked to prior knowledge.

The value of communication prior to the beginning of the placement is that the student begins to become familiar with the practice setting, gets to know more about the clinical specialism and meets the mentor, and staff get to know the student as well. The aim of this would be to ensure that the clinical experiences that the student will encounter meet their learning needs and enable the achievement of their practice objectives.

Creating and Maintaining a Learning Ethos in the Practice Setting

Healthcare students acquire knowledge and competence at universities that are seen as well-established learning environments. The value of work-based learning (WBL) in enabling healthcare practitioners to achieve fitness to practise was referred to briefly in Chapter 1. However, to what extent are practice settings learning environments?

Activity 4.2   A learning ethos in the practice setting

Using your current and past experience of factors that are significant in creating an effective learning experience for students during practice placements, make notes on the following: Who are the key people who are role models for learners (undergraduate and postgraduate, other) in practice settings? What are the factors that are important for the creation of a positive learning environment (including research-based factors) for everyone within any particular practice setting?

To be a role model for anyone can be a sobering prospect for most people. In response to who the role models in practice settings are, you would have identified a range of qualified healthcare professionals and probably even some unqualified staff involved in practice-based learning, including:

- everyone acting as a mentor
- ward sisters/charge nurses
- team leaders
- specialist nurses (e.g. pain specialists)
- PEFs
- other RNs on pay bands 5 to 8
- allied healthcare professionals (e.g. physiotherapists, occupational therapists)
- link lecturers

- other students
- senior doctors, mainly consultants
- outreach workers
- clinical managers
- healthcare assistants, for specific skills
- everyone who works in the practice area.

The concept of role models was examined in Chapter 1, which includes health and social care professionals being practitioners of best practice in patient or service user care. However, poor care and neglect of patients were reported in the recent Francis Report (2013) at one English NHS Trust. A number of actions are being taken in response to the report, of which the three main ones are:

- enhancement of patient safety
- staffing levels, 'to ensure the right people, with the right skills, are in the right place at the right time' (NHS England National Quality Board (NQB), 2014: 1)
- more openness and transparency, by providing information and acquiring feedback from patients and their families or friends.

These standards have to be met by the service provider to qualify as a practice placement for health and social care profession students. Similar recommendations were made in the Willis Report (RCN, 2012), as noted in Chapter 2.

Practice settings as learning environments

In response to Activity 4.2, that is, identifying the factors that are important for the creation of a positive learning environment, you might have noted friendly and knowledgeable staff, positive attitude and allocated time for teaching. Good communication is of course essential, as is the learner feeling that they are part of the team. Team members with up-to-date knowledge of the latest research in their specialism generally make a positive impression. The availability and accessibility of research literature in the working environment, stocked in a learning resources section or in a resource room, also create a positive image.

Furthermore, you might have noted that staff showing some awareness of students' likely learning needs and their stage of knowledge and competence development also create positive impressions. The enthusiasm of team members with responsibility for teaching in practice settings, and the input of PEFs/CHEFs, generate the impetus for learning. Constructive comments on skill performance in an appropriate environment are usually appreciated by learners. A culture in which clinical staff are open to new ideas and share new learning from courses also presents healthy perspectives, as does good staff morale.

Numerous research studies have been conducted on the effectiveness of practice settings as learning environments over the years, and new research in this area continues as the dynamics in practice settings evolve. A study by Newton et al. (2009), for instance, revealed that a supportive social and cultural arena that enables the student to become part of the clinical team is very important. From their study of nursing homes as learning environments, Carlson and Idvall (2014) report with conviction that the 'supervisory relationship' (that is between mentor and student) has the greatest impact on student nurses' learning, and recommend that the work of mentors in the independent sector should be fully recognised and that they should be supported through collaborative activities (for example, university-led workshops, mentor updates).

More than three decades ago, Fretwell (1980) coined the term 'clinical learning environment' (CLE) as her research concluded that key components of 'ideal' learning environment include 'anti-hierarchy', effective communication and teamwork between all those involved in the specific practice setting, and the availability of trained nurses to enable learners to meet their learning needs. Fast-forward to today, when the acronym CLE is extended to CLES+T (S signifying supervision, and T signifying additional input from academics and professionals other than the named mentor), and CLEI (I signifying inventory) discussed shortly.

Another study conducted in the Fretwell era was an RCN-sponsored research carried out by Orton (1981), which concluded by identifying the characteristics of wards that showed 'high student orientation' and those that reflected 'low student orientation'. In high student orientation wards, respondents stated, for instance that:

- 'All staff treated students with kindness and understanding and showed willingness to teach us.'
- 'Everyone got on well.'
- 'Each patient had individual total care however long it took.'
- 'Every nurse was made to feel important.'

However, in low student orientation wards, 96 per cent of students said that they learnt more from other students than from qualified staff, and that:

- 'The atmosphere was not very relaxed which made you worry about asking questions.'
- 'The ward sister did not respect us at all and gave us ten jobs to do at once.'

Clearly Orton's focus suggested that practice settings should have positive attitudes towards students who come to their workplace to learn skills that ultimately benefit patients or service users.

Activity 4.3   Creating a learning ethos in the practice setting

1 Based on the perspectives and ideas discussed above on practice settings being CLEs, make a list of your own of the factors that you consider make a good learning environment in the healthcare practice setting.

(Continued)

(Continued)

2 How far does your own practice setting meet with the recommendations and factors that you have identified?

3 Identify areas in which your practice setting is weak or could benefit from further improvement.

The responses to studies on clinical learning environments could be categorised as factors that promote learning in the practice setting and those that can hinder, a number of which are identified in the box.

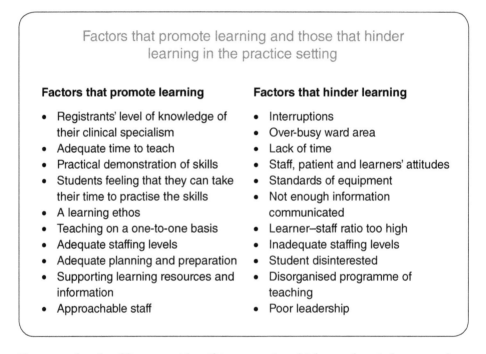

Factors that promote learning and those that hinder learning in the practice setting

Factors that promote learning

- Registrants' level of knowledge of their clinical specialism
- Adequate time to teach
- Practical demonstration of skills
- Students feeling that they can take their time to practise the skills
- A learning ethos
- Teaching on a one-to-one basis
- Adequate staffing levels
- Adequate planning and preparation
- Supporting learning resources and information
- Approachable staff

Factors that hinder learning

- Interruptions
- Over-busy ward area
- Lack of time
- Staff, patient and learners' attitudes
- Standards of equipment
- Not enough information communicated
- Learner–staff ratio too high
- Inadequate staffing levels
- Student disinterested
- Disorganised programme of teaching
- Poor leadership

Due to a dearth of literature identifying ways in which non-hospital areas such as primary care settings are CLEs, Gopee et al. (2004) make the following recommendations for enhancing these settings as learning environments:

- mentor–mentee matching in accordance with seniority of practitioner and the student's particular learning needs
- management support to enable designated time to be given for mentoring, so that students and mentors feel time spent in this way is valued by their seniors
- raised awareness of the need to integrate theory and practice
- ensuring student practice outcomes are achievable, for example carrying out dressings might not be available in, say, placement with school nurses
- prior notices of placement and appropriate timing, for example not allocating student to school nursing placement during school holidays

- ongoing professional development for all grades of staff
- more effective communication at all levels, and trust–university–mentor partnership
- all mentors (and practice teachers) ensuring that they maintain the relevant NMC standards
- access to clinical supervision for all qualified staff.

The need to ensure adequate staffing levels to safeguard patients and provide effective patient care was highlighted in the Francis Report (2013) as noted earlier in this chapter, and subsequently also by the CNO for England (NHS England National Quality Board, 2014: 45), who indicates that all 'nursing, midwifery and care staffing levels, and key quality and outcome measures should be discussed at Trust Board in a public meeting'. For this to happen, the Board has to receive monthly report of 'actual staff available on a shift-by-shift basis versus planned staffing levels' (ibid.). NICE (2014a) has also published guidelines on staff capacity and capability with its own perspectives on the issue.

Clearly, staffing levels have been a cause for concern for some years, and without sufficient and capable staff to provide safe and effective care, time might not be available to mentor students and learners. Additionally, the CNO has continuously emphasised the need to ensure a culture of compassionate care prevails, with concomitant staff education in this area (Department of Health, 2012b) (discussed in Chapter 5).

Stepping back from research and policies, Stuart (2013: 148) identifies the logical elements that are necessary for a practice setting to be an effective learning environment as well, which are: (1) the people in the team (including students and PEFs); (2) the learning opportunities that prevail in the setting; (3) staff commitment to teaching and learning; and (4) material resources.

A wide range of research studies have been conducted over the years on what contemporarily constitutes an effective CLE as the character of practice settings evolves with the times. On exploring the experiences of a group of pre-registration mental health nursing students during practice placements, for example, Wood (2005) found that students experience 'conflicting pressures', while their mentors experience difficulty supporting them because of high clinical workload.

Henderson et al. (2010) explored the organisational culture of practice settings that influence learning, which they discuss under the headings:

- Recognition of learners and learning in the organisation
- Accomplishment, i.e. acquisition of new knowledge and skills
- Affiliation, i.e. feeling part of the organisation, the team in the practice setting
- Influence, i.e. feeling safe to express opinions and suggest ideas.

Later, Henderson et al.'s (2012) research on CLE revealed that students tend to value 'task accomplishment' highly, but although the practice settings valued safe practice, they were 'not readily open to innovation and challenges to routine practices' (ibid.: 299). Thus, with continuing research and recommendations for enhancement of practice settings as CLEs, more positive findings are also reported. For example,

Sundler et al. (2014) found that students had positive experiences in the setting with regard to the 'premises' where nursing activities take place, the teaching and learning ethos, and leadership style of the ward manager. Students emphasised, however, that the supervisory relationship with their mentors was particularly significant in their achievement of their practice objectives.

Based on the above accounts of the subject area, a clinical learning environment can be defined as a practice setting that manifests a psychosocial ethos and culture, with related supportive resources, that fosters mutual learning amongst all healthcare professionals, learners and clientele, and where care and treatment are founded on evidence-based practice. The recommendations from earlier and recent studies regarding aspects that constitute good and effective learning environments form key components of annual educational audit documents.

Educational audit of practice placement settings

After Fretwell's (1980) and Orton's (1981) research, later studies on clinical learning environments (for example, Rotem and Hart, 1995) focused more directly on exploring the factors that can be identified as the necessary criteria in educational audit documents (or tools) that are used for identifying and monitoring the continuing suitability of practice settings for student placement. The criteria for suitability include evidence of a systematic approach to care delivery and holistic care (and the practice setting's philosophy of care). Orton et al. (1993) focused specifically on educational auditing, and asked qualified staff and students the same questions separately in relation to:

1 orientation to the placement
2 theory and practice integration
3 supernumerary status
4 staff attitudes and behaviour
5 mentors
6 progressive assessment.

Thus, having gathered data on the views of key players under the above-mentioned headings, Orton et al. (1993) then designed an educational audit tool with specified criteria that they referred to as 'ward learning climate indicators' to ascertain their suitability for student placement. It is an NMC (2013a) requirement that annual educational audits are carried out for each practice setting where students are placed for learning clinical skills (some can be done every two years).

More contemporarily, Newton et al. (2010) go a step further by empirically testing the recently advocated 'Clinical Learning Environment Inventory' (CLEI) (Chan and Ip, 2007), which comprises 42 criteria grouped under the sections: personalisation, student involvement, task orientation, innovation, and satisfaction and individualisation. They conclude their test by suggesting modifications to the inventory, and by recommending further research to establish the consistency of the modified inventory, which implies that even in 2010 the best educational audit tool had not yet been established.

Based on the various research on CLE like those cited above, each university, in partnership with the local healthcare trusts, devises its own research-informed educational audit tool. These audit forms contain a range of criteria for determining whether a practice setting is suitable for practice placement of healthcare profession students. Evidence needs to be available to auditors to demonstrate how each criterion is achieved.

The CLEI is designed to measure students' perceptions of the placement practice setting as a learning environment, and in doing so, Brown et al. (2011) found that there are significant differences between the students' perception of their 'actual' CLE and their 'ideal' CLE. The other prevailing educational audit tool that measures the practice setting as a learning environment from the students' viewpoint is CLES+T, which stands for clinical learning environment, supervision and nurse teacher, consisting of a total of 34 criteria under five sections (Johansson et al., 2010).

Activity 4.4 Strengths and weaknesses of your work base as a learning environment

Locate a copy of the current completed educational audit document for your workplace, a copy of which is usually lodged in the practice setting as a paper copy or electronically. If you cannot find the form, ask the ward manager or the PEF where the form can be found.

Then peruse each item or criterion in the document to decide for yourself whether the item has been fully achieved in your practice setting or otherwise. This exercise will comprise your own professional judgement of areas of strengths and areas where improvements can be made to your practice setting as a learning environment. Discuss your impressions with a peer if you have the opportunity.

Can you do anything about the weaker points? In fact, can you devise a SMART (specific, measurable, achievable, realistic and time-limited) action plan to make tangible improvements to the weaker areas/audit criteria?

Alternatively, view the CLES+T scale in Johansson et al. (2010: 2091, table 2), or in Saarikoski et al. (2008: 1235–6, table 1). The scale is designed and worded in such a way that it endeavours to measure the students' perception of the practice setting as a learning environment. Yet another alternative is to use the table related to CLEI in Chan and Ip (2007: 680, table 1). Using any of these three articles, peruse each item in the same way as indicated above for the educational audit document. (Full details of the articles are given in the References list at the end of this book.)

Further research on the CLEI and CLES+T evaluation scales continue. As noted, CLES+T has 34 criteria under five sections, which are: (1) supervisory relationships; (2) pedagogical atmosphere on the ward; (3) the leadership style of ward managers; (4) premises of nursing; and (5) the role of nurse teachers. Warne et al. (2010) conducted a multinational European study using the CLES+T scale of factors that enhance students' learning experience during practice placement, and found that student learning 'requires both significant time being spent working with patients and a supportive supervisory relationship' (ibid.: p. 809).

The educational audit document usually includes a section for recording the qualifications of each member of staff, of particular significance being which part of the profession's regulatory body's register they are on, and also whether they have a mentoring qualification and have been attending annual update sessions on mentoring. Other post-registration qualifications are also recorded. Template 4.1 shows the content of the section of the audit form that contains key information that identifies the particular practice setting.

TEMPLATE 4.1   Placement details page of educational audit document

XXX UNIVERSITY
Department of Nursing, Midwifery and Healthcare
Multi-Professional Practice Environment Profile

Placement Details

Name of NHS Trust /Healthcare Organisation:

Location/Address:

Name of Ward/Department/Unit/Team:

Placement Area Telephone No:

Contact Email address:

Name of Placement Contact Person (e.g. ward manager):

Type of Service Provision/Speciality:

Work/Shift Patterns:

Date of Review:

Date of Previous Review:

Names of Reviewers/Review Team:

Name of Academic Link Lecturer:

Name of Practice Education Facilitator:

Name(s) of Academic Institutions Placing Students (University/College of Further Education/Other):

Maximum number of students that the practice setting can support at any one time:

Other:

Naturally, each item in this section of the audit document is important. The document also tends to have a section for clinical staff to identify and to list all the formal and informal teaching and learning opportunities that are available in the particular practice setting.

Activity 4.5   Formal and informal learning opportunities

Identify and make two lists, one of all the formal learning opportunities that are available in your own practice setting, and one of the informal ones. You might find it useful to discuss the activity with a colleague in the same practice setting.

For formal learning, you might have mentioned lectures by the clinical nurse specialist, for instance; and for informal learning opportunities, you might have mentioned when you explain to the learner why the doctor has changed a patient's medication. There are likely to be various teaching and learning opportunities in your workbase setting. Maybe one of the consultants holds regular formal teaching sessions for junior doctors, which all healthcare professionals in the particular area are welcome to attend. Maybe pharmaceutical or medical devices company representatives give talks and demonstrations on their products in the practice setting. Further examples of teaching and learning opportunities that tend to be identified when completing educational audit forms are presented in the box.

Formal and informal learning opportunities

Formal teaching

- Lectures by senior doctors
- Assessment-related teaching
- Student interviews – initial, mid-placement and final
- Teaching while carrying out patient care, i.e. work-based learning
- Setting learning tasks to students
- Practice development manager's guidance
- Teaching by PEFs
- Cascade trainers
- In-service/postgraduate training
- Observing RNs, physiotherapists and other AHPs, or doctors performing clinical interventions

Informal learning opportunities

- Learning from patient with new condition
- Change in patient's condition discussed at handover
- Asking questions informally
- Reflection-in-action and reflection-on-action
- Informal chat in the staff room during coffee break
- Updating procedures and clinical guidelines' folders and learning resources
- Access to computer databases

If preferred, the resources for learning available in the practice setting can be grouped as human and non-human resources. Formal learning opportunities, such as teaching sessions and skill demonstrations, require human resources and include interprofessional learning. Non-human resources include printed instructions on how to use equipment, learning about medications, ventilator monitors or 'care programme approach'. Many of the resources needed to deliver patient care can also be used for learning and for achieving clinical and managerial objectives. Other learning resources include a room that can be used for teaching and learning, with Internet-enabled computers, whiteboard or flipcharts, for instance. The learning resource files containing project or research reports compiled by individuals in the team, research articles, etc. are also usually available for consultation and learning.

Interprofessional learning (IPL)

As for interprofessional learning (IPL) in practice settings, the concept is promoted in various authoritative documents (for example, DH, 1999, 2001c; UKCC, 1999; NMC, 2008a). Successful education programmes and projects (for example, DH, 2008; Goldsmith et al., 2009) are documented on the Internet and presented at conferences. The NMC (2010a: 5, 'Explanation of terms') states that 'interprofessional learning is: 'An interactive process of learning which is undertaken with students or registered professionals from a range of health and social care professions who learn with and from each other.'

The basis for IPL is multi-professional working, in that to resolve the individual patient's or service user's health problem (or to avert it), a group of different healthcare professionals such as nurses, doctors, dieticians, physiotherapists and speech and language therapists input their own areas of professional expertise as appropriate. Multi-professional working can involve different healthcare professionals attending to the patient, delivering their clinical input and withdrawing. These actions can be fragmented and inadequately coordinated and recorded.

Interprofessional working implies better coordinated patient care with fuller communication, verbal and written, between different healthcare professionals. Interprofessional learning extends the concept to the exchange of knowledge, understanding and clinical skills. Lloyd (1999) and Pirrie et al. (1998) have also similarly distinguished between multidisciplinary working and interdisciplinary working.

IPL also comprises informal and formal learning. Informally, for instance, the nurse explains to the occupational therapist the plan of care for a particular patient and the rationales for each action. In turn, the occupational therapist designs a plan of action and explains the rationales from their perspective. This could also form the basis for work-based learning, which is explored in some detail shortly.

Formal IPL involves attending structured learning programmes, such as courses that are designed for specified healthcare professionals, covering the physical, social and psychological basis for health and illness and the clinical skills that aid recovery. Some courses (or part of them) are designed for shared learning by, say, nursing and medical students (for example, Reeves and Pryce, 1998; Morrison et al., 2004;

Hood et al., 2014). Others, such as a course on counselling, might be designed for nurses, social workers and specific allied health professionals.

Informal IPL refers to all modes of unstructured, incidental or opportunistic teaching and learning between different professional groups, while interprofessional education (IPE) refers specifically to university-designed courses that result in students being awarded diplomas or degrees. Interprofessional education is defined by the Centre for Advancement of Interprofessional Education (CAIPE) (2014: 1) as follows: 'Inter-professional education occurs when two or more professions learn with, from and about each other to improve collaboration and the quality of care.' It indicates that IPE includes such learning in academic and work-based settings before and after qualifying.

Another definition of IPE is provided by Buring et al. (2009: 59) as: 'Inter-professional education involves educators and learners from two or more health professions and their foundational disciplines who jointly create and foster a collaborative learning environment.' They indicate that IPE results in positive outcomes on patient satisfaction, teamwork, error rates and mental health competencies. Pirrie et al. (1998) conclude that there are considerable benefits associated with multi-professional education in healthcare, although it needs to be adequately resourced and its success depends on the commitment of all staff involved.

An alternative to IPE is IPL that is a more holistic term that encompasses all manner of interprofessional learning, while IPE refers specifically to learning by students on formal courses.

IPL and IPE

Consider to what extent IPL occurs in your work setting. In those settings where it does occur, is it linked to IPE?

Reflection Point 4.1

Interprofessional learning has been explored for some time as either IPL, IPE or shared learning by, for example, Long et al. (2001) and Miller et al. (1999). A report by Hughes and Marsh (2006) for the Creating an Interprofessional Workforce programme presents a structure for implementing interprofessional working, which also identifies a number of themes and issues related to IPL. In a study of post-qualified students undertaking an interprofessional studies programme, Salmon and Jones (2001: 18) found that skilful facilitation of learning was particularly important, and involved gaining an 'understanding of the knowledge bases, aspirations and values that underpin those (healthcare professions') roles'. Some of the issues related to IPL are as follows.

Hean et al. (2006) report on a study that concluded that different AHP students saw themselves as distinct from other professional groups. This is healthy as it enables them to establish their professional identity prior to exploring commonalties between them. However, when they identified the characteristics that made them different – for example physiotherapy students indicating that they believe that being a team player made them different – other groups also stated having this characteristic. This suggests that many of the characteristics of each AHP group are probably very similar.

Naturally, their areas of clinical expertise have different focuses. Reeves and Pryce (1998) found that medical, dental and nursing students revealed inconsistencies in their stereotypical attitudes towards the status of their intended professions. The authors suggest that these observations provide early evidence of key cultural, professional and institutional issues that need to be considered in planning and implementing interprofessional curricula.

Education programme planners need to be aware of the issues with IPE, such as those just highlighted, so that they can make relevant adjustments to retain teaching effectiveness. However, healthcare learners benefit from IPL. One way that the care and treatment of particular patients are planned and delivered interprofessionally is through integrated care pathways. These in turn can form the basis for constituting learning pathways for students.

Additionally, as for interprofessional assessment of clinical (or practice) skills, this can be implemented to a certain extent, bearing in mind the concept of 'due regard', which the NMC (2008a) uses to indicate that summative assessment of competence can only be legitimately performed by a mentor whose name is in the same part of the NMC's register as the mentee, i.e. in the same field of practice.

Holt et al. (2010: 264), for instance, report on a project that explored ways of assessing communication, team working and ethical practice, which are three essential competences for all health professionals at five HEIs and in 16 professional groups in the UK. They took into account the stance of 'professional statutory and regulatory bodies', practice-based and academic staff, and service users and carers on assessment of these skills, and reported that multi-professional assessment is feasible in the endeavour to 'accurately and fairly measure capabilities to help students develop into proficient and effective practitioners' (ibid.: 264).

Utilising learning pathways

The student's placement could in many settings beneficially incorporate patient journeys and patient care pathways that are concepts that have also been identified by the Department of Health (for example, 2002a, 2009). 'Care maps', 'collaborative care pathways', 'multidisciplinary pathways of care', are all terms that are used interchangeably. Once the care pathway for a particular patient has been formulated, it can be included in the student's learning pathway whereby the student can track the patient's journey through healthcare, and thereby gain knowledge of the interventions undertaken and underpinning rationales for them in order to enable the patient to recover from their health problem. The student's learning can then be supplemented by pre-arranged lectures and workshops held at the university or within healthcare trusts, and by self-directed study.

In *Liberating the Talents*, the Department of Health (2002a) noted that 90 per cent of patient journeys begin and end in primary care. The Department of Health (2007: 1) defines a patient pathway as:

the route that a patient will take from their first contact with an NHS member of staff (usually their general practitioner [GP]), through referral, to the completion of their treatment. It also covers the period from entry into a hospital or a Treatment Centre, until the patient leaves.

The word *integrated* is added to care pathways to signify interdisciplinary input.

The definitions of care pathways include that by Overill (1998: 93), who suggests that integrated care pathways provide 'locally agreed, multidisciplinary practise-based guidelines and evidence where available, for a specific client group'. Care pathways specifically designed for particular illnesses are well documented in healthcare literature. Examples of this include van Wijngaarden et al. (2006) on thrombolysis in acute ischaemic stroke, and Bowker et al. (2005) on the type 1 diabetes mellitus. Several care pathways are also available on the Internet, for example from the National Institute for Health and Care Excellence (NICE) (2014b) website.

Research on care pathways includes a quasi-experiment conducted by de Luc (2000), who found that the use of care pathways resulted in increased patient satisfaction and its ability to make staff focus more on the clinical care they were providing. A literature review of end-of-life care pathways for dying people and their families also revealed positive potentials in terms of enhancement of the quality of care provided to patients and their families. Furthermore, an evaluative study of patient journeys conducted by Baron (2009) found various benefits of this approach, including greater patient involvement in their recovery from illness and more effective interprofessional working.

A student on practice placement could encounter a patient whose relatively straightforward journey through healthcare takes them along the pathway identified in Figure 4.1.

Another example of 'patient journey' is identified by the DH (2009) that tracks the patient pathway for an adult visiting their GP with alcohol-related problems, whereupon, following a systematic set of actions, an alcohol treatment pathway is devised for him or her, a journey that includes all the stages that lead up to treatment, including outpatient consultations and diagnostic tests and procedures. Integrated care pathways continue with the care and treatment required by the patient to the point of maximum recovery from the health problem.

The student can follow a patient's care pathway through the healthcare system closely to gain knowledge and understanding of the care and treatment required in particular illnesses. The student's learning pathway through the practice placement would involve exposure to, and engagement with, selected patient care pathways, supplemented in various ways, for example by practice-based teaching by the mentor and other healthcare professionals.

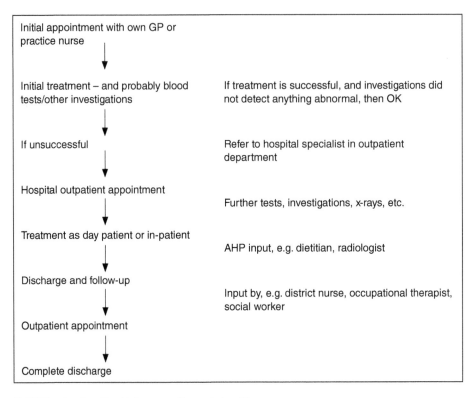

FIGURE 4.1   A patient's journey through healthcare

HEIs work in collaboration with local trust clinicians to develop and implement learning pathway programmes in healthcare course curricula based on patient journeys, with web-based scenarios for students to investigate. A suitable definition of learning pathways related to healthcare students' learning is difficult to locate. Essentially, a learning pathway constitutes a combination of retrospective and prospective case interventions that are determined by the beginning of the patient's health problem, current state of the problem and how it progresses. Furthermore, as care pathways incorporate involvement of an appropriate combination of nursing or midwifery, medical, social work and AHP staff, learning pathways are increasingly being referred to as 'interprofessional learning pathways'.

Pollard and Hibbert (2004) report on a project on enhancing student learning using patient pathways, and conclude that patient pathways constitute one way of turning students' learning during practice placements from an ad hoc set of activities into logical and organised experiences. Using patient pathways therefore offers a more structured approach to learning as opposed to relying on unplanned, opportunistic and therefore possibly erratic learning.

The learning pathway for a student on an Emergency Department placement could include the student starting with a day with the ambulance services, following a patient with a suspected fracture to the X-ray department, spending time working with plaster technicians and so on. Furthermore, if the same patient also suffers from say type 1 diabetes or displays aggressive or even violent behaviour, these themselves present instances for further learning for the student, the management of which can be explored up to maximum patient recovery.

Learning pathways have been identified as beneficial by Hutchings and Sanders (2001), for instance, who describe a successful project in which the development of learning pathways achieved its aims, which were to improve the quality of learning for the student, as well as being enjoyable, and promoting high-quality patient care. Students and clinical staff worked in partnership and had equal responsibilities for improving the quality of learning.

The effectiveness of learning pathways in making learning more comprehensive was also explored by Anderson (2009: 835), for instance, who conducted a qualitative study, which revealed that the use of learning pathways enabled students to develop 'a greater awareness and understanding of the delivery of healthcare in primary care settings and they expanded their nursing knowledge and skills'. However, Anderson also notes that some students felt that learning pathways fragmented their learning in the base placement area.

The fragmentation of learning downside needs to be heeded as the subjects of Anderson's study were final placement student nurses who felt that their priority in this placement was to consolidate their clinical skills. This can clearly also impact the achievement of sign-off proficiency by students during the final practice placement, which is an NMC requirement for them to register their qualification with the NMC.

It is useful to note, however, that the notion of learning pathways is found in at least another two contexts. One of these is the arena of adult education in which individuals who have missed education opportunities during compulsory education years are enabled to learn through NVQ routes and so on (for example, McGivney, 2003). The notion of learning pathways also belongs to neurophysiology when new learning can be identified along neuronal paths (for example, Brown et al., 1999).

Increasingly, one model of learning pathway is being favoured widely, with some useful developments that can counteract the above-mentioned weaknesses of learning pathways identified by Anderson (2009). The model is referred to as the 'hub and spokes' model. The hub is the base placement setting to which the student has been allocated, but from where the student can accompany the patient or service user to whichever department of health or social care personnel he or she has been referred.

Nonetheless, a spoke visit by a student on practice placement cannot be downplayed as 'just for a change of scenery', for instance. In fact, to optimise learning from the spoke experience, the student should articulate in writing, preferably on a page of the practice competencies booklet, one or more aims of the spoke visit against the name of the spoke to be visited – see Template 4.2.

TEMPLATE 4.2   Record of learning from spoke experience

Date of visit to spoke area	Name of spoke	Aim(s) of visiting spoke area	Summary of learning from spoke	Named mentor's comments (optional)

After the visit the student needs to write down specific learning acquired from the spoke visit. A number of studies have already been conducted on the hub and spokes model, which include Roxburgh et al.'s (2012) research that in conclusion identified the beneficial effects of using this model of placement learning as a mechanism that promotes deep and more meaningful person-centred learning than the concept practice placement that can imply that the student has to spend most or all of the placement time in the placement area itself.

Work-based learning (WBL)

Learning professional skills in the workplace is also referred to as work-based learning (WBL), except this term applies to learning in the workplace in all professions, and is equivalent to the term 'practice placement' in nursing and midwifery and to 'internship' in some university-linked programme such as business studies. Thus WBL is an overarching term, which has been defined by several people, including Barr (2003) who indicates that WBL is learning that takes place at work or learning that takes place away from work with the objective of improving performance at work. The definitions of WBL imply that, in addition to apprenticeship-type learning in workplaces, learning is supplemented by some classroom-based lessons or skills laboratory-based learning.

If the WBL is a component of a university-based programme, then it also awards credit points or CATS (credit accumulation and transfer scheme) points, the number depending to a good extent on the duration of the placement, such as whether it is for eight weeks or year long. An extensive study of WBL by Moore (2010) revealed that managerial support in workplace development is crucial for WBL to be successful as a learning activity.

In nursing, Rattray et al. (2006) report on the evaluation of a critical care module that incorporated WBL and resulted in various benefits such as module credibility through its clinical focus. Waddington and Marsh (1998) explored work-based shared learning with a multi-band, multi-skilled group of qualified nurses and healthcare assistants, and found that the perceived benefits included increased professional awareness of issues relating to standards and quality of care with enhanced communication and morale within the team.

Marshall (2012) reports on the beneficial effects of a work-based learning module in midwifery, writing that it enables participants to improve multi-professional collaboration and the consequential further development of maternity services within the local Trusts; it is efficient and cost effective to employee and employer and serves in increasing the link between higher education and the workplace; and also helps to bridge the theory–practice gap, which all in all has the potential to influence directly the development of global midwifery education and maternity services and ultimately benefit mothers, their babies and families.

However, Mallik and McGowan (2007) report on a multi-professional 'developmental project' on WBL that indicates that an inadequate supply of mentors results in inconsistency in the amount of mentoring that students receive. Spouse (2001b) notes that successful WBL requires an organisational environment that supports learning through investment in staff, with staffing structures in organisations and trusts that free up people to work and learn collaboratively in a climate of trust, where investigations and speculations are fostered and where time is protected for engaging in discussions about practice.

Becoming a learning organisation

In line with the general acceptance that various forms of formal and informal learning occur in the workplace and can be recorded on educational audit documents, and also the increasing trend towards interprofessional learning in practice settings, Holland and Lauder (2012) suggest that practice learning should be part of the wider concept of 'communities of (learning in) practice', and that healthcare providers should become 'learning organisations'. The concept of 'communities of practice' has prevailed for some time, and Lave and Wenger (1998) for example explain that they constitute groups of people who share a common passion for something, about which they extend their learning together, whereupon some of the learning may also be incidental, i.e. unintentional.

As for the whole of the healthcare provider, for example an acute NHS Trust, becoming a learning organisation, this can only be healthy so that all its practice settings as well as all departments that are not practice settings have learning and open-mindedness structured within their culture. This ethos is usually well established in UK hospices and university-linked healthcare providers.

Ward and McCormack (2000) suggest that as organisational factors have a major influence on learning, the term 'clinical learning environment' is increasingly being seen as connected to the concept of 'learning organisation'. They indicate that the development of a learning culture needs to be a dominant theme in the strategic plans of healthcare organisations. This arises from a drive to improve standards of practice, bridging the perceived theory–practice gap and creating the means of integrating learning with practice. There have been many initiatives to create such a change, including CPD, reflective practice, clinical supervision and WBL.

'Learning organisation' is a term that is part of a trio of notions that also include lifelong learning and learning society. It evolved with the development of various non-healthcare organisations such as banks, supermarkets and so on as learning organisations, on the basis that they all learn from customer feedback and actively engage in ongoing staff training. However, de la Harpe and Radloff (2000: 169) note that a learning society comprises a society in which 'every person has the opportunity to be educated to the level of achievement of which they are truly capable'.

A learning organisation is defined as one that 'facilitates the learning of all its members, and consciously transforms itself and its context' (Pedler et al., 1997: 3). The concept of a learning organisation is consistently becoming a feature of healthcare settings, as lifelong learning is not merely 'keeping up to date', but encompasses a flexible and enquiring approach to the development of a culture of learning as an important part of the work setting. The key features of a learning organisation, which also applies to health and social care providers, are identified by Wilkinson et al. (2004), for example, as one with:

- celebration throughout the organisation of success of individuals and teams
- absence of complacency, that is always seeking improvement
- tolerance of mistakes and failures, and learning from them
- belief in human potential for creativity and innovation
- recognition of tacit knowledge
- openness and sharing knowledge, and learning across teams
- trusting staff to work towards corporate goals, without close monitoring
- outward looking at competing organisations, and potentially learning from them.

You might wish to check for yourself how far your employing organisation demonstrates the above-mentioned features of a learning organisation, and maybe you will be nicely surprised.

Guidelines, policies and standards for practice placements

In *Helping Students Get the Best from their Practice Placements*, the RCN (2002) specifies the responsibilities of various stakeholders, that is, those of the student, the HEI, service providers, personal tutors and mentors, for ensuring effective learning during placements. The responsibilities of the student encompass those before, during and after the placement. The student's responsibilities before the placement include:

- reading the practice competencies that must be achieved by the end of the placement, and comprehending them
- recognising the purpose of the practice placement experience, that is to learn nursing or midwifery care

- contacting the placement
- acting professionally with regard to punctuality and attitude, and dress according to the local uniform policy.

During the placement, the student's responsibilities include being proactive in seeking out learning experiences. After the placement, the student has a responsibility to take stock of their achievements, evaluate the placement itself, ensure that all practice placement documentation is completed by due dates and reflect on the experience after completing the placement.

For mentors, the RCN publication states that good mentoring depends on well-planned learning opportunities and the provision of support and coaching for students. It lists and explains several actions that the mentor should take to fulfil their responsibility, which include:

- contributing to a supportive learning environment and quality learning outcomes for students
- being approachable, supportive and aware of how students learn best
- having knowledge and information of the student's programme of study and practice assessment tools.

In a subsequent publication that constitutes guidance for mentors, the RCN (2007) addresses how to mentor. This includes mentors helping students get the best from practice placements, including students with special needs, areas of accountability for mentors and support for mentors.

The underlying principles of the DH (2001b) guidance document *Placements in Focus* include the need for a dynamic and proactive approach to the organisation, provision and assessment of practice experience. It indicates that HEIs and service providers have to think creatively about how to plan and provide practice placements that meet the needs of the NHS, the wider healthcare sector and developments related to public health. Planning and provision should both take into account and value ideas and suggestions from students and draw on the experience and knowledge of other stakeholders. The guidance is intended to constitute a model of good practice. It focuses on four key aspects of practice placements, namely:

1 providing practice placements
2 practice learning environment
3 student support
4 assessment of practice.

For the practice learning environment, the DH (2001b) indicates, for instance, that:

- The practice area should have a stated philosophy of care that is reflected in practice and in the curriculum aims.
- Care provision should be founded on relevant research and evidence-based findings where available.

- Students should gain, where possible, experience as part of a multi-professional team.
- A learning resources area with relevant materials should be available for learning activities in the practice environment.
- Student feedback should be actively sought.

It also identifies how each component will be achieved by different parties, such as placement providers, HEIs and students. Another authoritative body that provides guidelines on placement learning for quality assurance is the Quality Assurance Agency (QAA) (for example, 2006a). Mulholland et al. (2006) make further recommendations under the *Making Practice-Based Learning Work* project.

Issues Related to Practice Placements

One of the issues related to pre-registration nursing students is their supernumerary status (discussed at the end of Chapter 2), accompanied by a relatively small bursary. The latter is a reason for a number of students holding down part-time jobs. This, along with some students having a family to support, may result in their learning being compromised to some extent. Consequently, the student is likely to need extra structured support while on practice placement. Link lecturers can provide this support, which does not necessarily require their physical presence.

A study by Young et al. (2010) evaluated the use of short message service (SMS) texting between university staff and students as an additional means of support for healthcare students (including nursing, radiography and occupational therapy students) during practice placements. They found that texting can improve students' access to additional support when needed during practice placements.

One of the reasons for various guidelines on practice placements being issued by the RCN, the QAA, the DH (for example, DH, 2001b) and others at the turn of the last century is the research findings of Phillips et al. (2000), which document various worrying weaknesses with prevailing mentoring processes. As noted in Chapter 1, this study highlights several issues or problems experienced by both mentors and students that resulted in a redefinition of roles and a change in educational preparation programmes for mentors.

Another reason is the increase in the number of students due to the shortage of qualified nurses. This means that more learners were to be mentored by fewer RNs. This also coincides with other research findings that some mentors were not failing students (discussed in Chapter 7) who were incompetent, and that some newly qualified RNs were not 'fit for practice', that is, not clinically competent.

Furthermore, the Care Quality Commission (CQC) – which is an organisation that was set up by the government to regularly monitor the quality of care and treatment being provided to patients and service users by each service provider in England – can also decide whether a practice setting is suitable as a learning environment for students. If deemed unsuitable they have the authority to instruct the particular practice setting to stop having students on placement with them until the weakness identified is rectified. The CQC's (2014) national standards are reproduced in the box below, and details of outcomes (criteria) for hospitals, care homes and other providers can be accessed on the CQC's website. These criteria are components of its framework that is based on five key questions that it asks of services, namely:

- Are the services safe?
- Are they effective?
- Are they caring?
- Are they responsive?
- Are they well led?

The Care Quality Commission's National Standards (CQC, 2014)

1 You should expect to be respected, involved in your care and support, and told what's happening at every stage.
2 You should expect care, treatment and support that meet your needs.
3 You should expect to be safe.
4 You should expect to be cared for by staff with the right skills to do their jobs properly.
5 You should expect your care provider to routinely check the quality of their services.

However, the heightened awareness of evidence-based practice means that students are more inquisitive about reasons for each step within clinical interventions. Nevertheless, for various day-to-day reasons, some procedures are not performed exactly as the procedures' manual states and consequently the so-called theory and practice gap at times surfaces. From qualified healthcare professionals and their managers' viewpoint these still constitute competent practice because procedures are adapted in accordance with resource availability and patient circumstances.

For instance, if the moving and handling procedure or guidelines state that a hoist should be used to help a patient above a certain weight, but a hoist is not immediately available, then the RN could use alternative measures. The reason for this might not be immediately obvious to the student, and at times students refuse to participate in procedures that are not being performed precisely according to guidelines. They should be exploring how to adapt theories to practice instead.

Chapter Summary

As with other components in this book, creating and maintaining an effective clinical learning environment is also identified as a key component of the mentor role. This chapter has focused on the different ways in which practice settings can be effective as learning environments, and has therefore explored:

- Students' perspectives on practice placements such as their hopes and expectations; a ward orientation or induction programme; advanced preparation of learners; and ensuring that course practice competencies are achieved.
- Research on clinical learning environments, which underpins the development of the tool for annual educational audits of practice placement areas; learning resources (human and material), including interprofessional learning, and learning pathways; role models for learners in the practice setting.
- The part played by national guidelines, standards and current policy documents on practice placements.
- What work-based learning is and how it applies to learning nursing and midwifery practice; and how healthcare providers can become learning organisations.
- Some of the main issues related to practice placements for students.

Further Optional Reading 📖

1 For practical and contemporary guidance on how to enhance the quality of practice placements for healthcare trust-based professionals, including AHPs, that builds on previous work and on evidence about students' experience of practice, and prepared collaboratively by a number of statutory and professional bodies and the Department of Health, as well as a complementary element of quality assurance of NHS funded health professional education programmes, see:

   - Department of Health (2001b) *Placements in Focus: Guidance for Education in Practice for Healthcare Professions.* Available at: http://www.nmc-uk.org/Documents/ Archived%20Publications/ENB%20Archived%20Publications/Placements%20 in%20focus%20-%20ENB%20January%202001.PDF (accessed 23 April 2014).

2 For the QAA's stance on effective learning during practice placements, see:

   - Quality Assurance Agency for Higher Education (2006a) *Outcomes from Institutional Audit Work-based and Placement Learning and Employability.* Available at: www.qaa. ac.uk/en/Publications/Documents/Outcomes-institutional-audit-Work-based-placement-learning-employability.pdf (accessed 13 December 2014).

3 Expectation 10: 'Commissioners actively seek assurance that the right people, with the right skills, are in the right place at the right time within the providers

with whom they contract' (NHS England National Quality Board (NQB), 2014: 54) – for detailed discussion on plans for provision of adequate staffing levels to provide safe care, see:

- NHS England National Quality Board (2014) *How to Ensure the Right People, with the Right Skills, are in the Right Place at the Right Time: A Guide to Establishing Nursing, Midwifery and Care Staffing Capacity and Capability'.* Available at: http://www.england.nhs.uk/ourwork/part-rel/nqb/#pub (accessed 20 January 2014).

To access further resources related to this chapter, visit the companion website at https://study.sagepub.com/gopee

5

The Mentor's Role in Evidence-Based Practice and Clinical Practice Development

Introduction

Chapter Outcomes

On completion of this chapter, you should be able to:

1 Explain why evidence-based practice (EBP) and clinical practice development are essential components of the RN's/RM's mentor role.
2 Identify the meanings of the concepts 'effective care', EBP and 'clinical practice development', and demonstrate understanding of the inherent components that they encompass.
3 Ascertain and analyse the extent to which the mentor engages in, and disseminates EBP.
4 Critically evaluate ways in which the mentor participates in the effective implementation of research findings, in practice development and in the management of change.

The key dimensions of being a mentor in healthcare professions incorporate practising one's craft to the highest standard. This in turn implies being conscious of the quality and effectiveness of one's practice, continuously ascertaining the evidence base of all clinical interventions, and of the various factors that influence effective delivery of patient and service user care and treatment. Awareness of standards of practice involves being open-minded with regard to novel methods of clinical interventions, of developments in one's own specialist field of practice.

The NMC's (2008a: 56–7) mentor standards document indicates under the domain 'Evidence-based practice', that the mentor must: 'Apply evidence-based practice to their own work and contribute to the further development of such knowledge, and practice evidence base.' Under 'Context of practice', it states that the mentor must: 'Support learning within a context of practice that reflects healthcare and educational policies, managing change to ensure that particular professional needs are met within a learning environment that also supports practice development.' The outcomes for these domains are:

Evidence-based practice	• identify and apply research and evidence-based practice to their area of practice
	• contribute to strategies to increase or review the evidence base used to support practice
	• support students in applying an evidence base to their own practice
Context of practice	• contribute to the development of an environment in which effective practice is fostered, implemented, evaluated and disseminated
	• set and maintain professional boundaries that are sufficiently flexible for providing interprofessional care
	• initiate and respond to practice developments to ensure safe and effective care is achieved and an effective learning environment is maintained.

The concepts inherent within these requirements and outcomes are addressed in this chapter, and are predominantly key components of effective evidence-based practice, practice development and the management of change.

Evidence-Based Practice (EBP)

One of the crucial components of effective practice and quality assurance in healthcare is evidence-based practice (EBP), a concept and practice that has been gradually adopted in all areas of healthcare. As indicated at the beginning of the chapter, besides being one of the NMC's (2008a) competences for mentors, EBP is also usually a component of the codes of practice of healthcare professionals. So what is EBP?

What is evidence-based practice?

'Safe and effective care' is a phrase that is often mentioned by the NMC in its standards publications (for example, 2008a, 2010a). Safety of patients or service users in practice settings is a strand of nursing and midwifery's code of practice (NMC, 2015) and therefore obligatory – but what does the term 'effective practice' mean?

Effective practice

'Effective clinical practice' is a concept that is closely related to quality of care and treatment, and is also related to such concepts as clinical governance and audits. The word *effective* itself is an adjective, which according to the dictionary (Brown, 2002: 794) means 'capable of producing results or a condition, and having the function of accomplishing'. It can be used interchangeably with 'efficacious' and 'productive'. Effective practice therefore means that the clinical interventions that healthcare professionals perform do achieve the goals of the care and treatment that are part of the patient's or service user's care pathway (or care plan). For example, if certain actions are taken to reduce a patient's body temperature, and after a specified number of minutes the temperature does go down, then the actions were 'effective'.

Ways of achieving effective practice incorporate ensuring that practice is evidence-based and is developed based on new evidence, i.e. practice development, which will be examined in detail shortly. Effective care (NMC, 2008a) is therefore a concept that is an integral component of EBP and practice development.

Achieving the goals of care and treatment also belongs to the arena of *patient outcomes*. This term has been explored for several years and is defined according to the research that it is connected with, as documented by the RCN (2004). However, despite the logic in ascertaining patient outcomes, there is a lack of consensus with regard to how patient outcomes are gauged, and it therefore remains in the background as an essential notion warranting further research and refinement.

Related to the mentor role, the word 'effective' therefore implies that as a qualified healthcare professional the mentor accomplishes the goals in their patients or service users' plans of care and treatment, as intended in their individual care pathways. Effective care and practice development are also part of the work of the NHS Improving Quality (NHS IQ) (2013), whose remit comprises projects and rigorous testing of new ways of providing care in various areas, including long-term conditions, primary care, end-of-life care and mental health services.

Evidence-based practice and related concepts

Evidence-based practice is closely associated with evidence-based medicine (EBM), for which Archie Cochrane is renowned for being one of its principal initiators (Clarke, 1999). Sackett et al. (2000) are also well known for being advocates of EBP and, according to them, EBP is the conscientious, explicit and judicious use of current best evidence in making decisions about the care of individual patients.

The key reason for the adoption of EBP in healthcare is the endeavour to ensure that each action taken by the healthcare professional is an 'informed' action, that is, it is based on evidence of its effectiveness. It also comprises a shift from traditional or routine procedures to more objective scientific working (Dale, 2006).

Another term related to EBP is 'evidence-based healthcare' (EBHC), and EBP has also permeated various areas of organisational function in the form of evidence-based nursing, evidence-based management and evidence-based education. EBHC is defined by Gray (2001: 9) as 'a discipline centred upon evidence-based decision-making about groups of patients, or populations, which can manifest itself as evidence-based policy-making, purchasing or management'. Although they overlap substantially, EBHC can be distinguished from EBP in that the former tends to refer to groups of patients, while the latter can refer to single clinical interventions. According to Gray, there are five key elements of EBP, namely:

1 Decisions are based on best evidence.
2 The nature and source of evidence are determined by the problem.
3 Best evidence integrates research and personal experience.
4 Evidence is translated into action that affects patients/service users.
5 These actions are continually appraised.

Best evidence

EBP therefore refers to the use of 'best evidence' and is based on national and international standards. How do we know that every clinical intervention that we perform in our workplace is based on the 'best evidence' currently available?

Reflection Point 5.1

Research evidence is available from national computer databases. However, Gray (2001) indicates that although the best evidence of effectiveness of particular clinical interventions comes from well-designed research, other evidence of best practice – referred to as 'best evidence available' – needs to be seriously considered. There are several likely sources of best evidence of good practice, including:

- clinical guidelines (e.g. from NICE), and policy directives (from the Department of Health)
- specialist and research conferences
- professional journal articles
- overview of evidence on specific topics on computer databases
- textbooks
- suppliers' information
- unpublished research
- suggestions from patients with a long-term health problem/their family

- colleagues and peer contact – uni- or interdisciplinary professionals
- personal intuition
- trial and error
- personal experience.

How is EBP achieved?

There are various ways in which EBP can be achieved. Healthcare professionals can search for evidence of the effect of particular clinical interventions and best evidence on computer databases such as the Cochrane Library, MEDLINE or Cumulative Index to Nursing and Allied Health Literature (CINAHL), or they can do a manual search of targeted literature.

There are various organisations that store and provide systematically reviewed (or critically appraised or meta-analysed) research on different healthcare topics. The Cochrane Systematic Reviews Library (available at: http://www.thecochranelibrary.com/view/0/index.html), which stores research evidence that has been appraised or systematically reviewed, is one of these. The Cochrane Collaboration (2013: 1) defines a systematic review as 'a high-level overview of primary research on a particular research question that tries to identify, select, synthesize and appraise all high quality research evidence relevant to that question in order to answer it'.

The strengths of the assembled research literature can be classified as a hierarchy of levels or grades of evidence, in order of validity and significance. Hemingway and Brereton (2009: 7), for instance, classify 'Hierarchies of evidence' at five levels of evidence (and sub-levels), as follows:

- Level 1a   Systematic review of randomised controlled trials (RCTs)
- Level 1b   Individual RCT
- Level 1c   All-or-none studies
- Level 2a   Systematic review of cohort studies
- Level 2b   Individual cohort study (including low-quality RCT; e.g. < 80% follow-up)
- Level 2c   'Outcomes' research; ecological studies
- Level 3a   Systematic reviews of case-control studies
- Level 3b   Individual case-control study
- Level 4   Case series (and poor quality cohort and case-control studies)
- Level 5   Expert opinion without explicit critical appraisal, or based on physiology, bench research or 'first principles'.

You might not have encountered some of above-mentioned terminologies. If so, their meanings are easily found on the Internet.

Other organisations categorise evidence differently but they are essentially similar. Evans (2003) explored various such classifications and concluded that the appraisal of evidence should also include assessing the evidence's effectiveness, appropriateness and feasibility. Nonetheless, Sackett et al. (1996) and others indicate strongly that

RCTs must not be treated as 'gold standards'. Thompson (1998) and others indicate that EBP should take personal experience, intuition and patients' reports into account. The benefits of EBP are that healthcare professionals can (Kopp, 2001):

- instigate appropriate and up-to-date interventions
- inform or advise patients more accurately
- make better use of limited resources
- measure practice against appropriate guidelines or standards
- provide a more informed decision-making process to previously untreatable or more expensive treatments.

However, there can be barriers to the implementation of EBP. These barriers are similar to those that present as obstacles to implementation of research findings and are examined shortly. Kopp (2001) suggests that such barriers include a lack of awareness of evidence, and of self-confidence, peer-support or resources. Another perspective is forwarded by Sackett et al. (1996), who suggest that in case anyone feels EBP is overplayed, then they should be reminded that although 'practice risks becoming tyrannised by evidence, … without available evidence, practice risks becoming rapidly out of date to the detriment of patients' (ibid.: 71).

The difference between research-based practice and EBP is that research-based practice of clinical interventions usually only allows consideration of findings of quantitative research, while EBP also considers descriptive or qualitative studies, professional experiences, intuition and tacit knowledge (when we know more than we can evidence or tell) (Benner, 2001).

The York University NHS Centre for Reviews and Dissemination is another resource centre for EBP. There is also the quarterly journal *Evidence-Based Nursing*. The Health Technology Assessment programme (DH, 2010b) is a government-funded venture that appraises research information, including costs and effectiveness, and is made available to NHS workers. Typical headings for appraisal of a research study are:

- How clear and specific is the research question?
- Was the research funded by a particular organisation and, if so, does the researcher hold any allegiance to them?
- Is the research design the most appropriate to answer the research question?
- Are the sampling strategies the most appropriate?
- Precisely what was measured?
- Precise details and relevance of how the data was collected.
- How researcher effects and other intervening variables were controlled.
- Was the framework or method used for analysing the data the most appropriate?
- Are the statistical tests used appropriate and accurately documented?
- Are the conclusions drawn logically argued and is the generalisability statement justifiable?
- To what extent is the study relevant to clinical practice in the particular practice setting?
- Does the dissemination of the study indicate frameworks for implementation, including resources required such as costs?

Much more detailed appraisal considerations are quite well publicised, and guidelines for systematic reviews are provided, for example, by Gopee (2010). It is in the interest of the implementer of a particular component of EBP to examine closely and carefully the appraisal or systematic review already conducted by established organisations, who in fact are also likely to have accessed and appraised the original study report.

The mentor's role in identifying, applying and disseminating research findings

Identifying existing research on particular healthcare topic areas or components of clinical practice has become increasingly easier with the wide availability of electronic databases such as the Cochrane Library and NHS Evidence. However, the actual dissemination of research findings is often not as effectively achieved. Whether it is the findings of the healthcare professional's own research or those of studies encountered at conferences or on courses, the ultimate stages of research studies entail critiquing the study or studies, implementation, and then systematic dissemination of the findings.

Dissemination of research findings by a single avenue, such as presenting at a conference, has limited impact. Scullion (2002) suggests that dissemination is a vital yet complex process that aims to ensure that key messages are conveyed to specific groups via a wide range of methods such that it results in impact, reaction and preferably implementation. The range of methods of effective dissemination include:

- journal articles/editorials/short reports
- feedback to research subjects
- in-person support mechanisms
- journal clubs
- seminars
- conference presentations
- poster presentations
- publishing as books/chapters
- inclusion in curriculum
- newsletters
- designing educational materials.

Scullion also suggests that the main barriers to the dissemination process are: poor journal reading habits of nurses resulting in them being unaware of research findings, lack of time, lack of knowledge, negative attitudes towards research and information overload. However, to disseminate new research-based or innovative practice, Price (2010) provides guidance on specific strategies that can be used, such as planning for the specific audience, identifying objectives for the session and the use of artefacts (for example, plastic models of body parts).

Furthermore, even with effective dissemination, there can be obstacles to the implementation of research findings. Almost two decades ago, Hunt (1997) repeated one of her earlier studies that explored the barriers to research implementation in healthcare and found at the time that these included:

- lack of critical appraisal and research skills
- lack of time to undertake research
- not having access to the right resources
- an organisational and managerial ethos and culture expecting instant answers
- lack of power and financial control to make things happen
- lack of valid research on any one topic, or of user-friendly reviews and guidelines.

Barriers to implementing research findings

Consider Hunt's (1997) findings for yourself or discuss with an appropriate colleague, if, and how far, the findings are still prevalent in the context of present-day healthcare settings, both in general and in your own practice setting.

Reflection Point 5.2

Williams et al. (2015) conducted an extensive review of literature to ascertain the barriers to implementation of EBP, and identified the five most commonly occuring barriers as:

- Workload.
- Other staff/Management not supportive of research.
- Lack of resources.
- Lack of authority to change practice.
- Workplace/professional culture resistant to change.

A decade after Hunt's study, Morris and Maynard (2007) identified 'time' and 'cultural issues' as the most prominent barriers to developing EBP. Education curricula for healthcare professionals have over the years rectified these problems to a good extent by inclusion of research modules in their health profession courses. Of course, undergraduate healthcare education curricula have been required (e.g. by the NMC, 2009a; 2010a) to incorporate research appraisal and application of research knowledge and skills to care delivery regularly for more than a decade, and therefore some of the issues discussed by Williams et al. (2015) and Morris and Maynard (2007) may have been resolved by now.

> ### Activity 5.1   Barriers to implementation of research findings
>
> Re-read the barriers to implementation of research findings identified by Hunt and
> Williams et al. in the preceding bulleted lists, and consider what you see as barriers
> in your workplace, at ward or trust level, and make some notes on how they are,
> or can be, resolved.

Implementing changes to clinical practice is examined later in this chapter. With
regard to EBP, Palfreyman et al. (2003) explored nurses and physiotherapists' perceptions of barriers to EBP, and found that both professions have problems overcoming
the barrier of time, with nurses also rating themselves as poor in EBP skills.

Hunt (1997) suggested that barriers to research implementation can be resolved by:

- making research available and accessible through professional development
  programmes
- providing research advice and support
- providing nurses with the appropriate skills
- changing attitudes.

In their comprehensive analysis of ways of placing research utilisation in healthcare,
Pallen and Timmins (2002) concluded their study with a framework for systematic
research implementation in practice settings by first considering the four main barriers, namely (1) the healthcare professionals' attitude and knowledge of research,
(2) organisational factors such as funding, staffing and education, (3) accessibility to
research and databases, and (4) communicating research. In their framework, each
item under these four barriers is individually assessed in relation to the extent to
which each prevails, plans to overcome them and sets goals, implementing the plans
and evaluating them.

Thus, managerial and organisational input and support tend to be as important as
individual skills in implementation of research findings, except such implementation
needs to be 'managed', as discussed shortly in this chapter.

In the mentoring role, research-based practice is an inherent component. EBP can
be a permanent feature, and 'where's the evidence?' sounds like a confrontational
question. The healthcare trust's clinical procedure and guidelines, however, almost
always include the evidence base for practice. However, consider the following scenario that involves mentoring a student midwife and her perception of EBP.

....

Case Study

Mentoring a student midwife

Sarah is the mentor to first year student midwife Helen. A 'triad'* assessment is
being conducted with Helen by Sarah and Geraldine, the link lecturer. The topic
chosen is the examination of the newborn.

Helen states that she is very nervous. She provides a full clinical picture of the woman and the baby in whose care she has been involved. Having confirmed the woman's consent, she then concentrates on the examination, which she performs in a professional manner. There is, however, little communication with the mother. Helen has to be reminded of the need to complete the relevant documentation. Her hand is shaking as she writes.

Helen then produces and discusses an article regarding examinations of the healthy neonate. She needs some prompting when asked about the NMC's Midwives Rules and Standards and what she would do if she identified a deviation from the norm. When asked about her assessment of her performance, Helen is very self-critical and feels that she did not do very well.

What are the key issues in this assessment situation? What are the ways in which the evidence base of Helen's performance influenced her performance, and what are the questions that Sarah and Geraldine might want to ask?

*'triad' refers to a tripartite assessment of competencies in the practice setting that includes the assessee, their mentor and a midwife lecturer.

You do not have to be a midwife to ask relevant questions related to EBP, and in this case study a number of issues surface when this scenario is put to group discussions. In the context of the discussions in this chapter, all parties will question the strengths of the evidence that Helen seemed to have used during the procedure. They can be explored in the context of levels or grades of evidence available in relation to 'examination of the newborn'.

Clinical Practice Development

The two concepts of 'effective practice' and 'EBP' both potentially imply making changes to the ways in which care and treatment are delivered if the change benefits the patient or service user. Such changes are referred to as 'clinical practice development', which is also a key area of the NMC's (2008a) competences for mentors. This section explores what clinical practice development is, the different reasons for practice development and how these developments are managed, which links up to the third section of this chapter on management of change.

What is clinical practice development?

Clinical practice development implies changing the way in which particular care and treatment interventions are performed for the benefit of patients or service users. It has to do with improving and enhancing clinical practice where there is scope to do so. It refers to hands–on patient care interventions, that is patient contact. Which developments in clinical practice are currently happening in your particular area of practice? What changes can be made or have been made recently to specific care and treatments carried out in your practice setting?

Activity 5.2   Clinical practice development

Reflect on how care is currently delivered in your workplace and explore whether any aspect of the way in which care is delivered has changed recently – in the last few months or in the last year or two.

Next, identify an aspect of patient or service user care in your work setting that requires or could benefit from change, either in clinical care, patient teaching or organisation of care. State two examples of such potential changes.

So, changes can be made in different components or aspects of healthcare delivery, and the mentor can influence the nature and direction of these changes. Examples of changes in hands-on clinical practice include:

- implementation of early warning systems (EWS)
- no-lift policy
- a red jug of water next to a patient who is at risk of dehydration
- use of patient-controlled analgesia
- nurse-led specialist clinics
- cognitive behavioural therapy
- nurse prescribing
- using tympanic thermometers rather than glass thermometers
- cardiac output studies in intensive care units
- bedside handover.

Examples of changes in organisation or management of care include:

- introducing a new shift system
- team midwifery
- outreach work
- a quality assurance programme (e.g., patient satisfaction surveys)
- open-door availability of influenza vaccines to over-65s at the start of winter
- modern matron role in aspects of care (e.g. who does what to ensure hospital cleanliness)
- allowing parents to be present in the anaesthetic room
- clinical supervision for peer support and CPD (continuing professional development)
- a mechanism for reporting to colleagues from conferences and workshops.

Examples of changes in patient teaching include:

- health 'MOTs' conducted by practice nurses, SCPHNs (specialist community public health nurse)
- school nurses' advice to teenagers on sexual activity
- teaching self-relaxation
- teaching dietary control to a newly diagnosed diabetic
- advising older people on how to avoid hypothermia.

You could think of various instances of changes in teaching students and other learners, such as medical students, healthcare assistants, preceptees and inductees.

Practice development is defined by the RCN (2006: 1) as 'an approach that helps you, your team and organisation to provide care that patients feel is right for them'. This is a very brief definition. A more helpful definition is provided by McCormack et al. (2013: 4), which states that:

> Practice development is a continuous process of improvement towards increased effectiveness in patient centred care, which is brought about by enabling healthcare teams to develop their knowledge and skills, and to transform the culture and context of care.

According to Bryar and Griffiths (2003), practice development is taken to mean a broad range of innovations that are initiated to improve practice and the services in which that practice takes place. The term *innovation* differs from practice development in certain respects, especially in that the former refers to implementing something new and unprecedented. The dictionary (Brown, 2002: 1381) defines 'innovate' as introducing 'something for the first time, a new product, practice or method' and 'to make a change to something established'. Both activities refer to something developed necessarily in response to patient care needs, but development refers to a gradual progressive change and advancement. Innovation implies implementing a relatively radical new practice. Change as a concept, however, can mean substituting something with something new, a development or reverting to an older (but effective) practice.

Although nursing practice has been developing consistently over the years, one of the key stages in this is marked by the establishment of Nursing Development Units in the 1980s, which were practice settings where appropriate changes in practice were implemented and empirically evaluated.

Why clinical practice development?

One of the primary reasons that practice development is a mentoring role is that mentors are role models of good practice for their learners (NMC, 2008a; Billay and Yonge, 2004), which implies that they should always be reflecting on whether their clinical interventions are of the highest standard known, with a view to making them even more effective.

The two NMC domains clearly indicate that the mentor must continually question the evidence base and effectiveness of the care they deliver. However, clinical practice is only one of the components of the RN's role that can be developed, others being their education and management roles. Another categorisation of healthcare professionals' roles, each of which can be further developed, is by the Department of Health (2004a) in the *NHS KSF*, which identifies all patient care activities under six 'core dimensions', namely: (1) communication; (2) personal and people development; (3) health, safety and security; (4) service improvement; (5) quality; and (6) equality and diversity. All categories imply quality assurance, but service improvement in particular relates to making 'changes in own practice and offer suggestions for improving services' (DH, 2004a: 70).

Practice development is evolving continually, and the concept is taken further as some healthcare professionals develop their careers to become 'nurse entrepreneurs' (for example, Collinson, 2000; Faugier, 2005b). The term *entrepreneur* of course refers to people who engage in novel, unprecedented ventures on a substantial scale, and implies being innovators. Mooney (2009: 1), amongst others, reports on such developments but indicates that better support from colleagues and peers is required to allow nurses to innovate and become more entrepreneurial, in addition to the national level support that is already available.

The RN's teaching role starts soon after registering as a nurse with the NMC, and they have to be qualified for one year before accessing the mentor preparation course. Therefore, although the mentor needs to monitor the evidence base and effectiveness of their practice, the extent to which they can engage in practice development is variable depending on experience and clinical circumstances. Becoming a nurse entrepreneur is an even longer-term prospect.

Government directives that promote practice development include *Liberating the Talents* (DH, 2002a), a document that encourages primary care nurses and midwives to develop their practice. It indicates that the Chief Nursing Officer's (DH, 2002b) ten key roles for nurses provides a strategic framework for developing practice, and cites several examples of developments under 'setting up new services'. This is reinforced in various Department of Health documents, including *Modernising Nursing Careers: Setting the Direction* (DH, 2006).

Practice development is also propelled by RNs' expanded roles and senior nurse positions such as nurse consultants. Previously known as 'extended roles', 'expanded roles' refers to those clinical interventions that healthcare professionals engage in following relevant post-registration training and assessment.

With the implementation of the *European Working Time Directive* (NHS Employers, 2011) leading to a reduction in doctors' working hours, an increasing range of clinical interventions that were previously doctors' roles are now also performed by other healthcare professionals. These roles afford healthcare professionals greater autonomy and further scope for decision-making in holistic care, and therefore creativity and consequent practice development, as also noted by the RCN (2005).

However, clinical practice development is often triggered by a need for new actions to resolve a health problem. For example, falls amongst older people have presented as an issue for some time, and one of the actions taken by the NHS IQ ('NHS Improving

Quality', previously known as 'NHS III') (2013) is to publish case studies of good practice on preventing and managing falls, regarding which Ward et al. (2010) also report on novel interventions that are being implemented, namely:

- use of sensor alarms that alert nurses when an 'at risk' patient gets out of bed unaided
- identification of a falls team that is led by a matron, whose role includes staff training on the issue/topic area
- distraction therapy in dementia
- a new observation tool to identify the risk of falls.

Compassionate care

One mode of practice currently being developed with a high profile is compassionate care, which is a practice that was identified as lacking in healthcare provision in the Francis Report (2013). The report is the result of a thorough investigation into suspected malpractice in terms of patients being 'neglected', and concluded with approximately 300 recommendations, one of which refers to strengthening compassionate care in healthcare organisations. Compassionate care was also strongly recommended by the Chief Nursing Officer for England and the Director of Nursing for Public Health England (DH, 2012b), as well as in the Department of Health's (2013b) *The NHS Constitution for England*, and by the NMC (2010a). The publication by the above-mentioned nurse leaders discusses compassionate care in the context of their suggestion of 6 Cs that are required for modern care, which stand for: (1) care; (2) compassion; (3) competence; (4) communication; (5) courage; and (6) commitment (as noted on p.51).

> ### Activity 5.3   What does compassionate care mean?
>
> Discuss with a colleague/peer whom you trust whether you practise compassionate care in your day-to-day care delivery; and then explain in your own words what it is that you do that comprises compassionate care.

Compassionate care involves caring through a relationship that is 'based on empathy, respect, and dignity – it … is central to how people perceive their care' (DH, 2012b: 13). Your ways of providing compassionate care are the ways that your mentee is very likely to adopt for their future practice as RN or RM, as your mentor role incorporates being a role model. So, you are likely to incorporate acting with warmth and empathy, active listening, being sensitive and accessible, respecting dignity and privacy, etc. when interacting with patients or service users, which are characteristics also found by Bray et al. (2014) in their study of healthcare professionals' understanding of compassionate care.

Adam and Taylor (2014) suggest that compassion is developed through understanding patients' experiences, and approaching patients in gentle and respectful ways, and that the prerequisites of compassionate care include the ability to build effective working relationships with patients, and being able to feel secure and trusting of colleagues in the team.

Additionally, Adam and Taylor suggest ways of teaching students the ability to practise compassionate care that includes experiential learning and reflection. However, on exploring the RN's process of professional socialisation, Curtis et al. (2012) found that healthcare profession students' socialisation tends to drift towards the uncertainty of having time to practise compassionate care on qualification as an RN. Nevertheless, compassionate care does not always depend on time because it is an inherent component of most clinical interventions and can happen in the briefest of interactions with patients, and this is also where role modelling of mentors is so crucial in the mentee's learning.

See the Companion Website for more details of ways in which compassionate care can be implemented and learnt.

Management of clinical practice developments

Concept analysis of practice development

Moving on from actual examples of practice development and the two definitions of the term cited earlier in this section, in most instances practice is not developed or improved by individuals acting on their own, as it usually takes team effort to change to new practice. The team can be a small group of colleagues based at a specialist area (for example, day surgery unit, nursing home, intensive care unit), or a hospital level team (when a change is introduced at organisational level), or at national or supra-organisational level (as currently in the development of compassionate care).

Before implementing new ways of working, which is discussed in the next section under 'Managing change', another two perspectives of practice development need to be considered. One perspective constitutes exploring more thoroughly all that practice development entails, and one way of executing this is by a concept analysis.

Garbett and McCormack (2002) undertook a concept analysis of practice development based on an analysis of literature, focus group interviews with practice developers and telephone interviews with practitioners. A conceptual framework derived from the study comprises the purposes, attributes and outcomes of practice development (see box).

Purposes, attributes and outcomes of practice development

The purposes of practice development are to:

- Increase the effectiveness of patient care
- Transform care and the cultures and context within which it takes place

The attributes of practice development are that it:

- Requires a systematic and rigorous approach
- Is a continuous process
- Is founded on various types of facilitation

The consequences of practice development include:

- For users – improved experiences of care in terms of their sensitivity to the needs of individuals and populations
- For practitioners – increased capacity for thinking creatively and more broadly
- Greater awareness of the impact of organisations on practice

Contemporarily, McCormack et al. (2013: 5–7) provide a further dimension of practice development in indicating that it should be based on nine basic principles, which include:

- Practice development for achieving person-centred care and EBP.
- Practice development is gauged by the patient's experience of ways in which healthcare is provided.
- It integrates work-based learning.
- It integrates free thinking with creativity.
- It integrates evaluation that is always inclusive and collaborative.

Titchen (2003) identifies three overarching themes that form the basis for effective practice development, which she refers to as the practice development diamond. The themes are: (1) changing the practice philosophy; (2) the process of change in practice; and (3) investing in professional development.

The second perspective is that implementing a new way of practice (changing how a clinical intervention is performed), might require new resources in terms of new equipment, medical devices or disposable materials, the step-by-step procedure for performing the new practice. We also have to be completely clear about the 'purposes' and 'consequences' (Garbett and McCormack, 2002) of the novel practice. This perspective is captured by the Donabedian (1988) 'structure–process–outcome' model of implementing change, as also noted by Page (2001) and Gopee and Galloway (2014).

Thinking, for example, in relation to introducing patient-controlled analgesia (PCA), the 'structure–process–outcome' model constitutes the following.

- *Structure* refers to the material items required for implementing the new practice, such as new equipment, devices (such as PCA devices) and premises.
- *Process* refers to the step-by-step procedure for the new practice, such as the procedure for utilising the PCA device, and for teaching the patient how to use it, etc.

- *Outcome* refers to identifying clearly the results of the new practice, which in relation to PCA comprise, for example, pain relief in x seconds, saving staff time,
  quicker patient recovery.

The Donabedian model comprises a very practical framework for implementing and
monitoring or formatively evaluating (see Chapter 8) the progress and effect of a new
form of practice. The framework can be instigated or utilised by individual practitioners, as also noted by Page (2001), at team level, at organisational level (for example,
hospital) or at supra-organisational level (for example, within a clinical commissioning group's (CCG) healthcare providers) or nationally.

> ### Activity 5.3   Developing practice
>
> Based on the list of developments generated as a result of Activity 5.2, think of two
> aspects of practice at your work base that could be developed. Consider and make
> notes on how the framework presented by Donabedian (1988) can be utilised to
> change these two aspects of practice.

The practice development framework suggested by Donabedian should enable you
to take these developments further systematically if you so wish, and maybe within
the context of management of change (discussed next in this chapter). The RCN
(2006) also has a designated Practice Development Team that provides structured
help, advice and support in various ways.

The resources that can help healthcare professionals include the journal *Practice
Development in Healthcare*, and national conferences specifically on practice development. Several NHS trusts employ Practice Development Nurses or Facilitators.
Some have Practice Development Units that conduct experiments on new modes
of practice.

Managing Change

All healthcare professionals will have encountered changes in the way care and treatment are organised and delivered in various practice settings. It is therefore almost
inevitable that mentors will be involved as participants in change, and they are also
expected to initiate change as and when appropriate. Therefore, the mentor needs to
have knowledge and competence in managing change. It is important to distinguish
between the concepts of 'managing' change and 'introducing' or 'imposing' change;
the latter can be effected at short notice, but managing the change implies longer-
term, planned and systematic activities. Change is ongoing in healthcare delivery but
why do we have changes in healthcare in the first place?

Why changes in healthcare?

Activity 5.4   Changes in healthcare delivery

Consider the points made about practice development earlier in this chapter, and think of as many reasons as you can for changes that continually occur in healthcare at ward level, hospital level, and in primary and social care settings. Make notes on what you feel are the range of reasons for these changes.

The chances are that you will have thought of quite a few reasons for changes that you have observed in healthcare. They include government policy directives, such as *The National Service Framework for Long-Term Neurological Conditions* (DH, 2008), or action based on research for increasing productivity in healthcare (Smith and Rudd, 2010), care pathways for people with various long-term conditions (NHS IQ, 2013), the need to improve practice, and learning from 'near misses' or mistakes. These reasons can be grouped under seven areas, as noted in the box.

Reasons for changes in healthcare

1	Change in medical technology	• New medical devices and equipment; use of computer networks and easier access to information
2	New knowledge	• Research and audit findings; expert guidelines
3	Safer and more effective products	• Consumable materials and hardware being superseded by more efficient ones
4	The nature of the workforce	• Workers of different age groups and with domestic responsibilities; changes in qualified:unqualified staff ratio, e.g. healthcare assistants with different skills
5	Revised policies and strategies	• Use of devices and strategies to prevent injury to staff, or to avoid 'hospital acquired infections'
6	Quality-conscious consumers	• Consumer satisfaction surveys indicating the changes that should be made
7	Funding and budgets	• Availability and distribution of scarce resources

Consequently, change emanates from various sources, in addition to the mentor's role as evidence-based practitioner and practice developer. In fact, change is an inescapable feature of both organisational and personal life. The many sources of change that you thought of as well as those noted in the box above can also be grouped under those that are internal to the organisation (for example, efficiency measures) and those that are external (for example, legislative changes). However, some reasons can be both internal and external. For instance, if the quality of care is unsatisfactory, then the employees of the organisation will usually be aware of this and they will endeavour to rectify it, but the same issue might have been identified through external sources such as Care Quality Commission (CQC) audits.

Seven essential and interrelated factors for successful management of change have been identified by Gopee and Galloway (2014) as the seven-step Recognition, Analysis, Preparation, Strategies, Implementation, Evaluation, Sustaining (RAPSIES) framework for systematic management of change. The RAPSIES framework entails (in sequence):

1 **Recognition** of the need for change to solve a problem for instance, or to improve an element of practice.
2 **Analysis** of the available options related to the contemplated change, the environment or setting where change will be implemented and the users of the change.
3 **Preparation** for the change, such as identifying a change agent to lead the implementation of the change, education, defining intended outcomes and involving relevant colleagues.
4 **Strategies** for implementing the change.
5 **Implementation** of the change including piloting the change, timing of implementation.
6 **Evaluation** of the impact of the change against the intended outcomes.
7 **Sustaining** the change, i.e. how to ensure the change endures and is mainstreamed.

The change could succeed or fail, depending on the effectiveness of each of the seven steps in the framework. For example, if integrated care pathways (discussed in Chapter 4) are to be implemented, then has each of the seven steps been managed effectively? Further details on each of these steps are as follows.

Recognition of the need for change

The key attributes that are necessary in the innovation or change if it is to be implemented successfully, are:

● *Relative advantage* – the change must show that it should improve or enhance patient or service user care and has a relative advantage over the status quo.
● *Compatibility* – the proposed change must be compatible with existing beliefs and values of the group at philosophical as well as at pragmatic levels.
● *Communicability* – the ease with which the change can be understood.
● *Simplicity* – the ease or difficulty in the use of the innovation.
● *Trialability* – possibility of piloting the innovation, to identify and resolve unanticipated issues.

- *Observability* – the change must be observable.
- *Relevance* – the degree to which the change is relevant for the particular practice setting.

Therefore, if there is recognition of the need for change to integrated care pathways, then questions need to be asked about whether it is to the advantage of patients and service users compared to how care and treatment are currently delivered; whether the concept is compatible with the healthcare team's beliefs and values regarding care and treatment, etc. The specific meaning of the term 'innovation' was explored earlier in this chapter under 'Clinical practice development'.

Analysis of environmental and user factors

The second essential factor for effective implementation of change is whether the particular practice setting is suitable and ready for the change. It might not be 'ripe for change' if there is extensive resistance to change by the employees or in the team where change is to be implemented. An inappropriate time would be when there are too many unresolved issues or too many unfilled vacancies. There could also be barriers to change, which implies that organisational factors such as funding levels, politics or management are likely to present as obstacles.

In addition to the environment where change will be implemented, another essential component to consider for effective change implementation is the 'users' of the change. Rogers (2003) identifies six categories of users who are likely to be found in the organisation when change is envisaged. They are:

- *Innovators* – individuals who feel excited by novel practices that appear more effective and efficient.
- *Early adopters* – those who accept the change quite soon.
- *Early majority* – the first group to follow the early adopters.
- *Later majority* – other groups join the adopters of the change.
- *Laggards* – individuals who tend to lag behind.
- *Rejecters* – individuals who usually reject any change.

Innovators, laggards and rejecters

What, if anything, can practice managers do about each group of staff identified in the above categorisation of users of change?

Reflection Point 5.3

Healthcare managers can react or be proactive in specific ways towards each group of staff for managing the particular change effectively. For instance, with:

- *Innovators* – use the energy, allocate responsibilities; maybe appoint as change agent (leader of the change).
- *Early adopters* – recognise their motivation.

- *Early majority* – give sustained time and support.
- *Later majority* – reinforce by recognition and showing keen interest.
- *Laggards* – give extra support, prevent disillusionment.
- *Rejectors* – line manager to explore, as the individual might have evidence to the contrary, or might, for instance, be experiencing transient personal problems.

Preparation for the change

A change agent is usually appointed to advocate and lead the implementation of the change. He or she has certain fundamental functions such as:

- to have thorough knowledge of the change envisaged
- to identify the exact goals of the change
- to articulate the vision
- to develop strategies for introducing the change
- to disseminate relevant knowledge and strategies to appropriate individuals and groups
- to establish and maintain a working relationship with change users
- to retain big picture focus while dealing with specifics (integrative thinking).

Sullivan (2012) indicates that change agents have to be proactive at every step of the change process, and must be able to invest time, effort and energy. She suggests that some of the characteristics that successful change agents should cultivate and master are:

- well-developed interpersonal and human relations skills
- being a role model for the users of the change
- being trustworthy
- being flexible and persevering
- realistic thinking
- the ability to combine ideas from unconnected sources
- the ability to energise others
- the ability to handle resistance.

Thus, change agents have to demonstrate leadership abilities, and the transformational leadership style is particularly relevant for managing change. Some of the key facets of this style compared to those of the frequently demonstrated transactional style are presented in Table 5.1.

Transactional leadership involves the orderly breaking down of tasks but this often leads to loss of vision and energy. However, transformational leaders keep a distance, take a strategic or 'helicopter' view of the whole picture, lead by being passionate about the task in hand and empower.

Strategies for implementing the change

Strategies for change can be derived from existing models of change incorporating planned and systematic actions, based on underpinning beliefs and philosophies. As

TABLE 5.1 Transactional and transformational leadership

Transactional	Transformational
• Is task-centred • Has a short-/medium-term focus • Coaches and exercises sheltered learning • Rewards formally • Is comfortable, orderly • Separates home and work	• Empowers relevant others • Inspires by vision • Has a long-term focus • Challenges • Sees home and work lives on a continuum • Rewards informally, personally • Is emotional and passionate • Simplifies and clarifies

the change agent, there is a range of strategies that the mentor can choose from to implement change. One of the first steps in this venture is to do a SWOT or a 'force-field' analysis. SWOT analyses were introduced in Chapter 4, and an example of a forcefield analysis is presented in Table 5.2.

TABLE 5.2 Forcefield analysis – named nurse

Driving forces	Restraining forces
• Compatible with the government's patients' charter • Patient choice ascertained • Follow-up care – admission to discharge • Sense of responsibility and autonomy for nurses • Direction for nurses	• Could feel threatened • Shifts – practicality • Time factor • Staff disappointment, frustration • Patient may not like the nurse • Patients/relatives frustrated/ antagonised if nurse off-duty • Dissemination of information, e.g. at ward rounds

Activity 5.5   How is change managed?

Consider, maybe in a small group of healthcare professionals working in different specialisms, any one of the changes identified in response to Activity 5.1, for example self-rostering or integrated care pathways, one that approximates to a real change issue in the practice area of one of the group members. With the chosen change, do a SWOT or forcefield analysis in relation to your own practice area.

At times when a change that is to be implemented is contemplated by managers, an electronic (i.e. about by email) or paper copy about the change is sent to all those whom the change will affect. Generally, comments are invited from the prospective users of the change, and an open meeting might be held to enable users to ask for clarification. However, there are other well-documented systematic change strategies that are available to the healthcare professional to choose from, the most noteworthy of which are:

1 Lewin's three-stage process
2 empirical-rational strategy
3 normative-re-educative strategy
4 power-coercive strategy
5 action research
6 PDSA (plan–do–study–act)
7 combined strategy.

Each of these strategies is based on different assumptions held by the change agent about the people who have to accept and use the change. The appropriate strategies vary according to different situations, and a combination of strategies can be used.

1 Lewin's three-stage change process

Lewin's (1951) three-stage process of change involves unfreezing the situation, implementing the change, and then refreezing it. This is obviously an extremely simplistic explanation of activities that warrant careful planning and conduct. Unfreezing can be achieved by the SWOT or forcefield analyses just discussed. The implementation of the change is referred to as 'movement', and 'refreezing' refers to sustaining the change.

Following a SWOT or forcefield analysis, the actions that can be taken entail reducing the weaknesses and strengthening the driving forces. A format like the ones presented in Template 5.1 for introducing flexible hours, and in Template 5.2 for peri-operative visiting can be utilised for this.

TEMPLATE 5.1   Forcefield analysis – introducing flexible hours – and subsequent actions

Probable actions	Driving forces	Restraining forces	Probable actions
←	What people want	Long-term staff against	→
←	Retention issues	Fear of coming off worse	→
←	Encourage recruitment	'Unfair'	→
←	Staff morale	Difficulty fitting in with practical routine	→
←	Maximum use of staff time	Not feeling part of the team	→
←	Government favours this	Staff morale	→
←		Lack of communication	→

TEMPLATE 5.2 SWOT analysis – peri-operative visiting – and subsequent actions

SWOT analysis	Probable actions
Strengths • Reduces anxiety • Patient compliance up • Less post-operative compliance required • Patient articulates preferences to nursing staff • More interdisciplinary collaboration • Patient divulges more information • Continuity of care **Weaknesses** • Resources • Time • Possible lack of knowledge • Too many people disseminating information **Opportunities** • Role expansion • Specialist role • Education • Increased cost-effectiveness through patient compliance • Enhanced patient care **Threats** • Lack of continuity of care • Cost – funding • Patient information overload • Elitism – conflict	

2 Empirical-rational strategy

The empirical-rational strategy is used by the change agent by enabling the prospective users of the change to appreciate research findings or other evidence that indicates the need for change. It builds on the assumption that people are essentially rational, are guided by reason, and that if they can be helped to understand the reasons and processes of the proposed change, they are more likely to adopt it. Therefore this strategy is also based on empowerment through giving knowledge. Government health warnings are often based on this strategy.

3 Normative-re-educative strategy

Some change topics necessitate predominantly a re-educative approach in that if the users of the change are unfamiliar with the novel idea, then acquisition of new knowledge and skills will be a prerequisite for the change. This approach is also based on the belief that individuals and groups are inherently seeking and accepting of novel ways of practising their trade, based on evidence or research.

Change has to come from within the organisation, and if the bulk of the organisation's employees see change as a normal process (i.e. the normative strategy prevails) then this also comprises the bottom-up approach that includes the employees' active involvement in planning, implementation and evaluation of the process of change. Such involvement, in turn, leads to increases in motivation and personal growth, alongside commitment and cooperation.

4 Power-coercive strategy

Another strategy for implementing change is the power-coercive strategy, in which the change agent emphasises their position power by underlining political and economic dynamics to achieve the desired outcomes and, where necessary, the use of moral power, playing on feelings of guilt and shame. Coercion refers to very strong persuasion to accept the change and may incorporate potential threats and sanctions.

The assumption is that those in control of the organisation will identify the need for change, and people with less power will comply with their plans. If an empirical-rational approach does not work then a power-coercive strategy might be used but this does not usually prove as productive in the long term.

5 Action research

As noted earlier, one of the steps that could be considered in the management of change is trialability, i.e. whether a pilot project could be undertaken before full implementation. Change also presents an opportunity for research, meaning a more systematic implementation of the change along with a more rigorous evaluation of the impact of the change. Thus, practice development can be implemented and evaluated more systematically through action research rather than limiting the implementation at evaluation and sustaining stages of the RAPSIES framework.

6 Plan–Do–Study–Act (PDSA)

PDSA is a relatively recent notion that is advocated in the context of service improvement (Institute of Healthcare Improvement (IHI), 2014) in healthcare that is utilised as a strategy for implementation of change that acts as a spiral of continuous evaluation and improvement. Plan, do, study (or check) and act are cardinal steps in this strategy for managing change, and although this may initially sound like a simplistic framework, each step entails a number of structured action points. See also Chapter 8 for PDSA as a framework for evaluation.

Strategy for change

It is likely that during your early years as a newly qualified healthcare professional you were involved in some component of change. This encounter may have been deliberate or incidental. The change may have been initiated through internal or external forces. In relation to this, consider how:

- you reacted to the change
- you as an individual (or within a group) accepted or resisted the change
- you perceived any specific strategy used to bring about the change (e.g., power-coercive, action research).

7 Combined strategy

An appropriate combination of the above six strategies may be structured to suit the innovation, the environment, the users and the change agent.

The concepts of practice development, and change and innovations are widely discussed at national levels mainly at conferences, and through benchmarking. Binnie and Titchen (1999) refer to these activities as a series of journeys, implying that awareness of new ways of working and change management are naturally evolving dimensions within healthcare professions. They also identify a number of principles for practice development, which include components such as promoting and supporting a climate in which work is experienced as intellectually stimulating, growth is fostered and the relevant infrastructure is well developed.

Implementation of the change

Various factors need to be considered with regard to the actual implementation of the change, for example: the start date; the evaluation dates; the key staff; any specific paperwork required; if an action research strategy is being employed; how to deal with arising issues and infrastructure and whether all required resources are available; whether users have had the required training; and even if a buddying system is instituted. Dissemination of the impact of the programme is also an option.

Evaluation of the impact of the change

Naturally, an aspect of healthcare cannot be introduced without instant and continuing evaluation of its effects, and therefore the formative and summative evaluation points should be identified. Frameworks and models for evaluation are discussed in Chapter 8 of this book.

Sustaining the change

One of the key reasons why many new ideas fail some time after implementation is shortcomings in the resources needed to sustain the change. Staff motivation also needs to be sustained by reinforcement from the change agent or line managers. Personnel involved in ensuring success of the change should be explicitly recognised and rewarded as appropriate. The structure, process and outcome mechanism (Donabedian, 1988) should be kept firmly in mind in order to identify any weak spots in each of these components that need immediate action.

Mentors as Role Models of EBP and Practice Development

In summarising the discussion of the mentor's role as evidence-based practitioner and practice developer, it very much looks like one of the added values or knock-on effects of the mentor's activities as a practice developer is that it is a suitable dimension for the mentor to embody the qualities of a model healthcare professional. Being amenable to adopting changing modes of clinical intervention that benefit or enhance the health of patients or service users is a characteristic of a role model that mentees can emulate.

Price and Price (2009) support the argument that role modelling is an appropriate method or process for enabling students to learn safe and effective practice. The notion is based on Bandura's (1997) social learning theory that, as noted in Chapter 1, suggests that individuals learn behaviour through observation, mental retention of the procedure utilised, reproducing the behaviour and reinforcement. An analysis of role modelling was also presented in Chapter 1.

Wright and Carrese (2002) conducted a study to ascertain the characteristics of role models in a healthcare profession, and concluded that 'clinical attributes' is one of the most important characteristics, other characteristics being personal qualities (for example, positive outlook and interpersonal skills) and teaching skills. Paice et al. (2002) explored the significance of doctors as role models for medical students, and report that 'excellent' role models show:

- positive attitude towards junior colleagues
- compassion for patients
- integrity
- clinical competence
- enthusiasm for their clinical specialism
- communication and teaching ability
- understanding of the importance of the doctor–patient relationship
- consideration of psychosocial aspects, i.e. viewing the patient as a whole person.

Chapter Summary

This chapter has focused on the mentor's role in evidence-based effective practice and clinical practice development, as well as management of change, and has therefore examined:

- Effective practice and its relevance for the mentor role.
- Evidence-based practice, addressing what it is and how it is achieved; research-based practice, and the mentor's role in identifying, evaluating, applying and disseminating research findings, and how to overcome barriers to implementation.
- Clinical practice development, what the term means, including definitions and a concept analysis of practice development, the reasons for developing practice and how they can be managed effectively.
- Managing change, incorporating the key reasons for constant changes in healthcare, and the components necessary for effective change implementation utilising a seven-step framework for doing so systematically, which includes different strategies for implementing change.

Further Optional Reading

1 Various detailed examples of innovations (case studies) and practice development in healthcare are available on NICE's 'NHS Evidence' website, e.g.:

- National Institute for Health and Care Excellence (2014c) *Quality, Innovation, Productivity and Prevention (QIPP)*. Available at: www.evidence.nhs.uk/qipp (accessed 2 May 2014).

2 See the following book that asks: 'Is evidence-based practice really best practice?' The book presents a supplementary perspective to the scientific but often mechanical approach that evidence-based practice takes, and re-emphasises the humanistic values that must underpin the art of health and social care practice:

- McCarthy, J. and Rose, P. (2010) *Values-Based Health and Social Care: Beyond Evidence-Based Practice*. London: Sage Publications.

3 An excellent resource for the best ways of critically appraising research papers is:

- Greenhalgh, T. (2014) *How to Read a Paper: The Basics of Evidence-Based Medicine*, 5th edn. Oxford: Wiley–Blackwell.

To access further resources related to this chapter, visit the companion website at https://study.sagepub.com/gopee

6

Assessing the Learner's Knowledge and Competence

Introduction

Chapter Outcomes

On completion of this chapter, you should be able to:

1. Identify what assessments are, and the elements of healthcare courses on which students are assessed.
2. Enunciate a number of reasons for assessment of clinical skills and knowledge of students on healthcare profession courses.
3. Cite instances of various staff members who are involved in assessment, including the roles of self- and peer assessment.
4. Explain a range of strategies that mentors can utilise in the conduct of student assessments, and the various key principles of assessments that they need to abide by to fulfil this function.
5. Explain the role of 'ongoing record of achievement' and the requirements that the mentor has to fulfil to be able to sign off proficiency competently.
6. Explain the processes of the management of assessment of clinical competencies, and how assessments can meet essential criteria such as validity and reliability.

One of the most fundamental functions of the mentor is to assess students and other learners' clinical skills and associated knowledge. Assessment is an integral part of all credit-awarding healthcare courses, and one of the principal purposes of mentoring courses is to equip course participants with the capability to assess students on their placement competencies. At the end of each assessment, the mentor makes a decision regarding whether the student is competent to perform each skill independently, unsupervised and safely, and signs the appropriate section of the student's competency booklet as pass or fail.

There are a number of factors that the mentor needs to take into consideration to fulfil their assessment function effectively. These factors are explored in this chapter from the perspectives of what assessments are, why we perform them and when, who performs them, and the range of methods of assessment that are available. The specified procedures that have to be followed, and the validity and reliability of assessments are other components that are addressed. These points essentially comprise the principles and processes of assessments. Problems with assessments, as well as past and present criticisms and how they can be averted or resolved, are components addressed in Chapter 7.

In its specification of competence and outcomes for the mentor under 'Assessment and accountability', the NMC (2008a: 52–3) indicates that the mentor should be competent to 'assess learning in order to make judgements related to the NMC standards of proficiency for entry to the register or for recording a qualification at a level above initial registration'. The outcomes of this particular mentor competence are:

- To foster professional growth, personal development and accountability through support of students in practice.
- To demonstrate a breadth of understanding of assessment strategies and ability to contribute to the total assessment process as part of the teaching team.
- To provide constructive feedback to students and assist them in identifying future learning needs and actions, manage failing students so that they may enhance their performance and capability for safe and effective practice or be able to understand their failure and the implications of this for their future.
- To be accountable for confirming that students have, or have not, met the NMC competencies in practice, and as a sign-off mentor (SOM) confirm that students have met, or not met, the NMC standards of proficiency and are capable of safe and effective practice.

The concepts that are inherent to the principles of assessment implicated in the above NMC outcomes are therefore essential, and are addressed in this chapter. Just a note at this point about the sign-off mentor role, in that the role is different from the mentor's role, as discussed later in this chapter, and to achieve sign-off mentor status, the mentor is required to attend further training sessions (NMC, 2008a), which are often organised and run by PEFs.

What Are Assessments?

To begin to examine the principles and processes of assessments, it is useful to establish first what you as the healthcare professional already know about assessments of competencies.

Activity 6.1   What you already know about assessments

1 Think of the courses that you have already attended, and any one(s) you might currently be on. Think also of your contact with learners and students on various programmes of study. What are the various methods of assessment that are used to assess learners' knowledge and skills? Jot down as many methods as you can think of.
2 Consider what else you already know about assessments, which aspects of assessments you are unclear about, and what else you feel that you need to know about assessments. Make written notes of your responses.

So what do you already know about assessments? In response to Activity 6.1, you may have thought that assessment of clinical skills is best carried out by direct observation of the learner's performance, and some by reflective practice write-ups. Essays and written examinations are used for the assessment of theory. Most of these will be examined in this chapter under 'how to assess'. Examples of assessments of theory and practice in healthcare education programmes include:

- structured essays
- objective or multiple-choice tests
- profiles and portfolio, and reflective write-ups
- practice-based competencies
- care studies/case studies
- seminars
- written examination
- OSCE (i.e., Objective Structured/Simulated Clinical Examination)
- short-answer questions
- practical assessments in skills laboratories
- individually negotiated projects
- longitudinal studies.

Your response to what else you feel you need to know about assessments obviously depends very much on your experience, existing knowledge and understanding of the concept, and it varies between individuals. You might have felt, for instance, that you could do with knowing more about formative, summative, continuous, peer/self-assessment or about practice competencies.

What do we mean by assessments?

A number of assessment methods such as written examinations, practical assessments and projects have just been identified.

> ### Activity 6.2   Assessments that I've passed
>
> To explore this area further, first look back to a course that you attended, preferably recently, and make notes on the following:
>
> - A list of assessments that you had to pass in order to complete the course successfully.
> - When exactly during the course were you assessed, and on which components of the course?
> - Specifically what was assessed?

If you were assessed by continuous assessment, then you would have been exposed to a range of assessment components on different occasions, during both practice placements and in university skill laboratories and classrooms.

Definitions of assessment

The dictionary (Brown, 2002: 331) states that the word 'assess' originates from the Latin word *assidere*, which means sit by or beside, which implies a close relationship and sharing an experience. The word also means 'estimate the extent, value or worth' of something. Therefore, assessment tends to imply staying by the learner's side and observing them perform a clinical skill with a view to stating at the end of the performance whether the skill was carried out competently. It also seems to imply being supportive and identifying subsequent learning needs.

Taking a step back, however, it is important to note that an assessment is not an activity we perform only occasionally to fulfil our work role. We assess life situations all the time before we take any action, whether it is to do with assessing whether to wear a coat when going out based on the perceived weather and temperature outside, whether it is safe to overtake when driving, or whether we can treat ourselves to a delicious cake while bearing in mind the day's calorie intake. Such assessments do not result in someone awarding us a pass or fail but they still involve assessing stimuli or data, and then making a decision.

Assessment is also reflected in patient assessment, which entails collecting information and identifying actual and potential patient problems from the data, from which decisions are made regarding the actions to be taken. Student assessment, however, is related to collecting information as evidence of the student's ability to perform particular clinical skills or competencies. Some of the core skills necessary for assessing patients' needs and problems are also relevant for assessing learners. These are observing, measuring, interviewing and making decisions. These skills also apply to assessment of students' knowledge and skills.

For assessing health profession learners' clinical competencies and related knowledge, assessment can be defined as the purposeful observation and questioning undertaken to ascertain the learner's ability to perform particular clinical interventions in precise accordance with established or approved guidelines, and their knowledge of rationales for each action. Curzon and Tummons (2013) suggest that assessments involve collecting, measuring and interpreting information related to students' responses to the process of instruction.

Other definitions are provided by Nicklin and Kenworthy (2000), for instance, who define assessment as a measurement that directly relates to the quality and quantity of learning and is therefore concerned with students' progress and attainment. While quantity of learning could imply the number of skills or part-skills that the learner has already learnt, quality of learning refers to how thoroughly the skills have been learnt. The latter would also suggest progress and identifying areas of further learning.

What do we assess?

The NMC's (2010a) *Standards for Pre-registration Nursing Education* identifies the exact 'generic' competencies and 'field' (previously known as 'branch') competencies that each student needs to achieve to gain registered nurse status on the NMC's professional register. There are also 'specialist practitioner outcomes' for SCPHNs (NMC, 2004b), for instance, as there are criteria, competencies and outcomes for mentors and practice teachers (NMC, 2008a). Similarly, the HCPC publishes separate standards for pre-qualifying different AHP courses. These standards and competencies are reflected in the course and modules' aims and learning outcomes, in theory and in practice components.

The UKCC (1999) advocated an outcomes-based competency approach to education that encourages the development of knowledge, understanding, practical and technical skills, attitudes and values. Current pre-registration nurse education curricula thus contain generic and field (mental health, adult, child and learning disabilities) competencies under four 'domains': (1) professional values; (2) communication and interpersonal skills; (3) nursing practice and decision-making; and (4) leadership, management and team-working for entry to the professional register (NMC, 2010a), as noted in Chapter 2.

As we shall see later, it is absolutely vital for the mentor to establish very early on during the practice placement exactly which specific competencies they are expected to assess students on during that particular placement. Otherwise, the assessment may not meet the curriculum's requirements. In the notes that you made in response to Activity 6.2, you may have mentioned that the NMC or the associated university has already laid down the components that we need to assess in the form of competencies, but more detailed information can usually be found in a range of documents such as the student's course assessment booklet, the assessor's handbook and the course curriculum.

In addition to the NMC's (2010a) generic and field competencies, essential skills clusters (ESC) are incorporated into all pre-registration nursing education programmes, and the specific ones that form part of particular practice placement objectives to be achieved by students are discussed with them and their mentors before students embark on the particular placement. Over the duration of their pre-registration programme, mentors assess students on all competencies under the four above-mentioned domains, as well as on all ESCs.

All assessments of the pre-registration curriculum are mandatory, and those in the first year of the programme are set at academic level 4 (or level C – certificate level); those for the second year are set at level 5 (level I – Intermediate or diploma level), and those for the third year at level 5 or 6 (level H – Honours degree level) (QAA, 2008). Various other ways of differentiating between academic levels have also already been developed (for example, Steinaker and Bell, 1979; Krathwohl, 2002).

The competencies booklet that students bring with them to the practice placement contains other useful information such as the process of assessment, the roles and responsibilities of the mentor, those of the student and the university support available to them.

Optional activity – Pre-registration student assessment

Find out from your partner university all the assessments that the pre-registration student needs to pass for the field-specific part of the programme while on placement in your practice setting. You could access this information via the link lecturer, for instance, for your practice setting, or the PEF.

In addition to the placement competencies or practice objectives set by the university, students are encouraged to achieve as many other competencies as the placement can offer and thereby maximise learning. A number of clinical areas have their own clearly identified competencies or learning objectives that can be achieved during placement. A number of them are optional for pre-registration students but compulsory for newly appointed qualified healthcare professionals on induction or preceptee programmes.

Activity 6.3   Practice placement competencies

Obtain a copy of the staff induction pack for your practice area, one that contains all the clinical skills or practice competencies that RNs or RMs in your practice setting need to be able to perform to fulfil their duties effectively after the induction or precepteeship periods, and consider:

- Are these practice competencies separate from ward or team aims and objectives? If so, why?
- How far do the practice competencies give a clear indication of all competencies that students can learn during the placement?

The competencies are usually available in a 'learning resources' folder for students in your practice setting but it might prove useful to obtain a photocopy of this for yourself for revisiting if required.

In addition to the regulatory bodies' standards of proficiency, professional bodies such as the Chartered Society of Physiotherapy (CSP) (2002) publish further specific standards, such as those in the *Curriculum Framework for Qualifying Programmes in Physiotherapy*, for instance. This document identifies the nine outcomes that physiotherapy students have to achieve by the time they complete their preparatory programme, along with further guidelines. It specifies that, on successful completion of a recognised programme, graduates should be able to demonstrate their capacity to:

- practise within the core areas of physiotherapy
- manage themselves and work with others to optimise results
- enable people to optimise their health and social well-being
- deliver physiotherapy in response to individual need
- promote equality to all in physiotherapy practice
- demonstrate and apply knowledge and understanding to issues affecting physiotherapy practice
- engage in research and evidence-based healthcare
- respond appropriately to changing demands
- practise and promote CPD.

Why Do We Need to Assess Our Students?

We have already referred to some of the aims of assessments. Most individuals have mixed feelings about being assessed as, on the one hand, it creates anxiety but, on the other hand, on passing the assessment, the learner can be given permission to practise the particular clinical skill without close supervision. To begin our discussion on why we need to assess, consider what the range of purposes of assessments is, in addition to the (NMC, 2008a) requirement for mentors to assess learners.

Activity 6.4   Purposes of assessments

Think of all the methods of assessment that you noted during Activity 6.1, and of the reasons for assessing students and other learners. Make notes of these reasons for assessment. What did each assessment test?

As noted at the beginning of the chapter, according to the NMC, the mentor must indicate whether the student has achieved the NMC (2010a) standards for pre-registration nurse education and therefore whether they are safe and effective in practice, and thus the practice competencies are designed to test the student's ability to perform clinical patient care interventions. Structured essays test the student's knowledge and understanding of concepts in nursing, but mentors are not involved in marking essays as this is the remit of the HEI. In addition to these, assessments also ascertain learning in the affective domain (Bloom, 1956; discussed in Chapter 3), that is, values and attitudes. Several purposes of assessments are identified by different writers. In summary, we assess learners in order:

- To establish and then authorise them as developing health professionals to practise specific clinical skills without close supervision
- To inform the learner of their level of achievement at that point in time
- To determine the student's progress with the learning programme
- To ascertain the learner's overall competence and fitness for practice
- To motivate the learner towards new components of learning
- To judge the level of professional learning in the cognitive (knowledge and thinking), psychomotor (dexterity with clinical skills), and affective (attitude) components
- For the student to identify further learning needs based on self-assessment and mentor feedback.

As assessments also constitute an opportunity for identifying learning needs, this suggests that learning is an integral component of the assessment process, and not simply a means of measuring attainment. Students are encouraged to undertake self-assessment and to reflect on their learning. It could be argued that all assessments are learning situations, in that if the learner makes any error, then they are likely to be aware of it, or the assessor will point it out to them and identify learning needs. This notion also suggests that even if the student performs the skill competently, there is still scope for progressing from 'competent' to 'proficient' levels, for instance on Benner's (2001) skill acquisition continuum.

From the teacher's perspective, assessment also provides a measure of teaching effectiveness. It provides some feedback on the mentor and their colleagues' effectiveness at teaching particular competencies during practice placements. Naturally, the student will normally have had some teaching related to those competencies at the university beforehand. Assessments of theory also provide nurse lecturers with some measure of their university-based teaching.

In addition to the aims of assessments already mentioned, another function of assessments is to fulfil one of society's needs directly, in that they identify which healthcare professionals have acquired the necessary repertoire of knowledge and competencies for safe and competent practice, as a primary practitioner initially, and probably as a specialist later.

Who Assesses Learners?

As to who assesses learners, obviously it is qualified healthcare professionals who have completed a mentoring course who are given 'a licence' to assess learners' competencies. However, it is pertinent to consider the broader question of who else are the relevant personnel who assess competencies.

Who assesses?

Think about assessments that you and your colleagues have been involved in recently. Spend a few minutes thinking about who conducted the assessments, on what, on whom and how. Is it only the mentor who assesses the learner's competencies, or are other individuals also afforded this responsibility?

Perhaps an immediate response to this Reflection Point is that it is the mentor who assesses, or teams of mentors. However, the NMC (2008a) indicates that assessments are also performed by other registrants, practice teachers and qualified teachers. In fact, you might have concluded that all qualified healthcare professionals, including doctors, are involved in assessments, albeit often informally or indirectly. So, the answer to the question 'Who assesses?' could be everyone in the practice setting, and includes students' self-assessment, peer assessment and assessment by patients or service users. These are now discussed.

Student self-assessment

Self-assessment is one of the most valuable forms of assessment for students. It is almost always formative and therefore a learning exercise. As implied, the student uses a set of criteria or a checklist, written or mental, to self-assess their knowledge of a sub-topic area or of a specific competency. It also enables them to own the learning and to control the way they meet their needs. Self-assessment may be performed informally or more formally by the use of profiling documents or reflective diaries.

Much informal or subconscious self-assessment carried out by learners is based on their own individual aspirations, values and beliefs. These could be influenced by their views on patient or service user care based on their own personal and professional experiences.

Activity 6.5   Self-assessment

Take a critical look at the idea of self-assessment by students, and of the strengths and weaknesses of self-assessments, and identify as many of these as you can think of.

What is self-assessment? Falchikov (1986) states that in self-assessment, the learner judges their own performance against their own assessment criteria. According to Boud (1991), self-assessment is characterised by involvement of students in identifying standards and/or criteria to apply to their work and making judgements about the extent to which they have met them.

On examining the concept with groups of post-registration students, a number of areas of strengths as well as weaknesses were identified (Gopee, 2000). Strengths of self-assessment are seen as including:

- inspires a conscious effort to be honest with self
- opportunity to identify limitations of own knowledge, and of learning needs
- identifies where more practice/knowledge gain is required
- is less traumatic than traditional methods of assessment such as examinations.

As for the weaknesses of self-assessment, it was felt that some students can be too self-critical while others can be too lenient in their judgement of their own performance, some may not be capable of gauging the effectiveness of own performance accurately, and that self-assessment could worsen a student's poor self-image.

Peer assessment

The value and impact of peers and colleagues' impressions of our competence in various aspects of our roles cannot be underestimated. This is often informal, with colleagues, friends and even family members having different perceptions of our capability, based perhaps on their different professional experiences.

Because of its value to the student, increasingly peer assessment is being built into formal assessment processes. In distance and e-learning modes of education delivery, facilitators often encourage students to form their own 'learning sets' for the purposes of learning together, for discussions and questioning each other. In this case, peer assessment is not formal in that other students or colleagues do not usually award a summative 'pass' or 'fail' to the peer assessed. They do, however, provide valuable opinions and feedback on the individual's knowledge, which can be formally incorporated into a profile or a record of reflective learning. In this way, peer assessment usually presents an opportunity to verbalise uncertainties and reservations about one's learning without having to deal with the anxiety of examinations and pass or fail situations.

Assessment by peers, formal or informal, is increasingly becoming accepted as an educationally sound activity. Many of us may find assessing our peers uncomfortable. We either do not wish to appear to be over-critical, and therefore tend not to assess or voice our views fully, or we feel that as we have such good rapport with our peers, we could damage their self-confidence with our 'criticisms'. It is also important to recognise that being assessed by our peer group can be more daunting than being assessed by a qualified assessor. If it is done badly, peer assessment can quickly destroy students' confidence or make them feel unable to face their peers again.

Peer assessment, therefore, just like any other form of assessment, can benefit from the expertise of a facilitator if it is to be effective and help the student. Thus, peers who are doing the assessing, as well as the person being assessed, are helped by the facilitator to recognise the parameters of their roles. When one group of post-registration students were asked to list the advantages and disadvantages of peer-assessment, they felt the advantages include (Gopee, 2001):

- can confirm previously held belief in skills or lack of them
- chance to share colleagues' perception of the performance
- opportunity to identify one's weaknesses, which can later be worked on, to improve
- feedback from colleagues/students of equal status has impact
- is usually formative, so will not result in a pass or a fail for the course.

However, as with self-assessment, there can well be problematic areas related to peer-assessment in that some students can find it hard to take any criticism from equals, someone can be over-critical and destructive, the individual might not accept peers' views, it can destroy self-confidence and lead to deserting the course altogether, and there could be complete disagreement between peers.

Another related term is *peer review*, which involves seeking the views and impressions of peers in a structured or semi-structured way. When clinicians design a new protocol or audit tool, for instance, they may ask an uninvolved colleague who works some distance away but in the same clinical specialism to comment on it prior to finalisation for use. Lecturers usually engage in peer review by asking a colleague to observe their teaching on specified occasions and provide feedback against standardised criteria.

Patient or service user involvement in assessment of competencies

One of the judges of how competently a healthcare profession learner performs a clinical skill could be the patient or service user. User involvement in learner assessment and providing feedback on how competently the learner functioned in particular care interventions is increasingly advocated by regulatory bodies (for example, NMC, 2006b). In recommending user involvement in assessments, the NMC (2006b, 2010a) advises HEIs to explore ways in which lay people (including service users and carers) can be involved in the assessment of practice and supply evidence of this involvement, and that of clinical practitioners in Programme Boards/Boards of Study that establish the requirements for practice learning and assessment (Mott MacDonald and NMC, 2013: 46).

So, what are the specific ways in which the mentor can do this? Usually, the mentor gauges how content the patient or service user is with the care that they receive by observation, and even by casually asking them. The patient or service user can provide feedback to the mentor about the learner's communication skills, injection-giving skills and teaching relaxation skills, for example, which are competencies under the NMC (2010a) domains communication and interpersonal skills, nursing practice and decision-making, and leadership, management and team-working, respectively. User involvement in assessment of competencies under the domain professional values can be achieved by the mentor asking the patient or service user if they felt that their consent had been obtained by the student prior to the clinical intervention, if they felt that they were treated with dignity and whether confidentiality was maintained in the presence of others.

Evidence of effective service user involvement in students' learning and assessment prevails (for example, Gutteridge and Dobbins, 2010; Stickley et al., 2010), although it is acknowledged that it is a time-intensive activity that also requires additional infrastructure.

How Are Assessments Conducted?

Learners deemed competent in performing a particular clinical skill can move on to learn other skills identified in their practice competencies booklet for the placement. In this major section on how to assess, further principles of assessment are addressed, and comprise:

- ensuring the mentee has learned the clinical skill
- the assessor's essential interpersonal skills
- dimensions of assessment
- assessing different levels of competence
- fairness of assessment
- assessment criteria and pass or fail decisions.

Additionally, the process of assessment of competencies has to be managed, decisions made and feedback given to the learner. These latter points, along with how the mentor averts and resolves problems of assessment, are examined in Chapter 7.

Ensuring that the mentee has learned the clinical skill

An important prerequisite of assessment of a learner is to ensure that they have been taught the clinical skill systematically and given the necessary practice opportunities over time and under supervision prior to the point of assessment. What skills, competence and competencies are was discussed in Chapter 2, and how learners acquire the required competencies, including stages and levels of skill acquisition (for example, Fitts and Posner, 1973; Steinaker and Bell, 1979; Benner, 2001), in Chapter 3. But crucially and logically, before the student is asked to demonstrate that they are competent in any skill, they naturally need to learn to perform the skill according to approved procedures, and under the guidance of a registrant. The learning also has to be in the context of eventualities in the practice setting (i.e. situated learning, for example Phillips et al., 2000).

The assessor's essential interpersonal skills

Assessment is a role that has to be executed responsibly by the mentor, and to do so effectively, certain specific personal and interpersonal skills are essential to enable the student to feel at ease when they are being assessed performing clinical interventions. These skills are subsets of the NMC (2008a) mentor domain 'Establishing effective working relationships' that was discussed in Chapter 1 of this book.

Several communication skill items emerge when exploring in detail what and how the mentor communicates with the learner. The box lists many of the essential interpersonal skills that are required during assessments, identified by just one group of registrants on a mentor course.

Communication and interpersonal factors related to assessments

Generic communication skills

- Non-verbal communication – e.g. eye contact, facial expression
- Body language – posture, body orientation, proximity, attitude, behaviour, space
- Being non-judgemental – warmth, empathy, respect
- Always remaining calm
- Openness
- Questioning – open or closed questions
- Reflecting
- Active listening
- Verbal communication – pace, volume, tone, clarity
- Diplomacy
- Considering environmental factors
- Being enthusiastic, interested
- Making time, using silence
- Constructive criticism/advice
- Approachable and friendly, non-intimidatory

Specific interpersonal skills

- Putting the learner at ease
- Enabling learner to relax if anxious so that they can perform the skill to their potential
- Building confidence by positive feedback if necessary
- Giving clear directions
- Continuous feedback
- Being non-judgemental by not criticising verbally or non-verbally
- Giving prompts/clues if student's mind goes blank
- Allowing enough time for the learner to perform the skill fully
- Making time to listen, and to maintain rapport
- Preventing observer bias and observer effect
- Ascertaining level of understanding of terminologies/jargon
- Confidence – in the student/in self
- Reinforcing what has been discussed

Dimensions of assessment

There are a number of other essential facets of assessments that we need to consider to gain a more comprehensive picture of how to assess. Hughes and Quinn (2013: 245) and others identify what is generally known as 'dimensions of assessments'. Particularly relevant are whether assessments are:

1 continuous or episodic
2 formative or summative
3 criterion-referenced or norm-referenced.

Continuous or episodic assessments

Until the latter half of the 1980s, the assessment of pre-registration students used to take place at predetermined points during their course. The student on the general nursing course was assessed on their ability to administer medications in Year 1 of the course and to use aseptic techniques, and organise the total care of an individual or a group of patients or service users on specific subsequent occasions. They also had to pass written examinations at the end of the course. These are episodic assessments.

Obviously, students had to learn numerous other nursing skills necessary to function as a healthcare professional, which were identified in a competencies booklet and signed as appropriate. However, these snapshot assessments were not seen as representing the wide range of skills acquired during placements, nor were they seen as a genuine representation of how students usually delivered care, and they therefore fell into disfavour. They were replaced by continuous assessment and subsequently by modularisation of preparatory programmes, involving assessment of practice and theory on numerous occasions throughout the course.

Episodic (or intermittent) assessments therefore involve testing the student at specific times or occasions during an educational programme, such as at the end of a module, a placement or year. Continuous assessment aims to increase the quality and quantity of evidence gathered in relation to achievement of competencies by each individual student. It involves a continuing awareness by the mentor of the student's level of knowledge and competence, and is thus a cumulative judgement about progress and achievement.

Activity 6.7   Advantages and disadvantages of continuous and episodic assessments

Consider what you think might be the advantages and disadvantages of episodic and continuous assessments, and make some notes.

The principal reason for episodic assessments being discredited in nursing and midwifery in the past is that decisions about the student's competence were being made on the basis of one-off performances. This performance, be it excellent or otherwise, might be atypical. Another disadvantage is that some key skills can remain untested if they do not present themselves during the identified assessment episode.

Recently, following extensive consultation, the NMC (2010a) has introduced 'progression points' in the pre-registration nursing and midwifery education curriculum, when students are assessed and must achieve a 'Pass' on several key competencies before progressing to the subsequent stage of their education programme. These assessments can also be examples of episodic assessment, and students are required to demonstrate that they are competent in those competencies to be able to register subsequently with the NMC as an RN or RM.

Formative or summative assessments

Another dimension of assessment is whether the assessment is formative or summative. In common with the context of evaluation (which we discuss in Chapter 8), 'formative' relates to the developmental and improvement stages of something (for example, a clinical skill). The primary aim of the formative assessment of a professional practice skill is to promote learning so that the learner can perform the skill safely and effectively, and knows the rationales for each step of the intervention. The student's capability is thus developed under conditions in which they can reflect-in-action and think creatively without being too concerned about final pass or fail grades, and also has the opportunity to take time to learn the skill thoroughly with the support of mentors.

Formative assessment applies to assessment of theory as well as to practical skills. For the theory component of education programmes, the student thereby obtains feedback on the evidence they are presenting to the marker or lecturer on how far they are demonstrating knowledge of the subject area, critical analysis, general presentation of the paper, etc. Formative assessments are therefore instituted to provide feedback to the student on their progress, and their aims are to:

- maximise learning
- identify strengths/weaknesses
- inform the student of how they are progressing
- allow for individual development.

As a concept and an activity, formative assessment has been advocated for decades, but implementation proves erratic even today, which could be due to it being yet another extra requirement to create time for in busy day-to-day professional activities in both practice setting and HEIs. Thus it has resource and efficiency implications. It is, however, an educationally sound concept and students tend to be grateful for the feedback that they receive from it. On exploring the prevalence of its usage in nurse education, Duers and Brown's (2009: 658) study revealed that formative assessment has the 'potential to improve learning so that high quality, safe and effective nursing care to patients may be provided'. Koh (2010) also reports various benefits of formative assessment in nurse education.

'Summative' relates to a point in time during a unit of learning, for example a practice placement, when the mentor makes a decision about whether to declare the learner competent or otherwise on a specific component of learning. Summative assessments are conducted to determine whether the learner is now competent to work without direct supervision and, if so, then this is recorded in their competencies' booklet.

Summative assessments also constitute a periodic record of the student's achievement of the aims and outcomes of a course or module. The grade awarded for these assessments, along with those for coursework and examinations, contribute to the final classification of the student's university award.

It might prove useful to ask your mentee, or to look back on any long course you have done in recent years, and identify the range of formative and summative assignments incorporated in the programme. As to assessment in the practice setting, the student learning part-skills (for example, some of the skills required for administering an intramuscular injection) itself constitutes a formative assessment. The NMC's (2010b) 'signing off' of competencies point in the pre-registration programme constitutes a summative assessment.

In healthcare courses, summative assessments are concerned with patient or service user safety and standards of practice. They are also concerned with justice for the student and credibility of the university's awards. They must therefore meet the highest standards of reliability and validity, which are discussed in some detail later in this chapter.

Criterion-referenced or norm-referenced assessments

The third dimension of assessment we consider is norm referencing and criterion referencing. In norm-referenced assessment, the student's score, marks or grades are determined to an extent by those of other students in a given group or cohort. Programme Assessment Boards (also known as Award Boards) have the discretion to adjust the marks required by a particular cohort to achieve a particular grade if unusual circumstances have prevailed. Criterion-referenced assessments are different in that the score or mark given to a particular student for a particular piece of coursework is decided entirely on the basis of a predetermined set of marking criteria. Students will have been informed of these criteria long before the assessment date.

Norm- or criterion-referenced assessments

Think about some of the assessments that you have mentioned for Activity 6.1 and decide whether they are norm-referenced assessments or criterion-referenced.

Reflection Point 6.2

Occasionally, a criterion-referenced assessment can be marked on a norm-referenced basis at the discretion of the appropriate Programme Assessment Board.

Assessing different levels of competence

Student nurses tend to be taught and assessed at different academic levels during Year 1, Year 2 and Year 3. The NMC's (2010a) generic and field competencies noted in Chapter 3 are configured at different academic levels in the competencies booklets that students take to practice placements. Healthcare assistants studying for national vocational qualification are also assessed differently at different levels.

To teach and assess competencies at different levels of learning, a number of current nurse education curricula tend to use Steinaker and Bell's (1979) model (or taxonomy) of experiential learning. This taxonomy consists of exposure level, participation, identification, internalisation and dissemination. A broad guide to how the experiential taxonomy levels can equate with the QAA's (2008) academic levels is:

- Certificate level/academic level 4 – exposure, participation
- Diploma level/academic level 5 – participation, identification and internalisation
- Degree level/academic level 6 – identification, internalisation and dissemination.

This is a very simple classification and just a general guide that underpins specific wording of competencies to reflect the different levels. Alternatively, some programmes use Benner's (2001) stages of skill acquisition model, which was discussed in Chapter 2. Others use Bondy's (1983) five levels of competency, namely dependent, marginal, assisted, supervised and independent, usually in post-registration courses.

The assessment of theory of nursing at different levels, however, is usually based on Bloom's (1956) taxonomy of cognitive learning, which was also discussed in Chapter 3. You may wish to look back to the appropriate section to remind yourself of the details of this model, which comprises knowledge, comprehension, application, analysis, synthesis and evaluation. In both models of assessment, the first points, that is, exposure and knowledge, represent lower-level learning and the last points represent the higher levels.

Fairness of assessments

In assessments, we are measuring the performance of the individual student on particular competencies. Wouldn't you agree, however, that assessments have to be as objective as possible and must be fair to each student? What does 'fairness of assessment' mean?

Activity 6.8   Barriers to 'fairness'

Think about your own experiences of assessment (either assessing or being assessed) and consider instances that can make assessments 'unfair', and how we can make them 'fair'. Identify all factors that you feel interfere with the fairness of the assessment, using the three headings: (a) student factors; (b) mentor factors; and

(c) environmental factors. If you can't remember being assessed, then make some notes of your own ideas of what we should be aware of during an assessment to ensure that it is being conducted fairly.

It is conceivable that, on occasion, the demand being made on a student during assessment or the questions being asked may seem beyond the boundaries of what would generally be expected. Fairness of assessment refers to being aware of external circumstances that could influence the student's performance of the clinical skill. There are several factors that could hamper fairness of assessments. An unfair assessment could also mean that it might not be a valid assessment. Student factors that can make an assessment unfair include:

• expected level of knowledge is too high
• theory–practice disjunction
• not enough opportunities to practise the competencies
• last-minute delays or changes
• undeclared physical illness or fatigue.

You should be able to think of other student factors, including personal circumstances. Mentor factors include the mentor not working on the same shift as their mentee, bias towards or against the student, not having had educational preparation to become a mentor, overpowering attitude and lack of knowledge of the student's course. Some of the factors in the clinical environment that might unfairly affect assessments are interruptions, lack of resources in the practice setting (for example, equipment), suitability of placement and low staffing levels.

Assessment criteria and pass or fail decisions

Following a fairly conducted assessment, the mentor has to decide whether it's a pass or a fail for the particular competency. This decision may well depend entirely on whether the student closely followed the trust's approved procedure to perform the clinical skill, or the written (or unwritten) protocol. The procedure is the main form of 'assessment criteria'.

What am I looking for in the student?

Consider two examples of assessment of competence that you may have been involved in. This could be a pre-registration or a post-registration course competency.

• How did the mentor determine what criteria to use to pass or fail the learner?
• What influenced them to choose these particular criteria?

Reflection Point 6.3

The term *assessment criteria* (Hughes and Quinn, 2013: 397) refers to the predetermined set of components that are used for deciding whether the learner performed the clinical skill competently. They can therefore constitute a checklist of the step-by-step actions taken by the learner when performing the skill. These step-by-step actions are normally the trust's approved procedure or clinical guidelines for that skill, and are set down in two columns as 'actions' and 'rationales', and usually supported by references to make them evidence based. They are normally kept in the practice setting's 'Policies and Procedures' section for use and for reference purposes. There is likely to be a separate folder for clinical guidelines or protocols that refer to expanded role competencies.

However, for those nursing activities for which there is no identified step-by-step approved procedure, the performance criteria can be established by asking the skilled practitioner to describe to someone in detail everything that they would do to perform the skill competently. For instance, there might not be a procedure for assessing communication skills, for bed-making, for taking body temperature using tympanic thermometers or, say, for doing patient handovers. A set of performance criteria for patient handovers (or 'reporting on patients' progress') is presented in the box.

Case Study

Assessing a Learner Perform a Clinical Skill
(Peripheral Blood Glucose *Monitoring*)

Registered Nurse Adam works in an Endocrinology Unit, and as part of the mentor course that he is taking, he is required to assess a learner perform a clinical skill under the supervision of a qualified and experienced mentor (learning supervisor). Taking into account the content of the practice competencies document that second year student nurse Jenna who is on placement in the Unit had to achieve, and the learning contract agreed during initial interview in the first week of the placement, it was agreed that student mentor Adam will assess Jenna perform 'peripheral blood glucose monitoring' on one of the patients in the Unit.

Peripheral blood glucose monitoring is regularly performed at the Unit with patients who have diabetes, and the agreed plan was that Adam will assess Jenna by the end of the second week of the placement. They agreed on the clinical guidelines that all staff have to follow on the Unit to perform this clinical intervention, which also comprise the assessment criteria for assessing Jenna. Over the days leading up to the assessment, Jenna observed qualified staff perform the procedure, assimilated the rationales for each step of the procedure, and performed the procedure under supervision.

At the beginning of the assessment Adam briefly questioned Jenna about the reasons for performing blood glucose monitoring on the particular patient and the step-by-step action that Jenna was going to take to perform the procedure. The assessment was to be conducted by direct observation of Jenna and minimal questioning, in the presence of the learning supervisor.

Having initially gained the patient's consent, Jenna washed her hands according to agreed protocol, gathered the necessary equipment and performed the procedure. Unfortunately, Jenna was unable to obtain a large enough droplet of blood to cover the test pad, and the reading on the blood glucose monitor failed. During the procedure, Jenna didn't attempt to 'milk' the finger to assist with the formation of the droplet. At this point, Adam placed a gauze on the patient's finger and indicated that he would come back in 15 minutes to perform the procedure himself.

Jenna was very apologetic to the patient for the undue discomfort she had caused to the patient, and indicated that the procedure would be attempted again a few minutes later. The patient in turn was accepting of this. However, Jenna did not have the confidence to try the procedure again, seemed to panic about what to do next, looked visibly distressed and was physically shaking.

Student mentors are strongly advised to perform only formative assessments on learners, and in this instance after giving feedback to Jenna on her performance of the procedure, away from the patient in a private setting, Adam decided on a 'Fail' for Jenna in relation to this procedure. Adam's feedback was supportive and constructive in indicating that even the most simple-looking procedures are obviously quite complex and take several attempts to master, and also ways of getting more practice before being re-assessed sometime afterwards. The learning supervisor also gave feedback to Adam on his skills in assessment of student competence.

Assessment criteria for assessing competency – patient handover

- Have the right documentation, e.g. care plan/pathway, to refer to
- Have a good understanding of the patient's conditions
- State the procedures that have been performed, e.g. removal of drains, sutures
- Keep the information concise and focused
- Use an appropriate genre of English
- Pitch the amount of information imparted to the level of knowledge the handover recipients already have, e.g. more detailed information may need to be imparted if new staff or students are present, and vice versa
- Ensure that information that must be given, is given
- Inform of individual patient's overall progress
- Note any relevant communication from the patient's family or from members of the multidisciplinary team
- State any investigation results received, and any subsequent action prescribed
- State any changes in medication, and patient's reaction to them
- State the plan of care for the rest of the day
- Include patient's awareness of own condition, e.g. in mental health
- Observe confidentiality issues, especially for bedside handovers

For competencies for which there are no written assessment criteria in the practice setting in the procedures or clinical guidelines folder, they might be found
in, for instance, *The Royal Marsden Hospital Manual of Clinical Nursing Procedures*
(Dougherty and Lister, 2011). The criteria or procedure might also be available
from NICE, the World Health Organization, Scottish Intercollegiate Guidelines
Network and other reputable authoritative organisations via their websites, especially clinical guidelines, or from manufacturers' instructions. As in the trust's procedure, clinical guidelines are usually tabulated as actions and rationales in two
columns, and include a references list. However, from the time that a book or
clinical guideline is written to the time it is available for use, adjustments may
have been made to the procedure, based on more up-to-date evidence or research.
Trust-based procedures tend to have an addendum to reflect this.

As to keeping the information concise, handover reports are naturally time limited
as they could be seen as keeping healthcare staff away from direct patient care. On
noticing ineffective patient handovers practices, Davies and Priestley (2006) suggest
that conversation on irrelevant topics should be excluded from this activity. Furthermore, some commentators like Walsh and Ford (1989) see handovers as a ritual,
although in reality they comprise a necessary medium for communicating the effects
of care and treatment to staff on the next shift.

Depending on the clinical specialism, further specific information may need to be
imparted during handovers, for example resuscitation status or mobility levels in
rehabilitation services. Very importantly, often teaching and learning points arise from
patient handovers, for both students and clinically based unqualified staff and registrants. Thus, the assessment criteria for passing or failing a student on their ability to
do patient's handover can be quite involved.

Ongoing Record of Achievement and Signing-Off Proficiency

In its periodic review of pre-registration education curricula, the NMC (2006b)
found that mentors wished to have access to their mentees' progress documentation of preceding practice placements as evidence of skills that they are already
deemed competent in, prior to establishing the mentee's learning requirements and
needs in their current placement. In response to this, the NMC (2007a) issued
guidelines for universities to implement a systematic way of establishing a mechanism to achieve this.

This mechanism was initially termed a 'passport' but due to different interpretations of this term, it was changed to 'ongoing achievement record' (OAR) (it
retained at least one element of passports which is to have the student's photograph
included in the document). With the information in OAR and the placement's
competencies booklet that the student brings with them, a 'diagnostic assessment'
of competencies is made at the mentor–mentee meeting at the beginning of the
placement so as to establish the student's specific learning needs and objectives. The

OAR is a requirement for all students who commenced on pre-registration nurse education programmes in September 2008, following guidance provided by the NMC (2007a).

The NMC (2007a: 2) notes that the OAR is necessary for documenting continuity of assessment, to ensure safe and effective practice and 'enable judgement to be made on the student's progress'. Then, for the final placement of the pre-registration programme, the student is mentored by a sign-off mentor (SOM) whose role essentially is to ascertain and vouch that the student has achieved all NMC (2010a) practice competencies related to 'standards of competence', and sign and date the appropriate pages of relevant documents.

Signing-off proficiency

The SOM for the final placement will have received specific educational preparation as determined by the NMC (2008a, 2010c), and is required to utilise a minimum of one hour a week protected time with the student in addition to the 40 per cent of placement time that they are expected to work with the mentee. The SOM ascertains whether the student has achieved the competencies by a combination of means that includes the above-mentioned minimum student contact hours in order to facilitate the student's learning, and by assessing them on the competencies that they are required to achieve during the placement.

Other means include a review of requirements in the OAR document; the student's practice competencies booklets from all preceding placements; and any other relevant skill achievement document; certificate of attendance from additional study days/workshops, etc. The practice competencies booklet tends to have a section where the protected one hour per week is recorded – see Template 6.1 for an example of this.

TEMPLATE 6.1   Recording protected time for sign-off mentoring

Week 1	Notes on learning during this week:	
	Signature of student:	Date:
	Signature of sign-off mentor:	Date:
Week 2	Notes on learning during this week:	
	Signature of student:	Date:
	Signature of sign-off mentor:	Date:
Week 3	etc. ...	

Accurate recording of one-hour-per-week protected time with the mentee has several advantages. When evidence of this NMC requirement for the protected time is asked for, then the record will comprise proof of this provision. Recording protected time is also likely to act as a trigger so as to ensure that this contact time happens, and the contact time can also foster increased support for the student to achieve the necessary competencies. The contact must however be recorded straightaway, and not retrospectively.

The reasons for assessment of competence and signing-off proficiency during the final practice placement include ensuring safe and effective practice, achieving validity and reliability of assessments and fairness of assessments. Signing-off needs to be performed by an SOM who is on the same part or sub-part of the NMC's professional register as that which the student is aiming to enter (for example, NMC, 2008a). The NMC refers to this requirement as 'applying due regard'. Signing-off proficiency is required for:

- pre-registration nurse education programmes
- pre-registration midwifery education programmes
- post-registration specialist practice programmes
- SCPHNs courses
- return to practice course
- overseas nurses programme.

Midwifery mentors are different to nurse mentors in that all midwifery mentors have to be SOMs (NMC, 2010c), as they have to sign off student midwives' proficiency at the end of each year of their pre-registration course, that is at the end of each 'progression point'. Midwifery SOM status can be achieved as part of the initial mentor preparation course, but often as an extension to the course for practical reasons.

The NMC (2010c) provides further advice on the options available to enable prospective sign-off mentors to achieve SOM status, indicating that the mentor has to be supervised by an existing SOM (or PEF) on at least three occasions for signing-off proficiency. The first and second occasions can be realised using a range of methods such as simulation, e-learning and OSCE, and could be achieved as part of the local NMC approved mentor preparation programme, but on the third occasion the aspiring SOM has to be supervised assessing a finalist student in the actual practice setting.

Signing-off proficiency is also a role that can be fulfilled by practice teachers and NMC recognised teachers, but only if they have undertaken the additional educational preparation indicated by the NMC (2008a); and they will also be required to undergo a period of precepteeship (NMC, 2007b).

Signing-off proficiency entails declaring the student's 'fitness for practice' as an imminent RN, and is therefore a role that has to be performed responsibly and with full accountability. The box summarises the NMC's criteria for nurse SOMs.

Summary of the NMC's criteria for SOMs

- Must be on the same part of the NMC's register as that which the student is intending to enter.
- Successfully completed an NMC approved mentor preparation course, and is on the local mentor register.
- Working in the same field of practice as that in which the student is aiming to qualify, and has clinical currency and capability in the field.
- Has a working knowledge of the student's pre-registration programme requirements and practice assessment strategies.
- Has in-depth understanding of their accountability as a registrant and in the SOM role.
- Has knowledge of actions to take if the student is perceived to be underachieving/struggling.
- Has knowledge of all documents that comprise acceptable evidence of competence in the NMC's SOPs.
- Has been supervised on at least three occasions for signing-off proficiency by an existing sign-off mentor.
- Must be identified on the local register as a SOM.

The NMC (2008a: 6–7) indicates that the 'role of the sign-off mentor is to make judgments about whether a student has achieved the required standards of proficiency for safe and effective practice for entry to the NMC register', and to sign the relevant local documentation indicating that they have been achieved. When all evidence has become available to indicate that the student has successfully completed all theory and practice requirements, then the HEI informs the NMC accordingly, leading to the student applying to have their name entered on the NMC register as RN.

Research by Hutchison and Cochrane (2014) suggests that the SOM role tends to lead to a change in focus in the mentor role towards assessment of competence, as different from the teaching and pastoral roles that normally prevail in mentoring. Furthermore, Andrews et al. (2010) indicate that there can be problematic aspects to this role. For instance, how will inter-mentor consistency (reliability of assessments – discussed later in this chapter and in Chapter 7) be monitored? This question seems to imply that there should be a panel or peer group who can peer review the consistency and accountability of the SOM, although the designated PEF can monitor this to some extent. The peer group or a panel member can also provide support to the SOM with any issue or uncertainty related to signing-off proficiency, as also concluded by Durham et al.'s (2012) research.

Protected time for sign-off mentoring is an NMC (2007a) requirement. However, protecting the required time can itself prove difficult to achieve in a number of very busy practice settings or during particularly busy periods, as was also found by

Rooke (2014) in her study of implementation of the SOM role, and by Hutchison and Cochrane (2014). Furthermore, in midwifery practice, on reviewing current mentoring practices, Passmore and Chenery-Morris (2014: 92) conclude that there is no need for tripartite assessments (lecturer, mentor and student midwife) of students any more, because SOMs are now 'much better prepared to undertake this role'.

Moreover, if a student is awarded a fail on this final placement, then this can raise questions about the quality of mentoring and assessment of competence that the student has experienced over the preceding two-and-a-half years of their education programme. To resolve the 'challenges' of time, workload, responsibility related to the role and practicalities of the assessment of competence, Rooke's study participants suggested various possible solutions, including more concerted proactive forward planning of the off-duty to ensure that the student and the SOM work sufficiently on the same shift and co-mentoring.

Assessing AHPs, support workers, assistant practitioners

The mentor periodically gets allocated mentees who are students or learners on other health or social care profession programmes. This is of course fully acceptable especially in the current day's ethos of interprofessional learning, and endeavour towards a health and social care seamless service. This is also so that the underlying principles of mentoring and supervising learning comprise core knowledge and skills that apply to all professions. However, logically they might be required to undertake further courses to do so or to attend relevant workshops, in particular to comprehend the technicalities of their role towards learners from other specific healthcare professions.

For example, to supervise and assess support workers on NVQ courses, they would need to have successfully completed and achieved the A1 Assessor Award (previously D32 and D33). If the nurse mentor's mentee is a medical student, then they have to acquaint themselves with the competencies that the medical student has to achieve by the end of the placement.

Validity and Reliability of Assessments

The principles of assessment constitute further key considerations that are usually referred to as attributes or essential factors. There are four attributes that are absolutely crucial in all assessments of competencies. These are validity, reliability, discrimination and practicability (or usability) of assessments.

Validity

'Validity' is the most crucial aspect of an assessment in that it refers to the extent to which the assessment measures what it is expected to measure. A valid assessment is one that assesses the competency or learning outcome(s) it sets out to assess, and does not target other competencies that might not have been learnt adequately by the learner at that point in time. The five main types of validity are: content validity, predictive validity, concurrent validity, construct validity and face validity. However, some of these apply more to the overall curriculum and not necessarily to assessment of competencies in practice settings.

Content validity

'Content validity' refers to the extent to which the assessment adequately samples the content of the curriculum. Do the assessment question and assignment guidelines assess all the learning outcomes of the curriculum? Note that for various reasons, not everything that the student learns during the course can be assessed. Content validity is primarily addressed by the structure of the assessment in the endeavour to assess all module or course outcomes, and is monitored by the programme manager for the course.

Predictive validity

The extent to which the result of assessments can predict the future performance of the student is referred to as 'predictive validity'. It is important for the mentor to determine if the student's performance during, say, a particular practical assessment, can predict how far he or she will perform to the same standard in future situations, and also whether they can adjust the performance to different practice settings, for example from a ward setting to community care and to different patients.

Concurrent validity

The extent to which the assessment results correlate with those of other assessments administered at the same time is referred to as 'concurrent validity'. In other words, if two different assessments are designed to measure the same learning outcomes, then the student should do equally well in both, for example asking a student to talk through how they would perform a skill, and actually to demonstrate it.

Construct validity

Validity that refers to the extent to which the results of the assessment are related to impressions or evidence gained from observations of the individual's behaviour with regard to their attitudes, values and intelligence (which are also known as 'psychological constructs') is referred to as 'construct validity'.

Face validity

'Face validity' involves stopping to consider the overall impression about how competently the clinical skill was performed, and whether the student actually demonstrates the complex array of observational, analytical, interpersonal and technical skills required for the competency.

Types of validity

A first year student is being assessed on a surgical ward changing a patient's dressing using aseptic technique. The purpose of this particular episode of assessment is specifically to do with changing a dressing using aseptic technique skills. However, during the procedure, the patient makes some statements that clearly reflect marked disorientation, and the student is unable to respond therapeutically to disorientation. The aseptic technique is performed correctly. Should the mentor pass or fail the student? Which decision is the valid decision?

Reliability

In addition to validity, another key consideration of any assessment is its 'reliability', which is a term that is used to indicate the consistency with which an assessment measures what it is designed to measure. This means that if the assessment is conducted again, the same level of performance should produce the same result, provided other variables remain similar.

To take this a step further, reliability has to do with consistency in the grade or result awarded for a particular piece of work:

1 between different mentors
2 between different occasions on which the work is done, and
3 between different methods of assessment.

In all cases, the result or grades awarded should be almost or preferably exactly the same for the test to be deemed 'reliable'. Consistency in assessment of student competencies in this way is referred to inter-mentor reliability or inter-assessor reliability, and is discussed in detail in Chapter 7.

Reliability of assessments

Think about assessments you or your colleagues have been involved in recently. Then spend a few minutes thinking about how reliably the assessment was conducted. Decide why you think that the assessment was or was not reliable.

Generally, there are certain factors that might negatively affect reliability being achieved. These are practical issues, such as:

- individual biases
- halo effect
- insufficient time allocated for the assessment

- ambiguity of questions being asked
- competence as an assessor
- whether more than one assessor was involved, as two assessors could mean less subjectivity
- whether the assessment criteria had been agreed.

Discrimination

Discrimination in assessment refers to the ability of assessment to differentiate between different levels of competence demonstrated by students, such as Year 1, Year 2 or Year 3 students. Steinaker and Bell's (1979) taxonomy of learning is generally used to differentiate between these levels of competences. However, by and large, learners should be given the opportunity to demonstrate their true level of ability, regardless of the level that they are expected to reach at the particular stage of the course.

Discrimination also refers to the distinction between all learners. A healthcare assistant would be assessed against different criteria for a particular clinical skill from a medical student or from a student nurse, for instance, mainly because the level of theoretical knowledge expected of each is different.

Practicability (or usability)

The concept 'practicability' refers to whether the assessment can be conducted within the time, and with the resources, available.

Practicability of assessments

Think about your own practice setting. Have you encountered situations when you are required to assess a learner's competencies but felt that the time allocated was not adequate or that it was not practical to conduct the assessment comprehensively?

Reflection
Point 6.6

Mentors encounter problems of practicability of assessment when practice placements are too short, or when for some reason the assessments have been left until the last few days of the placement. In the study of assessment of competence by Phillips et al. (2000) several problems of practicability of assessment were identified, the more crucial ones of which will be explored in Chapter 7. However, despite effective assessments being complex and challenging, the validity and reliability of assessments remain the benchmark of rigour in the assessment of health and social care competencies (for example, Rowntree, 1987; Wilkinson, 1999).

A study conducted by Norman et al. (2002: 143) that examined the validity and reliability of different methods of assessment of competence of pre-registration nursing and midwifery students concluded that 'no single method is appropriate for assessing all clinical competence of nursing and midwifery students', and that a 'multi-method approach' should be taken.

Implementing Approved Assessment Procedures

Each university identifies clearly in their course documents exactly which assessments students have to pass to complete the course successfully. This is supported by further assessment guidelines and specifications on how students are to acquire the necessary knowledge and competence to do so. Examples of course assessments were cited at the beginning of this chapter in response to Activity 6.1.

The procedure for assessing practice competencies is detailed in students' placement booklets. These procedures, alongside other requirements for the course, will have been planned before the course starts, under the scrutiny of the university's quality assurance guidelines and protocols for designing courses and modules. Thereafter, they will have gone through a rigorous course approval process before being offered to students.

The pass marks for assessments may vary by a few points between different universities, as may the weightings between practical and theoretical assessments, or different assessment components. The number of assessments may vary, as may the number of formative assessments related to the summative ones. Each course and module is assessed on its learning outcomes, indicative content and competencies.

All universities are governed by identified boards and committees for addressing specifically designated functions related to the courses they offer. An example of a university-level board is the Academic Board and that of a committee is the Deferral Committee. Those at faculty, school or department level include the Board of Study and the Subject Assessment Board.

The functions of each of these committees – whose membership includes clinical managers, the subject librarian, the placement manager, for instance – and boards, are identified in their terms of reference. The Faculty's Board of Study for pre-registration courses, for instance, holds meetings each term to receive module and programme results, module and practice placement evaluations and issues raised at course consultative committee meetings. The mentor is not required to know in detail what each committee does, unless they are members of those committees, but some of the decisions made by these committees may affect mentoring activities with students during practice placement, such as extending the placement.

The university's Board of Study fulfils essential functions, in that it assumes ultimate responsibility for the effective delivery, evaluation and revision of modules, courses and the students' programmes of studies, some of the feedback for which it receives from relevant Faculty Board(s). It tends to have an overall monitoring role in relation to module or course assessments. During the planning stages, the modules will have been fully discussed by the Course or Module Curriculum Planning Teams. They will have been designed following the university's protocol. It would, for instance, have followed the university's protocol for writing modules and the university's Assessment Parity Rules, which include rules on word limits for coursework. They would then have been approved by an assembled panel of experts, which usually includes representations from the NMC, probably the Health and Care Professions Council (HCPC) and subject specialists from other universities.

Furthermore, in addition to the overall university assessment strategy, there are specific assessment strategies within each course and module, thereby ensuring that each programme is fully structured before students start on the course.

Policies and strategies for assessments

For assessment of practice, students' practice placement competencies booklets clearly identify the procedure for assessment of competencies. This entails an initial mentor–mentee interview when the competencies to be achieved are ascertained, and often a learning contract constituted. Approximately halfway through the placement, a mid-placement interview takes place so as to ascertain the student's progress with the contracted competencies. During the last week of the placement, a final interview is conducted for the decision on which clinical competencies have been achieved, and those that have are signed and dated accordingly.

A case study of a student for whom an action plan had to be constituted following the mid-placement interview is as follows.

A Successful Action Plan

Kayleigh is a 33-year-old third year mental health student nurse who is a new mother, and whose return from maternity leave was delayed due to medical reasons. On her return, she had two theory modules and the final practice module to pass in order to complete her pre-registration programme. For the practice module, Kayleigh was placed for 12 weeks at a 9–5 day services centre for working-age adults with mental health problems and who have been referred to secondary mental health services for further therapy and rehabilitation.

Although an initial interview with the 'sign-off' mentor took place in the first week, and the weekly one hour protected time was utilised to monitor progress with practice competencies, Kayleigh struggled to re-engage after the break from the course, and in subsequent weeks found it difficult to achieve the agreed competencies and was unable to express why this is to her mentor. Both mentor and the day services manager were very accommodating and supportive. The student failed various objectives at the mid-placement interview and an action plan was compiled in the presence of the student, sign-off mentor, link lecturer and day services nurse manager. The competencies that were identified in the action plan, which were related mainly to 'interpersonal skills', included:

(Continued)

Case Study

(Continued)

- Be consistently on time for shifts and planned activities, and thereby demonstrate reliability, punctuality and good time management.
- Take responsibility for meeting professional codes of practice and organisational policies whilst prioritising care of service users, and work with team members to promote health with high standards of practice, whilst acting with integrity.
- Take responsibilities that are appropriate for Year 3 students by demonstrating the ability to take the lead in reviews, admissions and group work.

The student felt disappointed, but had anticipated being given fails during the mid-placement interview and needing an action plan. The support that would enable Kayleigh to achieve the action plan objectives were identified as the mentor and the manager, and resources included the NMC's guidelines and codes of practice, as well as the trust's policies and procedures. The PEF would regularly contact the mentor to check on progress and offer any further help and advice that were required, and made himself available during the subsequent weeks for further support.

The student composed herself and with the above-mentioned support during subsequent weeks, put the required time and effort in, and went on to achieve the competencies in the action plan and the remainder of her practice competencies, and subsequently passed the practice placement.

If Kayleigh had not managed to achieve any of the objectives in the action plan, then she would have failed the practice module. However, students are usually allowed a second attempt at any fail component, which in this case could constitute extending the placement by four to six weeks, or changing to another placement for a similar period of time.

To assess students' competence during practice placements, various assessment strategies are advocated, such as direct observation of skill performance, writing a reflective account and questions and answers. It is usually up to the mentor to decide which NMC competency area can be assessed by each strategy. For example, direct observation can be utilised for assessing clinical skill, attitude, communication skill; and questions and answers for the rationale for each action taken, knowledge of the effects of medication, etc.

A variety or 'diversity' of assessment strategies is also recommended by the QAA (2006b) to enable students to demonstrate their capabilities and achievements of module or programme outcomes, and by the NMC (2010a). For assessment of theory components, critical analyses of key concepts and seminar presentations, written examinations are utilised. It is, however, well known that some assessment methods, for example written examinations, enable some students to demonstrate their capabilities more effectively, whilst other methods suit other students better. Garside et al. (2009) explored the feasibility and outcome of allowing students a choice of assessment methods, and found that this is achievable, as some students chose to be assessed by seminar discussions, others by poster presentations, others by essays, etc., to good effect.

Consequently, curriculum planners should be able to justify which mode of assessment tests which module or programme outcome more effectively, and complementarily the NMC (2008a) indicates that mentors should also be able to demonstrate understanding and ability to utilise a range of assessment strategies. Research on the effective use of assessment strategies is scarce. However, in a study that explored the extent to which mentors use different assessment strategies in Ireland, McCarthy and Murphy (2008) found that a limited range of these were in use. McCarthy and Murphy recommend further research on utilisation of assessment strategies, and further education of mentors on their use.

All aforementioned proceedings are documented as evidence of progress with continuous assessment, for the final summative assessment of the practice module and for legal reasons. The practice competencies booklets also identify the exact roles and responsibilities of the mentor and those of the student before, during and after the placement. They also contain a set of components related to the student's professionalism, attitude and their team-working, and which the student must demonstrate at a satisfactory level (related to construct validity). Usually there is also a section on actions to take regarding underachieving students, which is explored in Chapter 7.

Chapter Summary

This chapter has focused on the assessment of learners' clinical knowledge and competences, taking the approach of what assessments are, why we conduct them, who assesses, when and how, which encompassed:

- What the term 'assessment' means in the context of assessing professional knowledge and competence. This involved considering various definitions of assessments, and the exact competencies to be assessed.
- Why we need to assess our students and learners, that is, the exact purposes and aims of assessments, and at which particular points in students' programmes of study to assess.
- Who assesses learners, including student self-assessment and peer assessment, and patient or service user involvement in the assessment of competencies.
- How assessments are conducted, which includes ensuring that the mentee has learned the clinical skill, the use of essential interpersonal skills, the dimensions of assessments, namely continuous or episodic assessments, formative or summative and criterion-referenced or norm-referenced assessments.
- Assessing different levels of competence, fairness of assessments and the use of performance criteria.
- Validity, reliability, discrimination and practicability as essential aspects of assessments; and the role of approved assessment policies, procedures and strategies.

Further Optional Reading 📖

1 For an analysis of problematic aspects of assessment, the recurring danger of which usually looms, see:

- Rowntree, D. (1987) *Assessing Students: How Shall We Know them?* London: Kogan Page.

2 Access online or print: *Standards for Pre-Registration Nurse Education* or *Standards of Proficiency* documents from the NMC or HCPC website, either to gain an overview or for more detailed scrutiny of the standards and outcomes that pre-registration students have to achieve in order to be able to register in the relevant part of the Professional Register:

- Nursing and Midwifery Council (2010a) *Standards for Pre-Registration Nursing Education.* Available at: http://standards.nmc-uk.org/PublishedDocuments/ Standards%20for%20pre-registration%20nursing%20education%2016082010. pdf (accessed 7 January 2014).

3 For more detailed information on criteria and processes for achieving sign-off mentor status, see Sections 2.1.3 and 3.2.6 of:

- Nursing and Midwifery Council (2008a) *Standards to Support Learning and Assessment in Practice.* London: NMC.

To access further resources related to this chapter, visit the companion website at https://study.sagepub.com/gopee

7
Leadership and the Challenges of Mentoring

Introduction

Chapter Outcomes

On completion of this chapter, you should be able to:

1 Explain specific ways in which forward planning and prioritising work comprise important means by which the mentor exercises leadership.
2 Identify likely problems of assessment of competencies, and ways in which the mentor averts or resolves them.
3 Present an analysis of the responsibilities and accountability of the mentor in the assessment of practice competencies, along with related ethical and legal aspects of mentoring.
4 Cite various ways in which the mentor achieves and monitors intra- and inter-mentor reliability in the decisions that they make in relation to the assessments they conduct.
5 Establish the mentor's role in supporting the struggling or underachieving student, and the use of various lines of support that can be available to them, including resources and guidelines.

Mentors are generally informed of the student allocated to them well before the practice placement starts, to which the mentor responds by structuring a tentative plan of learning experiences for the student for the duration of the placement. However, research findings (for example, Phillips et al., 2000; Duffy, 2003; Gainsbury, 2010) highlight various day-to-day problems that could be encountered by both mentors and students in the assessment of students' competencies during practice placements.

That assessments are conducted 'on the hoof' by registrants that the student 'bumps into' and as part of 'multiple roles', were issues highlighted by Phillips et al. (2000). 'Failure to fail' was the main problem highlighted by Duffy (2003), as well as by Gainsbury (2010) as sometimes mentors award a pass to students without sufficient evidence of their competence in specific clinical skills.

Similarly, O'Driscoll et al. (2010) identify problems with mentoring such as the workload interfering with facilitation of students' learning during practice placements, and mentors feeling pressurised to take on the mentor role for their career development. The various problems that are likely to be associated with assessments make early and careful planning of assessment imperative.

Such problems can fully or partly be averted by the mentor's leadership, which includes accepting the role as a serious responsibility, and early, careful forward planning of their own workload and the mentee's practice learning. In their study of the mentor's leadership, Adelman-Mullally et al. (2013) identify various ways in which mentors exemplify leadership, including role modelling, providing vision and challenging the system or status quo. The NMC (2008a: 58), under the leadership domain, indicates that mentors should: 'Demonstrate leadership skills for education within practice and academic settings', the associated outcomes of which are:

- plan a series of learning experiences that will meet students' defined learning needs
- be an advocate for students to support them accessing learning opportunities that meet their individual needs, involving a range of other professionals, patients, clients and carers
- prioritise work to accommodate support of students within their practice roles
- provide feedback about the effectiveness of learning and assessment in practice.

These outcomes reflect the mentor's leadership skills in the context of planning for the placement, prioritising, supporting and giving feedback. As for planning 'learning experiences' and 'accessing learning opportunities', these components were discussed in Chapter 1 to a good extent, and in Chapter 4 in more detail. Prioritising is a key feature of the mentor's leadership role with regard to each of the other seven mentor domains identified by the NMC (2008a), for example leadership in establishing effective working relationships with mentees and other professionals whom they will encounter during the placement and for facilitation of learning. Leadership therefore also applies to planning and prioritising so that the mentee can achieve placement competencies in good time, and also to acting proactively to pre-empt and avert the likely contemporary problems of assessments, and dealing with those that do occur.

At the end of the placement, the mentor has to inform the student of their levels of achievement, and of a decision to award the student a pass or fail for those assessment components. It is in relation to assessment of competence that mentors encounter most of the challenges to their role.

The Mentor's Leadership in Managing Assessments

The mentor's leadership related to pre-registration and post-qualifying education in healthcare professions has been identified by research for some time (for example, Fretwell, 1980; Phillips et al., 2000; O'Driscoll et al., 2010). According to O'Driscoll and colleagues, personnel who are in a position to take the lead include clinical nurse specialists, modern matrons, nurse consultants, nurse practitioners, nurse managers and others of similar seniority, but their role in student teaching during practice placements is less well defined. They also found, however, that the ward manager's leadership is crucial in creating an environment for learning in the practice setting, and also that it is the mentor who exercises leadership in facilitation of learning more regularly and fully.

Leadership as a notion in its own right was referred to in Chapter 5 in the context of healthcare professionals acting as change agents in the management of change (see Table 5.1 for the approaches taken by transactional and transformational leaders). Several definitions of leadership prevail in management literature, most of which emphasise the leader's ability to *influence* the activities, behaviour or actions of their 'followers' towards goal achievement.

In the context of healthcare, Gopee and Galloway (2014: 65) suggest that 'leadership comprises the ability to motivate, inspire and energise individuals and groups to identify and achieve healthcare goals'. These abilities also apply to effective mentoring. For a thorough and up-to-date analysis of leadership as a concept that applies to most areas of society, the reader is referred to Kouzes and Posner's (2012) *The Leadership Challenge*.

Assessment of competencies at times involves one-off short episodes of direct observation of the learner performing clinical skills, but mostly it is a continual process occurring throughout the practice placement. One danger associated with this is that if interruptions do occur during episodes of assessment, then the mentor could miss vital steps in the performance of the skill, incorrect or unsafe practice can also be missed, and a pass decision (or fail) could be made, wrongly, with incomplete information.

Managing the process of assessment in the practice setting

Activity 7.1   Planning and managing the process of assessment of practice

This activity asks you to explore in detail how to manage an episode of assessment of students' competencies or clinical skills by direct observation. To do this, focus on the specified outcomes or competencies of a specific practice module of the

(Continued)

(Continued)

pre-registration course for your healthcare profession, or the NMC's (2010a) competencies for, say, second year students in your field of nursing, or the outcomes of a post-registration healthcare course. Practice module outcomes are normally found in the student's practice competencies or outcomes booklet.

You might choose to work on this activity with a colleague or course peer who is in a similar specialism as you. Identify in detail everything that needs to be done to begin and complete the assessment of these competencies, from the time that the student starts on the practice placement to when the student is signed as competent for particular competencies. Include everything, such as how you would ensure that the skills (or knowledge/attitude) have been learnt, as well as the organisational aspects that have to be considered to ensure the assessment proceeds as planned.

From your response to Activity 7.1, you would have verbalised various preparations needed to ensure that assessment of competencies is completed effectively and efficiently. Maybe the mentor can compile a teaching and assessment schedule that identifies which competencies will have been learnt by the student by the end of week two, three, etc., and at which points the mentor will have assessed the student on each of them, as also suggested broadly by Price (2007). The learning and assessment schedule of course needs to be flexible enough to allow for opportunistic or incidental learning, otherwise it needs to be adhered to as planned, and can form part of a 'learning agreement' (as explained in Chapter 1).

For all assessments, there are usually certain curriculum regulations that need to be adhered to, such as submission dates for practice competencies booklets and the procedure to follow if the student fails a competency. A number of key points specifically related to managing practical assessments are identified in the box.

Planning and managing the assessment process

In sequence	• Agree, during Week 1 of placement, the objectives/competencies that need to be achieved and assessed.
Prior to the assessment	• Ensure that the learner has learnt the skill, allocate registrants to teach the skill in accordance with agreed procedure or clinical guidelines. The skill is taught at the appropriate academic level. The learner is given sufficient practice opportunities and has been formatively assessed during the placement.
	• Mentor feels: (a) up to date with skills being assessed; (b) competent to assess/has attended mentor update course; (c) takes a supportive and positive approach.

	• Day of assessment – ensure that the student feels ready for the assessment, set time of day, consider 'practicability' and fairness of assessment issues. • Colleagues aware if and when they can interrupt (if necessary), give bleep/pager to another person. • Agree assessment criteria.
During the assessment	• Use appropriate communication skills (see box in Chapter 6 titled 'Communication and interpersonal factors related to assessments'). • Create a climate that enables the student to relax so that they can perform the skill to the best of their ability. • Indicate to the student to start the clinical intervention(s) when ready. • Safety issues – if the learner makes a mistake, consider the seriousness of the mistake, and intervene, or provide prompt/clues, as appropriate. • Responsive assessment (Neary, 2000b) – taking into account the patient's changing healthcare needs. • Situated assessments, i.e. in the context of available resources and clinical activities, for instance. • Consider predictive validity of assessments, i.e. whether the learner can perform as well in future and in other patient care situations.
After the assessment	• Need to exercise professional judgement throughout. • Decide on whether to award a pass or fail for each skill or competency assessed. • Give feedback according to established good practice (discussed next). • Ensure documentation is completed – for clinical intervention, student competency and of feedback given. • If fail is given, then the mentor needs to follow the university's procedure for subsequent actions to take, which normally includes informing the link lecturer or the PEF.

Making decisions and giving feedback to the learner

Following assessment of competency, the mentor has to indicate to the learner whether they have passed or failed after giving them feedback on their performance. Feedback is also a means of justifying the pass or fail result. Feedback can be: (a) *intrinsic feedback*, which occurs within the performer through self-assessment and reflection (the student often knows how well or not so well they did); or (b) *extrinsic feedback* (or augmented feedback), which is given by the assessor or peers and done concurrently during the skill performance and/or on completion of the performance. Some mentors find it difficult to give honest feedback on a weak or faulty student performance. This could be tricky for the learner as well, but feedback has to be given honestly, and is generally accepted more readily if given constructively.

It is useful to ask the learner how they felt they performed straight (or soon) after completion of the clinical skill, instead of telling them first how well or badly they performed. The benefits of asking the student are that this is likely to make them put aside any anxiety that they might still have about their performance, think more objectively and be more receptive to feedback. So, the mentor could ask, 'How do you think you did?' This constitutes self-assessment by the learner (which was discussed in Chapter 6), albeit usually only briefly, which should also give the mentor an indication of the learner's insights into their level of competence. Good practice guidelines for giving feedback to students are listed in the box.

Guidelines for giving feedback to the student after clinical skill performance

- Ensure privacy and that adequate time is allocated.
- Use the sandwich method, which entails starting with comments on the positive points or strengths, discussing areas for improvement, and ending on positive notes.
- Give feedback constructively, as the aim of feedback is to enable the learner to learn and improve.
- Be sensitive to the recipient's feelings and self-esteem throughout this exercise.
- Try to be honest and fair but never be destructive.
- Be clear and concise.
- Allow the recipient of the feedback time to discuss and ask for clarification.
- Do not allow anxiety levels to increase unduly.
- Gauge the impact of your feedback on the student's feelings and self-esteem throughout the exercise.
- Respect and treat the recipient as an individual, and focus on behaviour and skill performance rather than personality traits (i.e. it mustn't be perceived as a personal remark).
- Acknowledge good practice.
- Suggest measures to correct inappropriate practice.
- Remain calm and objective; do not respond in kind to anger, aggression and defensiveness.
- Motivate the recipient to consolidate strengths and address limitations through strategies such as action plans.
- Be empowering through encouragement of the recipient to comment and explain issues discussed.

Good general communication skills are essential when giving feedback, including non-verbal communication such as maintaining eye contact. Following feedback, action plans or learning points can be constituted and mutually agreed, as also suggested by the RCN (2007). However, in an ethos of self-directed learning, ultimately it is up to the receiver of the feedback to decide how much of it to heed and act upon, and when, and to be accountable for their decisions.

Good practice guidelines for assessments

This section builds on the important principles of assessment of clinical skills performance discussed in Chapter 6, and in some of the literature such as DH (2001b) and Rowntree (1987). A set of guidelines for the day-to-day mechanics of assessment is therefore constituted and presented in the box.

Good practice guidelines for the day-to-day mechanics of assessment

- Allocate registrants for teaching specific skill/knowledge to the student.
- Utilise opportunities for formative (or mock) assessments.
- Arrange time and date, and diary it; treat it as 'protected time' (e.g. DH, 1999; NMC, 2008a).
- Inform other staff to ensure that they do not interrupt (considering staffing levels of course).
- Inform patient and obtain permission for student assessment.
- Ensure that all equipment is available.
- Ensure that the learner has had the opportunity to practise the skill.
- Ensure that you are fully available and accessible as the mentor/assessor.
- Be sensitive to the student's self-confidence or lack of it.
- Be aware of any crises in the practice setting, e.g. staff sickness, stress.
- Plan the assessment, ensuring availability of procedures and guidelines.
- Take safety measures if required.
- Work in teams as this strengthens the reliability of assessments.
- Seek the opinions of colleagues who have experience of working with the learner being assessed, when feasible.
- Create the opportunity for the learner to talk through the procedure, if necessary.
- Always remain calm.
- If the learner displays awe of the assessor, give confidence.
- Beware of unachievable goals.
- Be and look enthusiastic and motivated.
- Allow the student to work at their own pace.
- Allow for holistic care.

(Continued)

(Continued)

- Ensure that the learner knows the assessment criteria for the skill.
- Allow reflection and give feedback.
- Use professional judgement.
- Beware of other factors, e.g. the learner being preoccupied with assignments.
- Heed criticisms of assessments, e.g. research findings such as 'failing to fail' (Duffy, 2003), and 'on-the-hoof' assessments (Phillips et al., 2000).
- Intervene appropriately if unsafe practice is about to occur.
- Do not be biased by occasional polarised instances of exceptionally thorough or poor practice.
- Document results in practice competencies booklet, etc.

Various viewpoints discussed so far suggest that appropriate documentation is vital to mentoring activities. In fact, documentation of assessments is crucial, considering the NMC's (2010d) position that recording comprises documentary evidence of actions taken.

Activity 7.2   The student's practice competencies

Look through your copy (mentor's copy) or the student's copy of the practice competencies booklet, and read the sections where it identifies the roles of the mentor, the link lecturer and personal tutor, and of the student during the placement.

A clause in the booklet usually states the actions that the mentor needs to take if the mentee is perceived as underachieving or 'failing'. They tend to entail drawing on the expertise of mentor colleagues, the link lecturer, the PEF or the student's personal tutor. There may also be a section on the appeals procedure. However, for each new course or module being offered, there would have been a briefing session for prospective mentors to familiarise themselves with the course requirements, the specific competencies to be achieved by students and to discuss issues.

If you are on a mentoring course yourself, it is very important that, on completion of the course, before you conduct any student assessment, you acquaint yourself with the student's placement competencies and preferably with the overall assessment strategy for the course. Furthermore, you should fully understand the particular summative assessment that you are going to conduct. The action to take in case of 'failure to achieve required standard' by the learner and the 'appeals procedure' are discussed later in this chapter. The importance of careful forward planning to ensure assessments of practice competencies proceed systematically during practice placement, to prevent problems surfacing, to maximise learning and to reduce the likelihood of the student experiencing undue stress, are all extremely important.

However, despite careful planning, unfolding day-to-day events could still disrupt the smooth running of assessments. The patient could refuse consent to students performing clinical interventions on them, staff sickness, unexpected emergency admissions or referrals might present as obstacles. Nevertheless, these do not always present as problems, as Neary (2000a), Phillips et al. (2000) and others recommend 'responsive assessment', which entails taking into account situational contexts such as prevailing resource issues, and the patient's current physiological or psychological state.

Intra- and inter-mentor reliability

On the mentor course, at mentor update sessions and at course reviews, on and off, the question is asked as to how we know that mentors are consistent in their assessment of students' competencies. That is, how do we know and monitor how consistent a mentor is in assessing students perform a specific clinical skill, and that they are consistent in their expectations and decisions when assessing different students at the same stage of their professional education perform that particular clinical intervention; and also how consistent different mentors are when assessing students perform the clinical skill? This is the arena of intra- and inter-mentor reliability, which is also referred to by Mott Macdonald and the NMC (2013: 48–9) as 'intra- and inter-rater reliability', and by the general literature on assessment of theory and practice as 'intra- and inter-assessor reliability'.

Increasingly, the quality of student performance in practice competencies is graded (for example, Donaldson and Gray, 2012), and for each competency the student may be given any grade between A and F, depending on how well they perform that clinical skill. Although grading practice normally requires further appropriate educational preparation for mentors, this activity should also enable the achievement of intra- and inter-rater reliability with more ease.

Furthermore, it is only fair to students that mentors are consistent in their expectations of the standard to which students perform clinical skills, the highest standard being the healthcare organisation's approved procedure, protocol or clinical guidelines for performing the particular clinical intervention.

Thus the term *intra-mentor reliability*, in the mentor's assessment role, refers to how consistently the mentor assesses particular categories of students on particular clinical intervention, that is, that they consistently use the same identified criteria for deciding on whether to give a pass or a fail for that particular intervention, within a responsive assessment approach. *Inter-mentor reliability* refers to the consistency with which all mentors assess a particular category of students on each clinical intervention.

Mentor preparation courses and annual mentor update sessions usually also incorporate an exploration of ways in which intra- and inter-mentor reliability are achieved and can be monitored after qualifying as a mentor, especially in relation to conducting assessments.

Intra- and inter-mentor reliability

Think of ways in which mentors can achieve and monitor intra- and inter-mentor reliability. What are the informal and more structured situations or opportunities that they can utilise to explore these?

As you would have sensed, intra- and inter-mentor reliability refer to all roles of the mentor, such as those enunciated in the eight NMC (2008a) domains, associated competences and outcomes for the mentor, although it is usually related to assessments. There are various ways of monitoring intra- and inter-mentor reliability. The mentor update study days and trust-based update sessions provide a suitable opportunity to explore how consistency within and across mentors can be achieved. Mentoring case studies can be examined in small groups, or these groups can be invited to discuss consistency in the context of situations that they have personally encountered as mentors. In these groups, conclusions can be drawn on consistency in assessments conducted by mentors, and with the help of the facilitator, benchmarks of good practice can be established.

However, monitoring intra- and inter-mentor reliability must not wait for update study days. Informal monitoring is undertaken continuously through discussions with peers or team members in the practice setting or unit, with one's line manager or the mentor's own mentor or clinical supervisor.

Further ways of achieving intra-mentor reliability are by:

- consistently using approved protocols/clinical guidelines
- ascertaining that approved procedures and clinical guidelines are up to date
- ensuring that their own competence and skills are up to date
- informal monitoring of their own pass/fail rates of mentees
- ensuring an appropriate environment for assessing (so that the learner is relaxed when performing the clinical procedure)
- ensuring that the learner is being taught to the same standard and protocol/procedure by different registrants/associate mentors
- student feedback such as evaluating how the student feels about the assessment process and decisions
- external feedback, from colleagues through reflections on assessments conducted
- ensuring that learners are aware of the level of performance expected of them
- reflection-on-action on assessment just conducted
- ensuring being aware of halo effect, being non-judgemental, for instance about the learner as a person; objectivity
- being consistent in own standard of clinical practice.

In addition to the above-mentioned ways of achieving reliability of assessments, inter-mentor reliability is achieved by:

- mentor meetings within ward/unit team – formal and informal
- involving PEF when uncertain
- consulting colleagues on same ward/unit as appropriate
- auditing mentor's performance of assessments (e.g., by negotiating peer assessment)
- student feedback about mentoring practices
- feedback from university following student evaluations
- monitoring attendance at mentor updates, trust based or university based
- knowing and consulting/informing link lecturer
- exploring mentoring issues at clinical supervision meetings
- monitoring mentors are up to date with clinical guidelines/protocols.

Averting and Resolving Problems of Assessments

Potential problems of assessment of practice competencies can be averted by careful planning, and this is the component wherein the mentor's leadership is absolutely essential. However, problems with assessments do occur and, when they do, they have to be treated as a component of mentoring, and resolved, and efforts made to learn from them.

Potential problems of assessment of competence

The aims or purposes of assessments are quite clearly identified by several writers on nurse education, as noted under 'Why do we need to assess our students?' in Chapter 6. However, how far and how smoothly these aims are achieved in reality varies. We also need to consider exactly what the problems that mentors encounter in the assessment of students are, and what the criticisms directed at assessments are, including those of written examinations.

Activity 7.3   Current problems of assessments

1 Think of the weaknesses of assessments and the reasons why assessments, even written examinations, are unpopular with students (assuming that they are). Make brief notes.
2 Identify the actual problems that tend to occur with student assessment of theory and practice in your healthcare profession, ones that you have experienced or observed, or that you feel could occur.

Mentors and learners could encounter various difficulties with assessment of practice competencies. For assessment of theoretical knowledge (for example, of human physiology) and numerical skills as in drug administration and nurse prescribing courses, written examinations remain a favoured method, particularly in higher education. The likely solutions to the problems that you have identified will be explored shortly.

A range of problems with assessment was identified by just one group of students on a mentoring course. Many of these are presented in the box.

Problems with assessment

- Leaving things to the last minute (i.e. poor time planning)
- Difficulty with integration of theory and practice, or ineffective application
- Personality problems/clashes
- Problems of organisation in the practice setting
- Lack of time
- Student disagrees with mentor
- Attitude problems – student's or mentor's
- Structure of learning programme (e.g. placement is too short)
- Mentor accountable and responsible for how student performs the clinical intervention
- Inconsistency of student performance
- Student absence
- Mentor's low morale
- Mentor changes or absence
- Student appears indifferent
- Student's level of knowledge
- Lack of resources (e.g. equipment)
- Non-cooperation or refusal of consent by the patient or service user

---

One of the most cited difficulties mentors face is insufficient time for mentoring activities. Cognisance of this recurrent problem necessitates more robust leadership on the part of the mentor in terms of forward planning, prioritising and proactive actions. The substantial empirical study on assessments by Phillips et al. (2000) highlighted various problems encountered by assessors, which include (see also Chapter 1 Companion Website):

- The quality of assessment varies enormously, depending on staffing levels and workload in the practice setting.
- Named assessors perform their assessor role as one of many other essential roles.
- Many assessments are performed informally by registrants whom the student 'bumps into' during the course of their duty (i.e. 'opportunistic' and 'piecemeal').
- A major part of registrants' practice involves solving the operational and ethical dilemmas that they regularly face in 'situations' with competing demands on their time.
- Mentors experience difficulty in ascertaining different levels in practice.
- Few assessors feel well prepared for doing assessments and most express a desire for continuing support after initial preparation, and consideration of adequate infrastructure for valid and reliable assessments.

Other problems with assessments have been identified by Rowntree (1987), Lankshear (1990) and Duffy (2003). Rowntree discusses some of the 'side-effects of assessments', referring to concepts such as 'self-fulfilling prophecy', whereby students who are expected to achieve low grades tend to achieve low grades, which might not necessarily be a reflection of their innate ability. However, many of these weaknesses could occur in healthcare courses, although actions have since been taken to rectify some of them. The findings of Lankshear's and Duffy's studies are discussed shortly.

Difficulties with assessment of clinical skill performance

Activity 7.4   Difficulties with student assessment

Think about current day-to-day potential problems of assessments and, considering them in the context of your own current place of work, first identify at least one clinical assessor who has already conducted quite a few clinical assessments. They do not need to be based solely in your workplace but should work broadly within your specialism. Your task is then to approach the assessor and ask them to explain precisely what steps they take in preparation for, and in actually conducting, assessment of competence with learners. Find out also from the assessor how they anticipate potential problems and avert them. Ask about some of the actual problems encountered, and the options that they had for resolving them.

At the same time or afterwards, reflect for yourself on such problems and decide how you would go about dealing with them if they occurred in your own practice setting.

Alternatively, think for yourself of all the problems that you might encounter in your assessment function as a mentor, and then the options that will be available to you to resolve each of them.

Problems of assessment include differences in the interpretation of the exact meaning of placement objectives. There might be problems in conveying depth of knowledge expected, or level of skill demonstration. Issues like these can be rectified by open discussion between all personnel directly involved.

Resolving problems with assessment

Activity 7.5   Resolving difficulties encountered by mentors

Refer back to the box titled 'Problems with assessment' and work on the difficulties faced by mentors by identifying a number of problems of assessment you could encounter with a particular group of students, and the probable solutions for each of them. This can be done by completing Template 7.1.

TEMPLATE 7.1   Criticisms or difficulties with assessments, and actions that can be taken to resolve them

Criticisms/difficulties with assessments	Actions that can be taken to resolve them
Leaving things to the last minute	
Difficulty with integration, or ineffective application, of theory and practice	
Personality problems/clashes	
Problems of organisation	
Lack of time for conducting assessments	
Student disagrees with mentor	
Attitude problems – student's or mentor's	
The service user or patient not consenting to student assessment	
Lack of resources (e.g., equipment)	
Structure of learning programme: variation of experience, e.g. allocation too short	
...... (etc.)	

The chances are that you will be aware of or have thought of yet other problematic situations encountered by mentors in the assessment of learners, for which similar steps can be taken. They might include passing a student because the mentor likes the student, or failing the student because they dislike them (at times referred to as 'halo' and 'horns' effects respectively), unqualified mentors signing up clinical competencies or misinterpretation of wording of practice competencies.

With some of these problem areas there could be instances when a mentor passes a student on a particular competency when they should be awarding a fail. This cannot be condoned, but failure to fail students has already been identified over the years by, for example, Lankshear (1990), Duffy (2003) and more recently by Gainsbury (2010). If a student is failing, the mentor's professional judgement comes into play, and action plans are constructed.

Action planning

A mid-placement interview during the practice placement is an important component of assessment of students' progress with their placement competencies. The competencies will have been agreed at the beginning of the placement, and might be in the form of a learning contract. The mid-placement interview is technically a formal formative assessment point, which involves dedicated time for a discussion on, and documentation of, the student's progress with placement competencies.

If the student has been progressing mostly as expected, then these are documented and the student continues as agreed in the learning contract. If the student has not been achieving as expected in knowledge, skills and attitudes components, then a negotiated action plan needs to be constructed, which both mentor and learner mutually agree on and sign. A PEF or an academic such as the link lecturer might also be present and sign the action plan accordingly. The important sections of an action plan are presented in Template 7.2 – it is usually laid out in landscape format.

Action planning involves specifying all components identified at the top of the template. If such an action plan was not constituted, then the student could have grounds for complaint and appeal if they were subsequently deemed a 'fail' for the placement. This point also indicates the importance of documentation of progress with achievement of placement objectives.

While there are some similarities between learning contracts and action plans, there are distinct differences between them in that the former are more learning centred and the latter are more assessment centred. The learning contract is a systematic but speculative plan of learning based on practice competencies to be achieved and projected learning opportunities, and may be adjusted during mid-placement progress discussions. The action plan is a 'must-achieve' device that identifies competencies that need to be achieved by an identified date during the practice placement, non-achievement of which would lead to a 'fail' mark being awarded.

Re-assessing the learner

Once the action plan has been agreed, it must be adhered to, in that the mentor (or PEF) and the student jointly ensure that the competencies are being acquired, continuous assessment is occurring and, when ready, the student is reassessed and the documentation signed as and when achieved. The action plan is regularly reviewed and on the agreed date a final review is conducted.

The components discussed in the preceding section addressed mostly the duties of the mentor. The next section considers the ethical and legal aspects of mentoring.

Ethical and Legal Aspects of Assessments

All registrants have to comply with their professional body's code of practice, and this applies to mentoring or supervising juniors and colleagues' learning as well. 'Professional values' is one of the 'domains' of generic and field competencies that addresses ethical and legal aspects that the NMC (2010a) identifies as components that student nurses must achieve for gaining entry to the professional register.

Therefore the mentor should already be knowledgeable about legal and ethical aspects of professional practice through their pre-registration preparation, while their mentees will be developing these through theirs. On exploring the ethics of

TEMPLATE 7.2 An action plan

ACTION PLAN		Mentee's name:		Mentor's name:	
Mentee's learning needs	Specific objectives to be achieved	Who will help mentee achieve the objectives and how?	Other resources required	Achieve by dates	Evidence of achievement of objectives
Risk assessment for falls	Ability to assess the likelihood of an older patient falling when mobilising unaided	Mentor, physiotherapist. By supporting learning in actual patient or service user situations	Local criteria and clinical guidelines related to falls	29 November 2014	Demonstrate ability to accurately assess the risk of an older patient sustaining a fall when mobilising
Medicines management	Ability to administer medication safely according to local drug policy	......	......	......	......
......	......	......	......	......	......

AGREEMENT OF ACTION PLAN

Mentor's signature: .... Date: 17 September 2014
Student's signature: .... Date: ....

ACHIEVEMENT OF OBJECTIVES

Mentor's signature: .... Date: ....

mentoring, Brown (2005) suggests that the mentor needs to be aware of their own values and ethical interpretations of clinical practice to enable mentees to develop 'ethical competence'.

Ethics refers to the social behaviours, morals and values of individuals and groups in relation to doing good for the greatest number, and to the impact, or end results, of clinical interventions (adapted from Brown, 2005). One widely accepted set of principles of ethics that apply to many spheres of life, including medicine, business and education, has been formulated by Thiroux and Krasemann (2014). These principles are:

- the value of life
- goodness or rightness
- justice or fairness
- honesty and truth-telling
- individual freedom.

These principles apply directly to instances of mentoring in the following way:

- *The value of life* – can refer to ensuring that mentees develop the necessary competencies for effective clinical interventions that would restore health and well-being. It can also refer to ensuring that mentees acquire the necessary knowledge, skills and attitudes to register as a nurse so that they can earn a living.
- *Goodness or rightness* – refers to the mentor doing good to mentees and patients or service users, and doing the right things.
- *Justice or fairness* – refers to ensuring that all mentees acquire the knowledge, skills and attitudes in appropriate detail and depth.
- *Honesty and truth-telling* – ensuring that incorrect information is not given.
- *Individual freedom* – means that mentees have some freedom in deciding on the amount and type of learning, and patients or service users have a say in the clinical interventions available, where possible.

Other principles of ethics include: (1) being trustworthy; (2) autonomy; (3) beneficence (doing good); (4) non-maleficence (doing no harm); and (5) self-respect. Furthermore, the British Association for Counselling and Psychotherapy's (BACP) (2013) 'ethical framework' for counselling encompasses values, principles and personal moral qualities. Values refer to respecting human rights and dignity, alleviating personal distress and suffering, and fairness. Personal moral qualities include empathy, sincerity, humility and competence.

Gallagher and Wainwright (2005), reporting on deliberations at the annual RCN Congress, however, indicate that much of nursing ethics are theoretical level academic discourses and do not translate into day-to-day practice and eventualities regularly encountered by healthcare professionals. They suggest that ethics is subjective, and competent ethical practice depends to a good extent on the integrity, honesty and moral behaviour of the healthcare professional.

Reflection
Point 7.2

Application of principles of ethics

Think of healthcare professionals whom you know personally, and consider in some detail how far you agree with Gallagher and Wainwright's (2005) suggestion that ethics is much talk and less application. Consider this also in the context of Thiroux and Krasemann's (2014) principles of ethics.

The codes of practice of healthcare professional regulatory bodies often incorporate ethical principles that registrants have to follow. As for mentors' relevant ethical practice in the assessment of competence, they should, for instance, not award a pass to a student for any particular competency if they are not completely sure that the student can perform the clinical intervention competently.

The NMC (2008a) standards for mentors emphasise effective mentoring practices through the competences and outcomes for mentoring that it has identified. For instance, under the domain 'Assessment and accountability', it specifies that the mentor must be competent to 'manage failing students so that they may enhance their performance and capabilities for safe and effective practice' (ibid.: 52–3). This competence implicitly suggests that mentoring practices must also comply with ethical and legal aspects of both patient or service user safety and care, and of facilitation of learning and assessment of learners' competence. Consequently, if an inexperienced mentor finds dealing with the failing student a challenge, then they need to recognise this, and seek guidance and support from more experienced mentors or the PEF or link lecturer, as per local guidelines (see Figure 7.1 later in this section).

One of the legal implications of assessments is that on being awarded a pass, the individual is being given a licence and the legal right to practise the skill unsupervised when they register with their professional body. Awarding a licence to practise to someone who is not competent is in breach of the law, and the NMC's (2015) code of practice clearly indicates that all registrants must keep to the laws of the country' (clause 20.4).

A feature that frequently surfaces when the legality of the actions of registrants is questioned is the documentation of the actions taken. The NMC (2010d) and various other authorities clearly believe that if an action is not documented then it cannot be seen as having been performed. For instance, Kendall-Raynor (2007) reports on the case of a registered nurse who had allegedly failed to supervise a mentee adequately, which resulted in the wrong dose of medication being given to a patient, who subsequently died. The case was dropped by the Crown Prosecution Service (CPS) 'because of insufficient evidence', although it was due to be heard subsequently by the NMC's conduct and competence committee. This is an example of when legal and ethical aspects of mentoring may reflect different perspectives.

The three professional bodies most directly involved in health and social care, namely the HCPC, NMC and GMC, either explicitly or implicitly incorporate into their codes of practice such ethical components as respect for patient or service user as individuals, obtaining consent prior to clinical interventions, protecting confidential information, and identifying and minimising risk to patients or service users.

The principles of ethics translate into current healthcare practice by addressing accountability, informed consent, confidentiality (including record keeping), professional misconduct, delegation and supervision.

Responsibility and accountability of the mentor

All healthcare professionals are accountable for delivering care competently (NMC, 2010a), and also for other components of their roles such as enabling healthcare learners and colleagues to develop their clinical skills. We are accountable to our patients, ourselves, our employers, our professional regulatory bodies, and in fact also to the general public.

To be responsible implies being answerable for one's actions, and it is a component of accountability. However, Stuart (2013: 20) notes that before the registrant can be accountable for their clinical actions, certain preconditions have to prevail, namely: (1) the ability (knowledge, skills and attitude) to decide and act on a specific issue; (2) responsibility; and (3) authority. In other words, before the health or social care professional can be held accountable for particular clinical interventions or their overall professional competence, they must have acquired educational preparation in the knowledge, skills and attitudes that underpin their clinical actions beforehand, as well as their employment endowing them with the authority and responsibility to perform those clinical actions.

One of the main thrusts of the mentor's accountability is that it is related to the rules, regulations, policies and scope of practice that govern assessments. These are usually detailed in the appropriate mentor's handbook issued by the associated HEI, and briefly in the student's practice competencies booklet for the placement. It is also related to specific eventualities in the assessment of professional competence, to implementation of assessment strategies, to personal and professional responsibilities, and to the relevant legislation. You would need to refer to the mentee's placement competencies booklet and to your professional regulatory body's code of practice for further clarification when needed.

The healthcare professional's mentoring responsibilities direct the spotlight on one specific area of their several professional roles, that of developing and improving the professional expertise of their mentees.

Activity 7.6   Teaching and learning as components of professional conduct

Refer to your professional regulatory body's code of practice and the partner HEI's mentor handbooks for your own profession, and ascertain how they express your responsibilities in terms of teaching (and assessing) others.

You will have noticed that a few clauses in the codes of practice directly identify registrants' teaching and own CPD responsibilities and roles. This is usually also a component of the healthcare professional's job description (or contract of employment) for the post they occupy.

Registrants may not transfer or delegate their accountability to another person. The mentor also functions under legal obligations to know the mentee's course curriculum and built-in assessment procedures and regulations set out by the relevant HEI, and the appeals system that the mentee needs to follow if they feel that they are being unjustly treated. Students have a right to appeal against the conduct of the assessment, but not against the mentor's decision to pass or fail, or their professional judgement about safe practice.

In accepting the role of mentor, the registrant is implicitly accepting responsibility and accountability for maintaining standards of supervision and assessment. The mentor's accountability for student learning is not fully clear, and instances of concern are investigated in their own right. However, the mentor must ensure that students gain the necessary clinical experiences to develop their professional competence and that the mentee does 'no harm' to the patient or service user, by teaching them the correct way of performing clinical procedures.

Rowntree (1987) indicates that there are times when the mentor might intentionally give permission to the learner to perform clinical interventions while supervising them unobtrusively, which can be expected, but at the same time assessing their performance without having specified this to them beforehand. This is sometimes referred to as 'hidden assessment', and could be another instance of unethical action by the mentor.

Furthermore, both initial preparation and continuing development are the joint responsibility of healthcare trusts and HEIs. Making professional judgements about the performance of students and their ability to provide professionally competent and safe care, constitutes an endeavour to achieve predictive validity and reliability in assessments of competence.

The NMC (2015) affirms that the interests of the patient or service user are paramount, that is, accountability to the patient or service user is more important than accountability to the student. However, the legal perspective can be, depending on individual situations, that the student is also answerable for incompetent interventions. Lack of experience or knowledge is not an acceptable reason for incompetent care.

On not being awarded a pass for a clinical intervention that was not performed competently, the learner might feel either merely disappointed or emotionally distraught. The mentor then needs to contact the PEF or link lecturer if further help and support are needed, but might also have to use basic counselling skills to help the learner. As for all professional skills, if the mentor has not had training in counselling skills, then they should refer the learner to an appropriate professional or department that does have those skills.

Supporting the Underachieving Student

As mentioned earlier in this chapter, the mentor's leadership includes careful planning of practice placement to ensure practice competencies are achieved. However, it is well appreciated that, for a number of reasons, some students could be seen as struggling or even failing to show consistent learning and progress during the placement. So what are the different reasons for a student failing to achieve as expected?

The underachieving student

From your own experience of students who struggle to achieve their clinical competencies, think of the different reasons for this happening during practice placements.

Reflection Point 7.3

Some students genuinely experience obstacles that intervene in their achievement of placement competencies. Could this be because they are working extra shifts to supplement their income, and are therefore unable to find sufficient time to work on their practice competencies? There can be work-based reasons, or other personal or domestic reasons. The RCN (2007) suggests a number of actions that the mentor should take if their student is not achieving the set objectives by expected dates, including meeting with the student as soon as possible to discuss this issue; informing the associate mentor and the designated PEF; constituting a realistic action plan; making provision for any extra support; clarifying the area of weakness and advising on how to progress; and keeping careful notes of all discussions and incidents.

The signs that suggest that a student might not progress as expected with the placement competencies can appear very early during the placement. Limited interaction with clinical staff, lateness, sickness, absent-mindedness, inconsistency in standards of care delivery are just a few of them, but when such signs are detected, prompt action should be taken.

Activity 7.7   Failing to fail students

So, for one reason or another, a student might not be progressing as expected, and the mentor is not convinced that particular competencies will be achieved. However, on occasion mentors still decide to pass the student, as found by Duffy (2003).

Consider the whole spectrum of reasons why you think that a mentor might award a pass to a student for a particular competency, even if the student has not demonstrated competent performance. List as many reasons as you can think of.

You should have been able to think of various day-to-day circumstances that might lead to the mentor awarding a pass to a failing student, none of which is likely to be a justifiable reason. These could include, for instance, pressure from the student, who indicates that it is the last week of placement and that they have passed all previous placement competencies, and that insufficient time was allocated for assessing competencies.

As indicated earlier, 'failure to fail' has been identified as a dilemma over a number of years, and can occur in other health and social care professions (for example, Sharp, 2000). At times, the mentor may have done all the planning for the student to achieve competencies, and yet on assessment they might find that the student has not reached the level of competence required to award them a pass for particular competencies. This could mean failing the practice placement. Consequently, the student's placement may have to be extended to allow them more time to achieve the competencies, and their course extended. Individual HEIs usually provide their own specific guidelines on the action to take to support the struggling student. The necessary steps in such guidelines are sketched out as a simple algorithm in Figure 7.1.

Although appearing to be a compact whole-story process, Figure 7.1 does constitute the action that mentors should take to facilitate learning and achievement for the underachieving student, each step or stage comprises a concerted intervention that needs to be handled carefully and professionally.

However, the question arises as to how confident mentors feel in their judgement and skill at giving a fail for a competency if the student is unable to perform the intervention competently. It is noteworthy that a study conducted by Mead (2011) using a convenient sample of conference attenders as the subject of the study, revealed that mentors had no problem with failing students if the latter could not demonstrate competence in particular patient or service user care skills. They felt that they had 'sufficient training to enable them to fail nursing students' (ibid.: 23).

However, Hunt et al.'s (2012) study findings were the opposite to Mead's in that they concluded by questioning whether the preparation and support that mentors receive is adequate for them to be able to fail incompetent students confidently. Nonetheless, Heaslip and Scammell's (2012) research on this issue revealed that just over half of the 112 mentors who participated indicated that they felt confident to fail students, and recommend that grading practice may contribute to making it easier because, instead of a pass/fail result, the mentor can give a better indication to the student as to whether their fail was borderline or a more serious fail.

Still, some students are likely to become upset or ashamed at failing the placement, or maybe they did all that they could but still did not achieve. The mentor will then need to draw on their helping skills to help the student further. Some registrants on mentorship courses may find the idea of having to use helping skill anxiety-provoking, and therefore need to know where they can seek advice and guidance if required (as discussed later in this chapter).

Helping and counselling the struggling student

The general and specific communication skills needed to establish a relationship and support the mentee develop and achieve competencies were explored to some extent in Chapter 1. In particular, the 'communication continuum' and related purposes and skills, and who uses them detailed by Scammell (1990) (also in Chapter 1) suggests

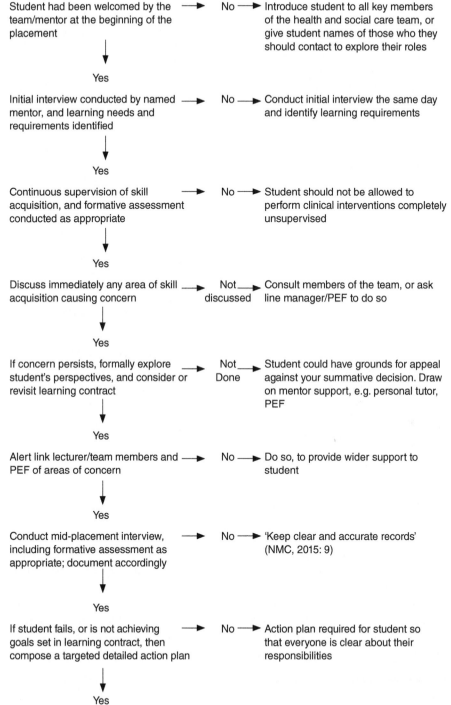

Student had been welcomed by the team/mentor at the beginning of the placement → No → Introduce student to all key members of the health and social care team, or give student names of those who they should contact to explore their roles

Yes ↓

Initial interview conducted by named mentor, and learning needs and requirements identified → No → Conduct initial interview the same day and identify learning requirements

Yes ↓

Continuous supervision of skill acquisition, and formative assessment conducted as appropriate → No → Student should not be allowed to perform clinical interventions completely unsupervised

Yes ↓

Discuss immediately any area of skill acquisition causing concern → Not discussed → Consult members of the team, or ask line manager/PEF to do so

Yes ↓

If concern persists, formally explore student's perspectives, and consider or revisit learning contract → Not Done → Student could have grounds for appeal against your summative decision. Draw on mentor support, e.g. personal tutor, PEF

Yes ↓

Alert link lecturer/team members and PEF of areas of concern → No → Do so, to provide wider support to student

Yes ↓

Conduct mid-placement interview, including formative assessment as appropriate; document accordingly → No → 'Keep clear and accurate records' (NMC, 2015: 9)

Yes ↓

If student fails, or is not achieving goals set in learning contract, then compose a targeted detailed action plan → No → Action plan required for student so that everyone is clear about their responsibilities

Yes ↓

(Continued)

FIGURE 7.1   (Continued)

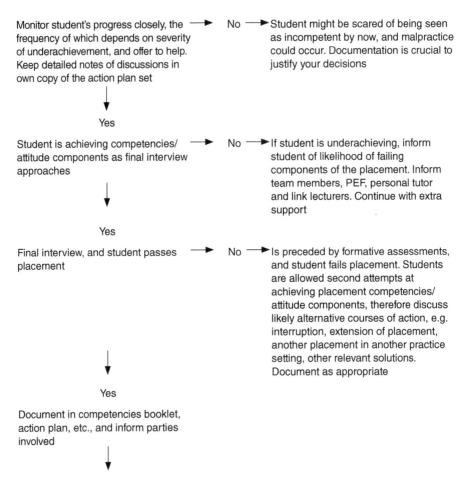

Monitor student's progress closely, the → No → Student might be scared of being seen
frequency of which depends on severity   as incompetent by now, and malpractice
of underachievement, and offer to help.   could occur. Documentation is crucial to
Keep detailed notes of discussions in   justify your decisions
own copy of the action plan set

Yes

Student is achieving competencies/ → No → If student is underachieving, inform
attitude components as final interview   student of likelihood of failing
approaches   components of the placement. Inform
                                          team members, PEF, personal tutor
                                          and link lecturers. Continue with extra
                                          support

Yes

Final interview, and student passes → No → Is preceded by formative assessments,
placement   and student fails placement. Students
                                          are allowed second attempts at
                                          achieving placement competencies/
                                          attitude components, therefore discuss
                                          likely alternative courses of action, e.g.
                                          interruption, extension of placement,
                                          another placement in another practice
                                          setting, other relevant solutions.
                                          Document as appropriate

Yes

Document in competencies booklet,
action plan, etc., and inform parties
involved

FIGURE 7.1   The underachieving student – action that the mentor should take

that specific communication skills are needed to help students who are struggling to achieve their clinical competencies, or who may be struggling with the nursing course as a whole and are even in danger of failing in their chosen career.

It is suggested at this point that you refresh your understanding of the communication skills (for example, those discussed in Chapter 1). In addition to the generic communication skills that are necessary for all effective relationships, specialist communication skills are also required by the mentor to deal with more problematic situations.

The special skill of 'counselling' is one of the roles of mentors and teachers (Hughes and Quinn, 2013: 374) and increasingly that of the mentor for the reasons just discussed. First, however, it is well recognised that for counselling to be effective, the process should be entered into voluntarily by the person being counselled (in this instance, the health profession student). Indeed, it is generally agreed that unless counselling is actively sought by the student, the interaction might not be as effective, even if the helper uses most of the skills used in counselling. Second, counselling is a therapeutic technique, requiring specialist training. Persons not skilled in its use will, at best, not help the student, and at worst potentially compound the student's problems. Therefore, unless they are fully qualified as counsellors, mentors and other teachers in healthcare are more likely to use helping or 'basic' counselling skills. For more intense mentee problems, referral should be made to specialist services such as the university's counselling service, which is often a section of student services provision.

The failing student

Bina is a pre-registration student on an eight-week placement at the end of the first year of her course. Her mentor has varied roles as part of their managerial functions, and has to cover extra shifts on days and nights due to staff sickness. However, Bina's placement has been marked by her frequent absence from the practice setting due to sickness and occasional tearfulness, claiming to feel depressed. She has been advised to seek help from the trust's Occupational Health Department, and has been made aware that she can access the university's counselling facility if preferred.

Shortly after the placement started, the PEF went on maternity leave, and it took a few weeks to install a replacement for her. The acting PEF contacted Bina's personal tutor to explain Bina's circumstances and was advised that, among other things, a mid-placement interview needed to be conducted to ascertain Bina's progress with practice competencies, and be documented accordingly. In particular, if these competencies were not achieved, then Bina would fail the first year and not progress to the field-specific part of the programme. The student is described as lacking in motivation and as 'a real struggle' by the acting PEF.

Due to Bina's continuing absence and health problems, the mid-placement interview only took place quite late in the placement, and an action plan was instituted as various practice competencies had still not been achieved.

Consider what would be the specialist helping or counselling skills that could be utilised in regular mentor–mentee contact if both Bina and her mentor were more available.

Case Study

The most important factor within a counselling situation is the relationship between the counsellor and the counsellee (for example, the mentor and the mentee). This was identified initially by Rogers (1983) and later by Rogers and Freiberg (1994). Both identified three key qualities (also known as 'core conditions' of helping) that are required for effective counselling. These key qualities, as detailed under student-centred teaching in Chapter 3, are: genuineness, trust and acceptance, and empathic understanding.

In addition to the generic communication skills, verbal and non-verbal, key help-ing skills include: self-awareness, attending, active listening, summarising, reflecting, questioning, and using silence. This set of skills can be used as a framework for check-ing how thoroughly you feel you dealt with these situations. By analysing your interactions with others you will develop a greater awareness of how far you, as a professional, are able to help others.

Dedicated time is required for a systematic approach to counselling. This is done by utilising a model of helping, such as Heron's (1989) six-category intervention analysis. This model indicates six possible interactions between the two parties as detailed next.

In the aforementioned case study, for instance, the mentor can help Bina by uti-lising components of Heron's framework. Instances of responses by the mentor to the student's account of his or her perception of the situation would therefore be as follows:

- *Prescriptive* – advise Bina to reduce less important life activities to concentrate on working to achieve her placement objectives as a priority.
- *Informative* – give information on professional and personal matters as appropriate (e.g. location of Occupational Health Department).
- *Confrontational* – ask Bina directly what she is doing or how she could behave differently for a more amiable experience.
- *Supportive* – allow Bina time and silence to think over the mentor's questions and suggestions.
- *Cathartic* – allow Bina to verbalise and explain in ample detail why she is strug-gling in this placement.
- *Catalytic* – the mentor acts as facilitator to enable Bina to meet her learning needs.

Activity 7.8   An underachieving student whom you have encountered

Think of a student whom you have known to have failed to achieve required prac-tice competencies resulting in the student being disappointed, upset or distressed. In case you haven't encountered such a student, think of a situation that you might encounter. Describe the situation in up to 75 words. Then, utilising Heron's (1989) six-category intervention analysis framework, identify the specific actions that you could take, using each of the categories to help the student.

Alternatively, consider Mel Alexis's situation cited in Chapter 1, and follow the above instructions.

One perspective on how mentors manage underachieving students ensues from a study by DeBrew and Lewallen (2014) that explored the thought processes that mentors go through in deciding whether to pass or fail a student on specific competencies. The researchers concluded that when mentors encounter these situations, they might still be wondering afterwards if they have made the right decision. To resolve this feeling, DeBrew and Lewallen recommend that they should afterwards engage in 'deliberate, intentional reflective practices' as a means of checking on the correctness of their decisions and possibly professional development. This sounds like a useful recommendation, although such reflective discussions may need to be facilitated by someone who is not closely involved with the mentor's practice setting, and of course the name of the student being discussed should be withheld.

Hawkins and Shohet (2012) suggest taking an inter-subjective approach that focuses on the relationship between mentor and mentee. This notion largely implies using empathy. Universities usually provide a counselling service for any student who is distressed about any issue that is affecting their progress with their course. To become a skilled counsellor, especially for dealing with particular psychological problems, requires several years of structured educational preparation. However, Hawkins and Shohet also provide a number of pointers on how supervisors can help, such as by developing 'the qualities of a good supervisor' in themselves, which are noted in the box.

Qualities of a good supervisor

- Flexibility with use of different concepts and intervention methods
- A multi-perspective view (i.e. being able to see the situation from different angles)
- A solid knowledge of the profession and orientation in which they supervise
- The ability to work transculturally
- The capacity to manage and contain anxiety, their own and that of the supervisee
- Openness to learning from supervision situations
- Sensitivity to the impact of wider contextual issues on the supervision process
- Ability to handle power appropriately
- Humour, humility and patience

Source: Adapted from Hawkins and Shohet (2012: 52)

Proctor's (2001) 'supervision alliance model' is widely accepted as a suitable framework for systematic supervision. As a model of helping that is also acknowledged by Hawkins and Shohet, it comprises three main functions or roles of the helper, namely: normative, formative and restorative (see the Companion Website for an explanation of Proctor's model of supervision).

Although the mentor is expected to exercise professional judgement and make pass or fail decisions on particular student performances, there are support networks that they can draw on whenever they are unsure. Informal or formal team mentoring and peer consultation frameworks might already be in place but, as indicated in this chapter, the mentor's copy of the practice competencies booklet normally contains full details regarding the procedure to follow in these circumstances, such as contacting the PEF.

This chapter has explored ways in which the mentor exercises leadership. However, it is useful to note that the leadership role is not just about taking action to avert problems. It is also about taking action to achieve aims and good practice. Sines et al. (2006) report on joint action taken by an NHS trust and the partner university in order to ensure that student nurses achieve fitness for practice by the end of the three-year undergraduate course. Most of the mechanisms instituted are not unknown, but several of them were planned in substantial detail. These mechanisms include:

- identifying core skill clusters
- adapted OSCEs
- enhanced clinical skills laboratories
- an additional training programme in assessment of skills for existing mentors
- regular mentoring updates
- appointment of PEF.

Chapter Summary

This chapter has focused on the mentor's leadership and the challenges of mentoring, particularly in relation to assessments, and has therefore explored:

- The mentor's leadership in careful forward planning of assessments, making decisions and giving feedback to the student after assessing them perform clinical actions. Good practice guidelines for assessments.
- Current criticisms, difficulties and potential problems of assessment of learners' clinical skills, resolving these problems, including action planning and re-assessment of the learner, and how these problems are averted.
- The responsibility and accountability of the mentor in ensuring that a pass or fail is awarded as appropriate, and relevant subsequent action taken.
- Use of professional judgement, and how intra- and inter-mentor reliability can be monitored and achieved; and the ethical and legal aspects of mentoring.
- How underachieving or struggling students can be supported using basic communication and helping skills, and more specialist communication skills, including counselling. They constitute skills that would also apply to student assessment situations, and include time management and proactive actions, and the use of support networks with peers, PEFs and academic staff.

📖 Further Optional Reading

1 For more details on the Duffy (2003) and the Gainsbury (2010) reports on 'failure to fail', see:

- Duffy, K. (2003) *Failing Students: A Qualitative Study of Factors that Influence the Decisions Regarding Assessment of Students' Competence in Practice*. Available at: http://www.nmc-uk.org/Documents/Archived%20Publications/ 1Research%20papers/Kathleen_Duffy_Failing_Students2003.pdf (accessed 18 March 2014).
- Gainsbury, S. (2010) 'Mentors passing students despite doubts over ability', *Nursing Times*, 106 (16): 1–3.

2 Ongoing international research-based accounts of leadership traits, theories, etc. are presented in:

- Kouzes, M. and Posner, B.Z. (2012) *The Leadership Challenge*, 5th edn. San Francisco, CA: Jossey-Bass.

3 For a more detailed account and analysis of leadership in healthcare, see Chapter 3 of:

- Gopee, N. and Galloway, J. (2014) *Leadership and Management in Healthcare*, 2nd edn. London: SAGE Publications.

4 For further guidance on the ethics of mentoring, see:

- Gopee, N. (2008) 'Assessing student nurses' clinical skills: the ethical competence of mentors', *International Journal of Therapy and Rehabilitation*, 15(9): 401–7.

To access further resources related to this chapter, visit the companion website at https://study.sagepub.com/gopee

8

Evaluating Mentoring, and Continuing Professional Development for Mentors

Introduction

Chapter Outcomes

On completion of the chapter, you should be able to:

1 Identify and elaborate on a number of reasons for evaluating mentoring activities such as facilitation of learning and assessment of competence.
2 Explain the nature and various features of evaluation, and who is involved in evaluating mentoring activities.
3 Identify different ways of evaluating clinically based and academically based teaching and assessment.
4 Justify the action that should be taken following evaluation and the likely difficulties and opportunities.
5 Explain how the challenges encountered by mentors also comprise opportunities for professional development, as well as for meeting the requirement for continuing learning and updating.

This chapter focuses on the evaluation role of the mentor, primarily because not only is evaluation of teaching, learning and assessment one of the eight domains of mentoring activities identified by the NMC (2008a) – the other seven domains having already been analysed in preceding chapters – but also because it can be a satisfying experience to receive positive feedback on your teaching, and to identify components for further improvement.

Evaluation of mentoring therefore includes mentors self-monitoring the effectiveness and quality of all their mentoring activities, and evaluation information forms the basis for progressive learning as it presents opportunities for further development, and thereby potentially also the mentor's own continuing professional development.

The chapter therefore examines reasons for evaluating mentoring activities, and the general nature of the concept of evaluation, which it does by addressing:

- precisely why we evaluate, what evaluation is, and what the mentor evaluates
- who should be involved
- how to evaluate, including frameworks for evaluation
- what to do with the evaluation data
- the mentor's CPD.

These areas are discussed in relation to both the mentor's practice-based facilitation of learning and assessment of competence roles, and university-based undergraduate and postgraduate course delivery.

Why Evaluate Mentoring Activities?

The reason for evaluating mentoring activities is that it is logical to do so to confirm that mentoring practices are, and remain, effective, and to identify likely areas for improvement. As registrants, we engage in evaluation of care and treatment continually during any span of duty, and therefore it is not an unfamiliar activity to us. The specific competence and outcomes under the domain 'Evaluation of learning' set by the NMC (2008a) for mentors are as follows:

- *Competence for 'evaluation of learning' domain* – determine strategies for evaluating learning in practice and academic settings to ensure that the NMC's standards of proficiency for registration or recording a qualification at a level above initial registration have been met.
- *Outcomes* – (a) contribute to evaluation of student learning and assessment experiences, proposing aspects for change resulting from such evaluation; and (b) participate in self- and peer evaluation to facilitate personal development and contribute to the development of others.

Activity 8.1   Why evaluate?

Consider the question of why we should evaluate what we do in the course of our duties anyway, and of what we can do with information gathered from evaluations. Make notes of your thoughts on this.

As noted above, evaluation is an activity that we engage in quite frequently, formally and informally, and at times without realising that we are doing so. Thus, with the problem-solving approach to health and social care, we engage in assessment of patient or service user health problems, plan care and interventions, implement them and continuously evaluate their effect. More widely, systematic approaches to most novel ventures entail evaluation of the plans implemented, and deciding on the action to be taken subsequent to evaluation.

There are a number of reasons for evaluation. If mentors do not evaluate their mentoring activities, then they are taking for granted that their actions meet their learners' learning needs. They are assuming that learners are satisfied with the learning provided, and that they are fulfilling their roles effectively. Formal evaluations provide evidence of the effectiveness of our activities, and often reveal unexpected findings, as the impressions of the recipients of mentoring might be different to those anticipated by the mentor. Hence, the NMC's (2008a) requirement for 'Evaluation of learning' is a necessary area of activity for the mentor.

In addition to identifying improvement points for subsequent mentoring activities, further reasons for evaluating mentoring are:

- To anticipate likely problem areas, and take preventive actions.
- To gauge whether the mentee's learning is pitched at the appropriate level and in appropriate detail.
- For continuing self-monitoring of competence in professional practice, which is often a requirement of employment, and a component of annual development and performance review.
- It is a component of the practice setting's quality assurance mechanism.
- To gauge progress made.
- It is professional 'good practice'.

Evaluation performed for the purposes of quality assurance can be done through looking at structures (for example, resources), processes, procedures, standards and consistency. It is performed for quality enhancement, which is for improvement through change and development. Evaluation can reveal any problematic aspect and which ones concerned the individual or group of students most, and it can identify areas of confusion or misunderstanding. Consequently, when problematic areas are uncovered, they also present opportunities for improvement, for creativity, and for novel structures and activities to be suggested and instituted.

Chelimsky and Shadish (1997) identify three approaches to (or levels of) evaluation, in that it is performed for: (1) accountability; (2) knowledge; and (3) development, namely:

1 Evaluation for accountability – i.e. to ensure that duties have been performed as required.
2 Evaluation for knowledge – i.e. to act on suggestions for extra components or experience to be included in the activity.
3 Evaluation for development – i.e. action taken based on evaluation results can constitute growth and improvement for mentor, team members and the organisation.

A fourth approach can be added– 'evaluation for management', that is, evaluation conducted as a management activity, with a view to identifying any professional development requirement. For university courses, course directors and module leaders evaluate to identify problems being encountered or foreseen by the students on the education programme, and solving those problems, or averting them. At times, what is seen as an issue by students just needs further explaining or justifying.

Before evaluation of any activity, it is important to ascertain what the purposes of the activity are. Thus if we are evaluating our teaching session, what were the specific aims of the session? The purpose of the teaching will have been to arm the recipient with relevant knowledge and to develop competence, and the purpose of the evaluation would be to check if this has happened. Considering the above-mentioned four approaches to evaluation: is your evaluation of your teaching for the purposes of accountability, to receive suggestions and explore associated idea for further development of your mentoring activities, or a management exercise?

Activity 8.2   Can evaluation of teaching improve learning?

Focusing on the mentor's teaching role, consider the evaluation of teaching that you have experienced, and identify at least two ways in which you can improve your teaching to enhance learning for your mentees.

Healthcare course lecturers are required to evaluate their teaching and act on the evaluation data. As for mentors, following evaluation of teaching, the mentor can follow up the teaching component by offering further reading materials or information to help students meet their learning needs. They can arrange further teaching sessions on topics suggested in the evaluation information, and can also adjust their subsequent teaching with a view to connecting more fully with the learner's learning needs.

What is 'evaluation'?

Most healthcare professionals are familiar with the concept of 'evaluation of care', as it constitutes a key component of a systematic approach to care and treatment, and is also an inherent facet of care pathways.

Activity 8.3   What does the term 'evaluation' itself mean?

Make brief notes on what you understand by the word 'evaluation'. What is it about?

Evaluation of the effectiveness of care given is important as the goal is to restore health, and we need to know if this has been achieved. Evaluation is also an essential facet of professional education programmes in healthcare in order to review or ascertain how effectively and efficiently the curriculum meets the stated philosophy, aims and objectives of the course. It is a part of the process that reviews the currency and value of the course or module.

The term *evaluation* originates from the French word *evaluer*, meaning to work out the numerical value of something. In current usage in English it means appraising or making a judgement about the worth of something (Brown, 2002: 871). Various definitions of evaluation have been offered by interested parties over the years. For instance, Roberts et al. (2001) indicate that evaluation is essentially about making judgements about the value and worth of something against explicit, justifiable and appropriate criteria.

Thus, evaluation is the process of systematically collecting and analysing information in order to form value judgements based on firm evidence. Furthermore, evaluation is also used as an empirical tool in the form of a research method involving in-depth exploration of the component being evaluated through data collection and analysis (Guba and Lincoln, 1989).

Reflection Point 8.1

What do we evaluate?

When evaluating care in clinical practice, exactly what is it that we evaluate, and what are the different ways in which evaluation information is obtained?

Evaluation of care plans and goals is obviously to determine the effectiveness of the plans, which can be supplemented by feedback from the patient or service user. Other terms that tend to have similar or overlapping meanings with evaluation are monitoring, quality appraisal and assessment. The term 'assessment', however, has a distinct and specific meaning in healthcare, referring to assessment of patients' health problems and of learners' competence. Thus, assessment refers to the collection of data against set criteria. It is therefore objective. Evaluation, on the other hand, refers to the values and personal judgement on whether action taken enabled the achievement of specified goals.

Returning to evaluation of mentoring, this can also be public or private, external or internal, continuous or episodic/intermittent and final (refers to timescale). Moreover, evaluation can be case specific or generalised/holistic or analytical (see box for a brief explanation of these modes and types of evaluation).

Who evaluates what?	
Public evaluation	Open evaluation of an activity by others
Private evaluation	Self-evaluation by the person who performed the teaching, for instance
External evaluation	Evaluation by others outside the organisation
Internal evaluation	Evaluation by departments or individuals inside the organisation
Continuous evaluation	Ongoing evaluation
Episodic/intermittent evaluation	Evaluation at set or specific times
Final evaluation	Evaluation at the end of one or a series of activities
Case-specific evaluation	In-depth evaluation of one particular instance of an activity
Generalised or holistic evaluation	Inviting and gaining overall impressions
Analytical evaluation	Detailed evaluation, may include numerical data

Furthermore, evaluation can be quantitative or qualitative. Generally, for new topic areas, qualitative evaluation is likely to elicit data that can enable further development of the topic. For more established topic areas, quantitative data are sought to monitor or ascertain the likely ongoing effectiveness of the activity.

The evaluation of patient or service user care and of teaching episodes is undertaken formatively and summatively. Formative evaluation of care is a continuous activity, the frequency of which is adjusted according to the dependency level of the patient/service user, or to the criticality of their condition. With some service users who require longer-term care, or those in the community, evaluation may be recorded at longer intervals at specific set periods. Summative evaluations are conducted at end points, i.e. retrospectively, for example evaluation of a practice placement experience or a module.

Evaluation is also one of the four stages of the regular development review process of healthcare professionals identified in the *NHS KSF* (DH, 2004a). The first stage is the joint review of the individual's work against the demands of the post. This is in the context of the six core dimensions of healthcare work. The second is the personal development planning stage (PDP), the third is the learning and development stage, and the fourth is the evaluation stage. At the evaluation stage, the individual:

- reflects on the effectiveness of their learning and development of their knowledge and skills
- identifies how their learning has improved the application of their learning to their post
- feed back to the organisation on how the learning and development can be improved.

Furthermore, job evaluation is another related concept that is a feature of banding of healthcare professionals' posts under *Agenda for Change* (DH, 2004b).

In the context of evaluating mentoring, this chapter addresses all the above aspects of evaluation except evaluation as a research method. Having examined why we need to evaluate mentoring activities and exactly what evaluation is, it is also important to consider who evaluates before moving on to how mentors evaluate their mentoring.

Who evaluates teaching and learning?

As mentioned earlier, evaluation can take different forms (see the box above titled 'Who evaluates what?'). Formative evaluation of practice-based teaching and learning is conducted through informal and formal mechanisms. It is a micro-level evaluation that the mentor performs informally when teaching clinical interventions, either in the clinical area or in university settings. It is a valuable internal mechanism for monitoring one's own competence through a continuous process of observation and sensory feedback.

There is also the formal evaluation mechanism that requires more concrete evidence to be gathered and reproduced when required. Formal evaluation mechanisms can manifest patterns of good or poor teaching delivery. These formal evaluation exercises take place periodically and allow scrutiny of the quality of theoretical and clinical learning. For instance, during the practice placement, the student also engages in a continuous process of informal evaluation of the extent to which the practice setting is also an effective learning environment.

Reflection Point 8.2

Evaluation of teaching in the practice setting

Who, in your experience, evaluates the effectiveness of teaching, both planned and informal or opportunistic, in the professional practice setting?

In general, it is the recipient of the teaching, that is, the learner, who is best placed to evaluate the effectiveness of the teaching. The result of the teaching will usually emerge as the knowledge and skill acquired by the learner and is ultimately reflected in the quality of patient or service user care they deliver. In addition to the mentor engaging in self-evaluation or self-monitoring the quality of their work-based teaching and assessment, quality and effectiveness can also be ascertained through peer evaluation.

Generally, there are at least two parties interested in the quality of a service or education provider: the provider, and the consumer or user (who is at times also the purchaser). The current purchaser–provider ethos has prevailed in healthcare since the NHS and Community Care Act (DH, 1990). The consumers of mentoring activities are the mentors' learners, and the university whose students they supervise, as well as patients or service users.

Activity 8.4   Who is interested in the evaluation of healthcare courses?

Think of all personnel and agencies that you feel are likely to be interested in the effectiveness and quality of healthcare courses at universities, and jot down specifically who they are.

The quality of healthcare courses is of interest to both purchasers and consumers of the provision. Purchasers of education are generally students who pay their course fees themselves. For healthcare profession courses, the purchaser is the NHS trusts for most undergraduate and post-registration courses, and individual students based in the independent sector (for example, private hospitals and nursing or residential homes). Other NHS trusts may be regular purchasers of certain courses, as are healthcare students from overseas, and professionals who qualified overseas but are seeking professional registration in the UK. The quality of courses is also of interest to ward managers and other qualified colleagues directly dealing with students and who have certain expectations of them during and after the course; and also the public who expect expert professional care.

For NHS healthcare professionals, Local Education and Training Boards (LETB) were established in 2013 to oversee funding for health profession courses. Their remit extends as far as specifying broad topic areas that educational programmes should cover, and to thereby focus on the health needs of the local population, as well as the clinical interventions that are necessary to address these needs (HEE, 2014a). They aim to fund courses which focus on ways in which on completion of the course, participants help to improve the quality of care for the local population.

There are thirteen LETBs in England, and they are supported by a number of Local Education and Training Councils (LETCs). LETBs utilise the Health Education England's (HEE) *Education Commissioning for Quality* (ECQ) framework (2014b) to review the achievement and impact of the quality standards ensuing from academic programme delivery.

Within the climate of purchasers and providers, educational establishments have to market their educational services and provide evidence of quality assurance measurement within their contracts for services. However, as professional learning takes place in clinical as well as university settings, learning is a partnership agreement between healthcare providers, education providers and students to enable learning that ultimately benefits patients and service users' health.

Other stakeholders interested in the quality of educational provision are the HEI's internal audit mechanisms, and externally the QAA, the NMC, HCPC and other regulatory bodies. Other universities who specialise in education in the subject being evaluated might also be involved, usually by invitation.

A number of ways of evaluating education programmes and the various agencies involved in evaluating learning, teaching and assessment are explored in the next section.

How Mentors Evaluate Learning Provision

Having ascertained why evaluate, what evaluation is and who evaluates, this section explores the different ways in which evaluation is conducted and performed. Broadly speaking, evaluation data can be obtained informally and formally. Informal evaluation can be performed by:

- direct observation of general state or appearance of a patient or situation
- direct observation of a class or group of students
- casual in-class evaluation
- anecdotal accounts
- information leaks through the 'grapevine' (the organisation's informal sub-groups)
- casual quasi-social conversation
- monitoring whether instructions are being followed.

Formal evaluation can be conducted by:

- assessments, written or oral examinations
- student surveys – national or local (i.e. at own university)
- module and course evaluation questionnaires
- asking the patient directly (or electronically, if this facility is available)
- measurements and pathology laboratory results
- focus groups.

The evaluation tools used, however, need to be 'fit for purpose', rather than just convenient tools that might be valid ones. 'Fit for purpose' means exactly what the term states, that is, the evaluation mechanism has to be appropriate for the activity being evaluated, and the criteria in the tool relevant and comprehensive. Furthermore, evaluation can also be conducted by individual professionals, by clinical teams or at the organisational level.

Quantitative and qualitative evaluation information can be obtained through the use of structured or semi-structured forms with selected headings. Such information can also be obtained through verbal or written means. Teaching sessions in practice settings can be evaluated from a number of viewpoints or conducted in various ways. As an internal evaluation mechanism, the teacher (i.e. the mentor) can decide which evaluation tool or model is the most appropriate to gain the necessary information. Some of these tools are identified in the box.

Methods of evaluation of teaching in the practice setting

- General discussion at the end of the session
- Verbal feedback – requested/volunteered
- Verbal question and answers
- Feedback from the university, probably through link lecturers or PEFs from the particular module leader
- Feedback from colleagues or peers, witness statement
- Quiz – on paper/verbal
- Observing how other teachers teach the skill
- Self-evaluation/reflection
- Using questionnaire(s)
- Observing/monitoring clinical skill performance – direct and indirect
- Continuous monitoring of student's general clinical competence and motivation to learn
- Checking whether objectives are being met
- Reflection/reflective account
- A short multiple-choice-type test
- Discussing booklet of competencies
- Asking the student to teach others, e.g. a patient or junior staff
- Service user feedback
- Using evaluation form(s)

However, evaluation is not always a favoured exercise as, according to Handy (1989), the highest quality service is not easily achieved, since it needs the right equipment, the right people and the right environment, which might not always be fully available. It engenders opinions from all interested parties, who might also set new personal or organisational goals for changing educational provision.

Evaluating learning using models of evaluation

There are several published or internally designed frameworks for evaluation that individuals or organisations can use for evaluating the quality of learning provision systematically. Maxwell's (1984) six elements or dimensions of quality, is one of them. The six dimensions are: accessibility, acceptability and appropriateness (3 As); and efficiency, effectiveness and equity (3 Es).

Healthcare course providers can develop their own criteria using Maxwell's model for formal evaluation of quality of learning by asking questions related to each of the six dimensions, such as whether the provision was appropriate or efficient. The education provider that aims and claims to offer a quality service should meet all these criteria. Some manage to do so explicitly, while others may be at different stages of development.

Another framework is provided by Lang's (1976) model of quality assurance. This model emphasises the process through a problem-solving approach. Yet another is the popular Donabedian (1988) model of quality assurance using standard statements, and structure, process and outcome components (for example, Page, 2001). This model was also discussed in the context of practice development in Chapter 5, and the evaluator may choose to evaluate all three components, or only the process component, or outcome.

Mentors, nurse lecturers and other education facilitators can use the Donabedian model to evaluate their learning facilitation. However, university modules and courses are generally evaluated using items under standard headings such as teaching, assessment and feedback, academic support, organisation and management, resources, personal development and any other comments.

Yet another model of evaluation, which is also utilised as a strategy for management of change, as noted in Chapter 5, involves a cycle consisting of: Plan–Do–Study–Act (PDSA) (IHI, 2014). PDSA comprises a useful framework for evaluation of any new activity in health and social care, and van Eps et al. (2006), for instance, demonstrate the use of a similar framework referred to as 'plan–do–check–act' to evaluate a mentorship programme. The model is usually presented as a cycle made up of four arcs, each beginning with one of the four steps, and thereby meant to represent a 'complete' circular model. Action research can also be similarly utilised.

Evaluating professional healthcare courses

Before starting to examine how healthcare courses are scrutinised for whether they meet quality and 'fitness for purpose' standards, it is useful to remember that the quality of patient and service user care itself is closely scrutinised regularly by appropriately appointed organisations. The exercise might be termed a 'review', an 'audit' or an 'inspection'. Such organisations, which are legally empowered to monitor and periodically measure the quality of service being provided, have their own framework and set of criteria for arriving at a decision as to whether the service meets the government's and the public's expectations.

Currently in the UK, health and social care services are 'inspected' through 'special reviews' by the Care Quality Commission (CQC) (2014), which judges quality of care utilising 'essential standards' as criteria, which was noted in Chapter 4 in the box titled 'The Care Quality Commission's National Standards'. However, for evaluating

educational preparation programmes for healthcare professionals, different headings
and outcomes are necessary.

Activity 8.5   Evaluating academic programmes

Consider education provision as a public service provided by a particular university
with which you are familiar. What criteria would you personally use to judge the
quality of their education programmes? Make a list of these criteria. Now try and
identify issues or aspects that constitute good quality education provision, say in
relation to a course you are interested in, in the health or social care department
of the university.

   If available, obtain local or national criteria, say from the Internet, that could be
used to ascertain the quality of this service. Do they match your own criteria of
quality, and do any of these standards match the services that are actually being
provided?

The QAA (2014) conducts 'Higher Education Reviews' (previously known as
'Institutional Reviews' or 'Institutional Audits') to scrutinise the quality and standards of universities' educational courses, including those of healthcare education
programmes. For these reviews, QAA 'Review Teams' utilise the QAA's own evaluation framework of 'core elements' and 'thematic elements' to report on standards
demonstrated by the HEI. The precise elements evolve and therefore change over
time, and for healthcare courses can include areas such as:

- quality of learning opportunities
- meeting employer needs
- maintaining academic standards
- the HEI department's self-assessment of quality enhancement.

As appropriate, the QAA engages with professional regulatory bodies such as the
NMC and HCPC in partnership, and involves NHS employers and funding agents
such as LETBs to carry out reviews of all NHS-funded healthcare education programmes, regularly. The QAA (2014: 1) indicates that it is 'entrusted with monitoring
and advising on standards and quality in UK higher education', and that its aims for
2014–17 are to:

- Enhance the quality and secure the standards of UK higher education wherever
  delivered in order to maintain public confidence.
- Provide leadership, through knowledge and resources, in assuring and enhancing
  the quality of higher education within the UK and internationally.
- Extend and enhance the value and reach of QAA's services within and beyond
  UK higher education.

Thus the QAA's focus is on ensuring high quality education provision, and further-more, its themes (or headings) and range of criteria can be used by universities for internal ongoing evaluation of programme provision in readiness for formal periodic QAA reviews. The QAA also publishes various guidelines documents that universi-ties can use to gain an impression of the QAA's expectations.

The NMC, however, performs regular monitoring reviews of nursing and mid-wifery education programmes through the quality assurance agency Mott MacDonald. In its *Quality Assurance Framework*, the NMC (2013a) provides detailed information on its quality assurance processes. Furthermore, Mott Macdonald and the NMC (2013) have jointly published a *Quality Assurance Handbook* that identifies full details of the criteria against which they determine the quality of the university's education pro-grammes related to healthcare. The criteria are grouped under five themes (Mott Macdonald and NMC, 2013: 33, 35–45):

- Resources – e.g. appropriately qualified nurse lecturers and mentors.
- Admissions and progression – e.g. considering health and character of applicants, accreditation of prior learning.
- Practice learning – e.g. providing suitable learning opportunities in practice settings.
- Fitness for practice – acquisition of required skills and proficiencies.
- Quality assurance – programme evaluation, involvement of external examiners, etc.

There are a number of subcategories under each theme for which Mott MacDonald will request information from the education provider (the HEI) and the practice placement providers (for example, the NHS Trust). During the monitoring event, the NMC will have discussions with various healthcare professionals who are involved in the delivery of pre-registration courses, when mentors and sign-off mentors are also expected to provide information on various aspects of the way in which they fulfil their mentor role, including the range of support that is available for students during practice placement.

A key component of these reviews of university courses is that the reviewers' remits include inspecting practice settings where students gain clinical experience, and this usually includes interviewing mentors and clinical managers. Evaluation requires openness and trust from both parties, a willingness to be open about expec-tations, and about the strengths and weaknesses in the organisation. Appropriate resources are required to meet the specified standards and consumer expectations and needs.

This chapter has so far examined the evaluation of teaching, learning provision and assessment. The next aspect to consider is the destination of the evaluation data. As for module evaluation, the academic who is the module leader collects informa-tion about the module from students against particular criteria, such as:

- staff – whether they were well prepared, accessible, gave constructive feedback
- teaching and learning methods

- assessment – marking criteria, feedback
- resources – teaching rooms, library support and online support
- the module itself – its relevance, difficulty level, whether the module was well organised, and achieved its aims and objectives.

The module leader has to present evaluation information at academic team meetings, together with the actions being taken to rectify any problem areas identified, and should highlight other key issues. As stated before, the module itself will have undergone quality scrutiny prior to delivery to students. Assessment questions will have been peer reviewed, approved by the relevant internal committee and then by the external examiner. However, flaws in the delivery of the module may surface due to, say, resource problems or problems with pass rates.

Usually, the module leader also has to report on the number of students who started on the course or module, how many completed on the first attempt, how many dropped out, and how many passed on resubmission. Internal moderators and external examiners report on quality of students' work, and consistency of marking is also considered.

Institutional evaluation issues are actioned or dealt with by heads of department or at Deanery level. Placement issues are jointly resolved by mentors and clinical managers, and university link lecturers. Senior clinical managers and higher-level university personnel may be involved in resolving more major issues.

Evaluating practice placements

Standards of teaching in practice settings are closely related to the quality of patient or service user care, the quality of student supervision and the expertise of mentors. For students' learning experiences during placements, the student may be asked informally at the end of the placement how good and useful they felt that the placement has been, maybe at the same time as the final interview at the end of the placement, or they may be given an evaluation form to complete after the final interview. On returning to the university for lectures after the placement, they are asked to complete a practice placement evaluation form, along with further verbal evaluation.

The written placement evaluation form asks students to give feedback on various aspects of the experience, such as whether they had adequate preparation for the placement and were given an orientation on the first day of placement. They may be asked to comment on whether a named mentor had been identified, whether their learning needs and placement objectives were agreed in good time, a range of learning opportunities identified, feedback on performance of clinical skills given, how often they worked with their mentor, and whether evidence-based practice was prevalent. There could also be questions on the amount and nature of personal support available.

Evaluation information on the quality of the learning experience is imparted to the placement areas by the university afterwards. The mentor may have obtained qualitative evaluation information from the student prior to the end of the placement. Placement evaluations also form a basis for communication between professionals in practice settings and university lecturers, and an additional benefit of the process is that training and development needs of clinical staff can be identified for both effective clinical care and for competent mentoring practice. Problems reported after the placement are generally investigated by PEFs and CHEFs.

Evaluation of assessments

The mentor performs numerous assessments of competencies in this role. How are the quality and efficacy of assessments performed by a mentor monitored? The mentor's professional judgement comes into play to some extent, as they have to be able to justify the decisions they make about the student's competence, in that the responsibility normally lies with the mentor to seek all information relevant to assessments and to keep their own professional competence up to date. Furthermore, if a student feels that the result of an assessment was unfair or incorrect, then they can appeal following appropriate procedures. This is usually only for the conduct of the assessment and any technical or practical interference during the assessment, but not against the professional judgement of the mentor.

Evaluation of assessment of theory is conducted through structured mechanisms. The pass mark for coursework or assignments for healthcare professional education courses is often 40 per cent. Assignments are marked by module teams, final projects are double marked, and then a stratified sample of scripts is internally moderated by another lecturer in the team, and then further scrutinised by external examiners. All are answerable to assessment or examinations boards and programme boards. Less clear student situations are debated, further advice is sought if necessary, and decisions are made using the university's rules and regulations and professional judgement.

Reflection Point 8.3

Evaluating assessments

Consider how the mentor evaluates the soundness of the assessments they perform. How do mentors ascertain that their own knowledge and competence in assessing students remain up to date, valid and reliable?

In response to Reflection Point 8.3, you may have felt that the mentor's accountability has a major role to play in ensuring that their own knowledge and competence in assessing students remain up to date, valid and reliable. This can be achieved by:

- discussions on mentor update study days regarding, say, intra-mentor and inter-mentor reliability
- team mentoring (including assessing)
- consulting link lecturer, PEF and/or senior colleague (e.g. ward sister).

Ways of achieving intra-mentor reliability were examined in Chapter 7.

Evaluation Results and Development Opportunities

Educational programmes are evaluated by the use of broader generalised forms that can be used for several different courses, by different authorities who use their own set of criteria, as well as by the course or module leader for 'micro-evaluation'. The latter, which Rogers and Horrocks (2010: 284) refer to as case-specific, and analytical evaluation, can reveal honest and more specific individual feelings related to the amount and relevance of teaching and learning, and the learning experience itself.

Accurate evaluation is a complex skill to acquire, especially if change is anticipated. It is also often an uncomfortable exercise as it may reveal unanticipated or perceived flaws, depending on the evaluator's own state of mind and general outlook. There might be other biased views stated or practical problems related to evaluation of teaching highlighted, whether the teaching should be clinically based or classroom based.

Following on from these observations, the next part of this chapter explores problems and the possible consequences of evaluations, and then their likely implications for CPD for mentors. Mentoring RNs on specialist practice courses, lifelong learning, support mechanisms for the mentor and the use of professional development plans are also discussed.

Problems and consequences of evaluations

As discussed throughout this book, the mentoring role of health professionals has various facets. Consequently, each facet involves a set of activities in itself, which requires relevant knowledge and competence. To ascertain how well each role is being performed, the mentor has to evaluate and self-monitor their performance, and also obtain feedback from mentees, peers and their own mentors or clinical supervisors. How much and how comprehensively does the mentor do this, and what do they do with the data obtained?

Mostly, this is not an issue because, as an accountable professional, the mentor continually endeavours to rectify any weakness in their performance and knowledge, and strives to enhance their practice at all times. However, there can be problems with the evaluation of mentoring.

Issues with evaluation

What do you feel are the likely problems associated with evaluation of the mentoring role?

Reflection Point 8.4

A possible problem area or danger related to the evaluation of a teaching session is that the criticisms of one's earlier teaching sessions may give the impression that you are not quite cut out for teaching. Despite this, teaching is one of the competencies of all qualified nurses and, like many other skills, can be learned and subsequently mastered with ample practice. It is also usually one of the items in the RN's job description, at times worded as 'contribute to professional development of other staff'. On self-evaluation of their mentoring functions – referred to by Rogers and Horrocks (2010) as post-hoc evaluation – they may encounter weaknesses that they may not wish to reveal to others and choose to rectify themselves by trial and error.

Practice placement evaluations could also highlight serious problems with mentoring, as was found by Phillips et al. (2000), for instance, that might not prove easy to resolve. The mentor needs to be able to differentiate between progress and levels of attainment by learners. All learners may be making progress but they could be achieving at different levels, depending on their educational background, efforts and time for study, and learning opportunities. Some of the likely problems of evaluation are as follows:

- Judgement pronounced can be aimed at influencing peers' opinions.
- Just one incident may colour statements about the whole session or the module/ placement experience.
- The teacher may be a perfectionist and may feel very disappointed if any weakness is pointed out.
- Points identified by students might not be seen as positive statements.
- May be seen as 'some you win, some you lose', and no action taken on suggested weaknesses.
- The person might genuinely not appreciate the weaknesses pointed out.
- Difficult to be entirely objective.

Research and ensuing recommendations have highlighted problematic areas of mentoring practice and aspects that need developing. For instance, Phillips et al. (2000) identified the role conflict that mentors encounter. Many of the challenges that the mentor encounters are related to assessment of practice objectives, and are predominantly due to insufficient time because of having to fulfil their various roles. Many of these issues were identified in particular in Chapter 7 (in the box titled 'Problems with assessment').

Furthermore, Gainsbury reports on a problem with assessment that was identified two decades ago by Lankshear (1990) and later by Duffy (2003), but that still prevails, which is that some mentors are failing to fail incompetent students. The NMC (2008a) responded to the Duffy report by issuing new standards and other guidelines for mentors; and to the Gainsbury report by reminding universities and their partner healthcare trusts of their accountability with regard to passing students signifying fitness for practice. Such issues may also present as further professional development requirements for previously qualified mentors.

Duffin (2005) reports that the NMC also remains concerned about the range of clinical expertise in the armoury of the newly qualified nurse, midwife or SCPHN, and is therefore considering relaxing the rules on 'skills labs', in which students carry out simulated procedures on dummies. Such laboratories have almost always been in use but the time spent in them is not generally counted towards the 50 per cent of time that nursing students are expected to spend on practice placements. This issue is addressed by the NMC (2010a) through its declaration that up to 300 of the 2300 hours of practice can be achieved within simulated learning environments, such as in skills laboratories.

In response, university deans of nursing indicated that there was 'evidence that students on placements are under extreme pressure' (Duffin, 2005: 4). The NMC engages with nurse directors and Department of Health officials on how to improve placements, and give mentors 'protected time' for mentoring activities. The NMC, however, would not wish to instruct trusts to introduce some of these measures, especially when there are major cost implications, but can recommend them.

Nonetheless, as indicated earlier in this book, new information related to the fitness for purpose of mentoring and mentor courses also emerge continually from research. For example, a study conducted by the National Nursing Research Unit (2014) concluded that there is growing and conflicting pressures on staff time that can affect the efficacy of mentorship, and also calls for a coherent strategy that includes mentorship programmes incorporating the recommendations of the Willis (2012) report as well as revalidation.

Students raising concerns – processes and outcomes

As noted earlier in this chapter under 'Evaluating practice placements', on returning to the university following a practice placement, some students may voice concerns in relation to aspects of the placement. This therefore forms a basis for further communication between university staff and those in the practice setting and can result in development needs of clinical staff being identified. Students of course do not have to wait till the end of placement to raise concerns.

Of course, when a conflict situation is reported, this can be due to misunderstandings between the two parties or to deficient communication.

Students voicing concerns

From your knowledge of dissatisfaction or complaints that students have voiced either directly in your presence or reported by others, what are the various avenues or media, informal and formal, that students are likely to use to voice their dissatisfaction?

Reflection Point 8.5

Dedicating just a few minutes to identify the various ways in which students offload their concerns unveils several powerful ways of doing so, but there are also some misleading avenues. It may well be that students at times just 'have a moan' with their close friends with regard to what they were unhappy about in relation to the placement, and the matter goes no further. Alternatively, students can report their concerns through various channels, such as:

- at workshops held by the PEF during the placement
- at post-placement evaluation, as mentioned earlier in this chapter
- to their university personal tutor or link lecturer
- through the Student Union department at the university
- at organised termly Student Forums at the University.

Some students may even resort to social media (such as Facebook). Other may even venture to mention their concerns at QAA or NMC periodic reviews when students are invited to meet reviewers to comment on their programmes of study.

The NMC (2013c) publication *Raising Concerns* and the NMC's (2015) code (professional standards of practice) provide guidance for qualified nurses and midwives on raising concerns, albeit at the level of broad principles that can be applied as felt appropriate in each situation. They also include information on legal protection to whistleblowers and information on organisations that nurses and midwives can go to for further advice.

As just indicated, evaluation of mentoring activities is likely to highlight areas that are problematic or those that warrant further development. The mentor also has a duty to be up to date in all eight domains of the mentoring role. Thus, of necessity, the mentor has to engage in ongoing learning and continuing professional development in relation to mentoring and other roles or dimensions. So, what is continuing professional development (CPD) and what is ongoing or lifelong learning, and how does the mentor participate in these?

Continuing Professional Development (CPD) for Mentors

The NMC (2008a) identifies registrants' four-stage roles in supporting learning on a continuum that generally progresses as follows:

1. Nurse or Midwife → 2. Mentor → 3. Practice Teacher → 4. (Qualified) Teacher

For RNs and RMs to progress from being a 'Registrant' to 'Mentor', as student mentors they have to demonstrate that they are competent at the twenty-six mentor outcomes specified by the NMC (2008a). To demonstrate competence they normally have to be assessed by experienced mentors in practice settings, and their competence recorded in a specifically designed workbook or portfolio. Intercalated between these qualification-based positions are likely to be various education facilitation and assessor of competence roles such as sign-off mentor, preceptor, clinical instructor, clinical education coordinator and lecturer–practitioner. These various stages constitute the mentor's own ongoing professional development. Therefore this final section of this examination of mentoring

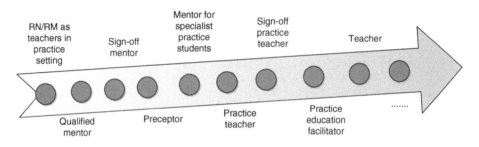

FIGURE 8.1   Progressive development of the RN's/RM's teaching role

and supervision focuses on the scope of the mentor's CPD needs as well as requirements. It suggests that, in addition to continuing to develop their own health or social
care practice knowledge and competence, a likely progression for nurses and midwives'
teaching roles is to advance from becoming a qualified mentor to a sign-off mentor to
a preceptor to a mentoring specialist and supervising advanced practice students to a
practice teacher and beyond (for example, nurse lecturer) – as illustrated in Figure 8.1.

A brief case study of a student mentor (studying for stage 2) who went on to become
a qualified 'Teacher' (stage 4) just a few years after is as follows.

....

Career Progression from Mentor to Nurse Lecturer

Straight after qualifying as an RN, Kelly took up a post as a community nurse as
she felt that in the community setting, she would be in a better position to provide
holistic care, see patients' health improve in their own home settings, and also advise
on preventing health problems recurring. This in turn enabled Kelly to build good
relationships with patients and families, and Kelly felt it was also a very rewarding job.

A condition of the post was that Kelly must attend an NMC approved mentor
course in a year's time because students are regularly on practice placement with
the community team. While on the mentor course, Kelly was alerted to the availability
of opportunities to teach student nurses in the university setting, which could entail
teaching specific clinical skills for a few pre-agreed hours periodically. On further
enquiry, approximately three years later, Kelly negotiated with the university to
participate in co-teaching taking manual blood pressure in the university's skills
laboratory. Despite some initial anxiety, Kelly realised that she enjoyed imparting
this clinical skill to student nurses. On further taking up such opportunities, Kelly
finally acquired a place on the postgraduate certificate in higher education course.
Eighteen months after her successful completion of the course, Kelly took up an
appointment at a UK university's Faculty of Health as a lecturer in clinical practice
and simulation, and is loving the experience, and is also hoping to engage in
research on simulated learning in the very near future.

....

Case Study

Attending annual updates and triennial reviews for mentors as well as being a lifelong
learning healthcare professional are the more immediate next steps.

Professional development of mentors as sign-off mentors is dependent on whether
the mentor will be required for supervising final placement students and assessing
their 'standards of proficiency'. The signing-off proficiency role of the mentor was
examined in some detail in Chapter 6.

The mentor may be required to take on the preceptor role for newly qualified
RNs or RMs who are new to the clinical specialism (the preceptor role was discussed
in some detail in Chapter 1). They might benefit from availability of clinical supervision. The mentor may also be required to facilitate learning and to assess competence
for RNs on post-qualifying clinical short courses. Naturally, they will need to hold

the same post-qualifying short-course qualification themselves in the first place. However, to facilitate learning and assessing students on specialist or advanced practice educational programmes, they will need to hold the particular specialist or advanced practice qualification themselves, and also have successfully completed an NMC approved, HEI-based practice teacher course.

Nevertheless, before moving on to these roles, the mentor needs to continue to develop mentoring knowledge and skills, and keep up to date with the latest developments related to the NMC's (2008a) competence and outcomes for mentors. All mentors are required to attend annual updates to remain on the university or trust's local register (or database) of current mentors, and most HEIs and trusts already have a partnership agreement for such ongoing development of their mentors. This constitutes a programme of learning for qualified mentors, which can incorporate e-learning mechanisms and reflective learning. Mentors who complete these programmes may be eligible for academic credit points. Furthermore, self-evaluation, along with personal research and clinical audits, can highlight issues that can present opportunities for further development for mentors.

As for the mentor's own ongoing professional development, a brief overview of what are continuing professional development and lifelong learning is provided next in this chapter, along with the specific CPD requirements of annual updating and triennial reviews.

Theories of continuing professional development (CPD)

Continuing professional development (CPD) is a concept that is an inherent component of lifelong learning, and is defined by the HCPC (2012b: 1) as 'a range of learning activities through which health professionals maintain and develop throughout their career to ensure that they retain their capacity to practise safely, effectively and legally within their evolving scope of practice'. CPD therefore reflects a responsible and proactive approach to one's own professional learning and, as McGill and Beatty (1998) note, it involves an attitude to life and work that allows for creativity in one's professional activities.

At the practical level, Wallace (1999: 28) sees CPD as a 'term given to the learning which takes place in a professional's career after the point of qualification and/or registration'. Wallace prefers to see CPD as identified and intentional learning rather than learning that only comes from the experience of professional practice.

The means and framework for CPD is also explained by Madden and Mitchell (1993), who suggest that organisations implement one of two main models of CPD: the sanction model or the benefit model. The employing or regulatory organisation that uses the sanction model tends to penalise the individual for not engaging in the necessary CPD. However, the organisation utilising the benefit model does not threaten with sanctions but reinforces and, where possible, rewards individuals for voluntary or suggested CPD.

Alternatively, Wallace (1999) suggests the statutory, mandatory and permissive types of CPD. Statutory CPD is that which is undertaken as a result of statute or legislation. Mandatory CPD has a similar meaning, in that it is instigated by an official command or instruction by an authority (such as the NMC), and is therefore compulsory. Wallace identifies the mandatory CPD model as one that suggests that CPD is a mandate by employers or regulatory bodies, which has to be executed but no penalty is attached directly to the individual if not fulfilled.

Permissive CPD is the type of CPD in which the individual has choice, and in this context, research by Lee (2011) revealed that although learning needs are often identified through personal development planning and appraisal, it is CPD based on the 'individual personal drive and enthusiasm of practitioners' that results in helping practice change, while policy driven factors and national health targets are secondary.

Most healthcare professions or regulatory bodies have instituted some form of sanction or mandatory model of CPD. The NMC (2011), for instance, indicates through post-registration education and practice (PREP (CPD)) that every practising nurse, midwife or SCPHN must declare that they have undertaken a minimum of 35 hours of learning activity relevant to their practice during every three-year cycle to be able to renew their registration. The registrant must also have worked in some capacity by virtue of their professional qualification during the previous three years for a minimum of 450 hours. The GMC and HCPC have similar requirements.

The learning activity for meeting PREP requirements has to be in relevant areas of practice and can be in one or more of the key components of healthcare interventions, aptly categorised in the *NHS KSF* (DH, 2004b) as the six core dimensions – as noted in Chapter 5 – and apply to all NHS employees (except doctors, dentists and some board-level managers).

The *NHS KSF* also identifies 24 specific dimensions under *health and well-being, estates and facilities, information and knowledge* and *general*, which apply to some but not all jobs in the NHS. More specific details on each of these dimensions of healthcare interventions are presented in the *NHS KSF* document.

However, as the NMC only requires registrants to declare that they have engaged in the required amount of learning activity, PREP in itself does not constitute a guarantee of up-to-date clinical competence. The CPD advocated by the NMC is the minimum requirement for safe and competent practice, but it is recognised that the practitioner generally engages in substantially more learning than this minimum. Relevant university-based courses normally meet the NMC requirement adequately.

Furthermore, self-directed or peer-based learning can also easily contribute to these requirements, as identified in the second outcome under the 'Evaluation of learning' NMC domain noted at the beginning of this chapter. Self-directed learning is explained in detail in Chapter 2 under andragogy and the work of Knowles et al. (2011) and Rogers and Horrocks (2010). Peer learning is also well documented, in particular in the context of human and social capital (see, for instance, Gopee, 2002a).

However, from December 2015, the NMC (2013b) anticipates being able to introduce a system of 'revalidation' that will replace PREP. While the precise details are yet to be made available, one of the changes that the NMC intends to institute is that the registrant will have to provide evidence of having sought and received confirmation that they are 'fit to practice' for their name to stay on the NMC register.

Annual updates and triennial reviews for mentors

In addition to educational preparation for the mentor role, the NMC (2008a) requires all mentors to attend annual updates to ensure that they remain up to date with contemporary healthcare as well as mentoring practice, and with technical details of the pre-qualifying educational programmes being followed by their mentees, along with their roles and responsibilities within them. The NMC (2009b: 3) indicates that annual update sessions 'must include the opportunity to meet and explore assessment and supervision issues with other mentors/practice teachers (face-to-face) and explore as a group the validity and reliability of judgements made when assessing practice in challenging circumstances'.

Activity 8.6   Mentor's annual updates

- Following completion of a mentor preparation course, you need to be aware of your own CPD in the mentor role. Consider how you can keep yourself up to date with new developments in professional knowledge and competence within your profession in relation to both clinical practice and mentoring. Discuss this with a colleague or your clinical supervisor.
- What would mentors themselves wish to see covered in the annual update study day?
- Think of a number of types of evidence that you as a mentor can provide at the triennial review. Are there any other types of items that other mentor colleagues can provide?

Mentor annual update events are usually one-day or half-day events, conducted by PEFs/CHEFs within the healthcare trust premises or at universities. At the annual update sessions, issues related to reliability and validity of assessments should always be discussed so that a certain level of parity is achieved in the locality or, better still, examined in small group workshops, which could include group activities to explore the exact ways in which intra- and inter-mentor reliability are achieved and monitored. The NMC (2008a) makes some suggestions of activities to include on annual update study days, such as ensuring:

- knowledge of current NMC approved programmes
- discussion on the implications of changes to NMC requirements
- opportunity to discuss issues related to mentoring, assessment of competence and fitness for safe and effective practice.

Support mechanisms available for dealing with 'failing students' could be explored, as well as any new NMC rules and guidelines related to supporting learning in practice, and their implications. The NMC (2008a) requires placement providers to hold and maintain a register of current mentors, which is annotated to indicate which mentors are also sign-off mentors and practice teachers. The register also includes evidence of placement areas having sufficient numbers of up-to-date mentors to support learning for students on NMC approved education programmes.

In addition to annual updating, the NMC (2008a) also requires mentors to be subject to 'triennial reviews'. These include ascertaining during the development and performance review meeting whether the mentor has engaged in mentoring activities and kept themselves up to date. Mentors should be prepared to provide evidence to their employers and NMC quality assurance agents of how they have maintained and developed their knowledge, skills and competence as a mentor, in particular, and evidence of having:

- mentored at least two students with due regard within the three-year period
- participated in annual updating
- explored as a group activity the validity and reliability of judgements made when assessing practice in challenging circumstances
- mapped their ongoing development against the current NMC standards.

Placement providers can therefore consider such evidence of updating as part of the triennial review, for which mentors can compile a portfolio of their mentoring activities, both as a means of effective record keeping and as evidence of meeting the requirements of triennial reviews. Generally, if a mentor has mentored a specified number of students in the preceding three years, regularly participated in annual updates and is currently on the NMC's professional register, then these could be treated as sufficient evidence for meeting triennial review requirements.

Some healthcare trusts conduct workshops to facilitate building and presentation of portfolio evidence of mentoring activities and updating at triennial review events (for example, Gover, 2010). In such workshops, attendees can work in groups to identify a range of activities that comprise items that are pertinent evidence of mentoring activities (third bullet point in Activity 8.6). In addition to annual updating, evidence could also include annual performance review objectives, achievement of personal development plans (PDP) objectives, evaluation or feedback from any related presentations (in-house, or at local or national conferences), any EBP initiative implemented or disseminated, etc.

Mentoring RNs on specialist practice courses

Post-registration students on specialist programmes have particular learning and assessment needs, a dimension that is not usually addressed on standard single-module mentor preparation courses. In the past, before the advent of the current mentoring courses that ensued from the Phillips et al. (2000) study, teaching and assessing programmes were twice as long. For specialist community nursing students, assessments were conducted by Practical Work Teachers and Community Practice Teachers (CPT), the educational preparation for which was one academic year.

After the implementation of the novel mentor preparation course, whether mentors are at degree or Master's level, it was soon realised that it was not sufficient to prepare them to assess the specific competencies of students on some specialist community courses (Stevens, 2003; NMC, 2005b). The NMC (2008a) therefore identified the practice teacher role as a role that mentors had to be educationally prepared for supporting practice-based learning for students on these courses, including those on SCPHN programmes. Gopee (2010) translates in detail how practice teachers can fulfil their role effectively, which includes a thorough under-standing of all NMC standards and outcomes for practice teachers and related knowledge bases.

Furthermore, the NMC (2007b) recognises that there is likely to be limited opportunity to assess sign-off proficiencies more than once during the practice teacher course, and therefore they recommend a period of preceptee status for newly qualified practice teachers.

Mentor support with CPD

Usually, all university–healthcare trust partnerships already have an infrastructure of mentor support that has been established. Mentor support implies a network of per-sonnel and other resources that the mentor can access to discuss and sound out the decisions that they are about to make on their mentee's performance of clinical skills, or to consult. Such support is available from peers and colleagues within their prac-tice setting or department, and also from PEFs, link teachers and the student's per-sonal tutor, which invariably results in further learning. Further support can be gained through professional networks, some of which are formed informally at conferences, and when exploring issues at annual update study days.

Clinical supervision is another mechanism that mentors can draw on for regular structured support and for identifying learning. However, one of the key sources of mentor support for CPD is the PEF team, and the study days and workshops that they offer to mentors. Lecturers who teach on the mentor course at the partner university and reflective practice are other mentor support mechanisms.

Various sources of funding have been available for all registrants to undertake CPD related to their employment, although the funding has usually been meagre. Health Education England is the organisation that has taken responsibility for educa-tion, training and CPD of healthcare staff since April 2013. For further details see *Liberating the NHS: Developing the Healthcare Workforce from Design to Delivery* (DH, 2012c) at the HEE website and subsequent documents.

The mentor as role model of lifelong learning

To be a role model for mentees, mentors have to be lifelong learners in both professional practice and mentoring. The concept of lifelong learning has been examined with intense attention in university education departments since the 1970s, and in relation to healthcare professionals' CPD for a couple of decades. The NMC (2004c: 3) sees lifelong learning as 'more than simply keeping up to date … (but also incorporate an) enquiring approach to nursing and midwifery', and currently discusses the concept in the context of PREP and revalidation processes (NMC, 2013b).

Activity 8.7   Why lifelong learning?

List as many reasons as you can think of, for healthcare professionals being required to be lifelong learners. How can healthcare professionals achieve lifelong learning? What are the probable problems with lifelong learning?

The NMC (2004c) provides several reasons for healthcare professionals being lifelong learners, including increasing technological advances in treatment and care, and expanding roles. Furthermore, lifelong learning differs from lifelong education in that, while lifelong education refers to learning activities directed by established education institutions and that normally leads to a qualification, lifelong learning refers to all forms of learning – formal, informal and incidental.

Mentors continue to learn and become even more effective as mentors through attending formal annual updating events after successfully completing the initial educational preparation programme to become a mentor and, informally, through consulting and advising colleagues such as during peer mentoring, as well as by incidental learning. This means that the healthcare registrant not only has a responsibility to facilitate the learning of others, but also to continue learning themselves.

The learning activity undertaken is of course also based on self-assessment, and members of healthcare professions need to be responsible for identifying their own learning needs. Indeed, the NMC's (2015) code of professional standards states that as registrants we must keep our knowledge and competence up to date through regular learning and professional development activities (clause 22.3). Thus, healthcare professions explicitly either dictate or encourage all registrants to continue the process of learning, asking us to reflect on and question the ways in which we deliver care, and to engage in continuing development of our competence and improve our performance.

De la Harpe and Radloff (2000) explored the characteristics of lifelong learning students, and found that they had:

- self-knowledge, self-confidence and persistence
- a positive view of the value of learning

- good self-management skills, such as being well organised and managing time effectively knowing when and how to seek help and when to collaborate with peers
- motivation to learn
- positive feelings about themselves as learners
- the ability to manage their feelings during highs and lows of learning
- developed a set of learning strategies (e.g. when to dedicate time to study and where to learn; and skills such as note-taking and summarising).

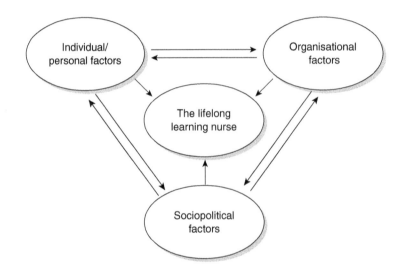

FIGURE 8.2   A conceptual framework for lifelong learning in nursing

Source: Gopee (2005)

Livneh and Livneh (1999) explored the characteristics of qualified teachers in the USA who regularly participated in learning activities, and found these to be self-motivation to learn, external motivators, as well as situational support and social/environmental resources. A later study of lifelong learning in nursing by Davis et al. (2014) identified several characteristics of lifelong learners, the most common ones of which include: enjoys learning, avails self to learn, self-motivated, reflective, asks questions and tracks down answers.

As to a systematic approach to facilitating lifelong learning, Gopee (2005) con-cluded from a qualitative study of nurses' perceptions of lifelong learning that a model (or framework) of lifelong learning in healthcare comprise three groups of factors, as presented in Figure 8.2. In brief, these comprise:

- *organisational factors* (e.g. time and release from work to attend CPD courses, work-based learning)
- *sociopolitical factors* (e.g. social group influences in the practice setting, clinical supervision)
- *individual factors* (the healthcare professional's professionalism, learning as a natural human activity).

The above-mentioned characteristics of lifelong learners are obviously 'individual factors', and as for the other two groups of factors identified by Gopee, naturally, there are numerous ways in which healthcare professionals can and do engage in CPD and lifelong learning, which range from university-based degree-awarding courses or modules, informal much shorter trust-based study days and workshops, to self-directed learning.

Personal development plans

Systematic CPD and lifelong learning for health and social care professionals can also be effectively supported through the utilisation of PDPs. PDPs have been advocated for over a decade in the UK through key NHS and education policy documents such as *Making a Difference* (DH, 1999), *NHS KSF* (DH, 2004a), *Guidelines for HE Progress Files* (QAA, 2001) and *The Dearing Report* (NCIHE, 1997). The *NHS KSF* advocates the use of PDPs by all NHS healthcare professionals for their professional development throughout their careers. Other than education and health policies, influential writers on self- and staff management such as Pedler et al. (1997) and Megginson and Clutterbuck (2005) also advocate the use of PDPs.

PDPs provide individuals with the opportunity to focus attention on their career aspirations, and comprise a mechanism for recording and reviewing career decisions periodically. However, Pedler et al. indicate that PDPs should not be part of the annual development and performance review process that is seen as a management control mechanism, but as agreements that are not centrally recorded. PDPs are instead a component of an effective learning organisation (a concept discussed in Chapter 4).

Nevertheless, a PDP is also often an NMC requirement for reinstatement to the professional register where a registrant's competence has been in question, and it suggests that in future, PDPs could be linked to PREP and revalidation. However, a PDP is not a punitive activity, and despite Pedler et al.'s assertion, they can be utilised in conjunction with annual development and performance reviews (Liefer, 2002; Duffin, 2003). It is feasible to implement PDPs so that they are discussed as part of annual development reviews, with only an agreed selection of objectives being incorporated into the performance review and the remaining PDP objectives being supported by clinical supervision.

The QAA (2001: 2) defines a PDP as 'a structured and supported process undertaken by an individual to reflect upon their own learning, performance and/or

Template 8.1 A professional development plan

Name: .... [Other relevant details, e.g. clinical supervisor's name]

Objective and development need/interest	Relevant dimension of my work and career	Hours required and date objective to be achieved	What I will do to achieve this development need/interest. Resources and support required	How I will apply this learning to my work	How I will know I have completed the development activity successfully	How I will share this learning with relevant others
1. Establish protected time for mentoring	Teaching learners	One hour every week, achieve by end of mentee's practice placement	Off-duty planned in advance. Team members aware. Two alternative protected times identified each week	Spend the protected time focusing on mentoring activities. Monitor and record use of protected time	An appropriate record of mentoring activities	Item on team meeting agenda. Present at local conference
2. Gain practice teacher qualification	......	......	......	......	......	

achievement and to plan for their personal, educational and career development'. Thus, PDPs can be separated as either personal or professional development, except that for most individuals these two components are either intertwined or experienced on a continuum in day-to-day activities. An example of a PDP for mentors – which has been constructed from prevailing guidance and other literature on the topic – and can be constituted in landscape or portrait format, is presented in Template 8.1.

The two development needs mentioned in Template 8.1 are part of the education component of nurses and midwives' roles, other components being clinical practice, research and management, as noted at the beginning of Chapter 3. Various components of required knowledge and competence can be acquired through in-house and in-service training, but for paid time for study, funding and support from managers for HEI-based courses, this can be an issue (Liefer, 2002) and therefore needs forward planning.

Chapter Summary

This chapter has focused on the evaluation of the whole range of mentoring activities, and having completed this chapter you will have examined:

- Why we should evaluate the effectiveness with which mentors facilitate learning and assessments, while they also fulfil other mentoring activities and roles.
- What evaluation is, i.e. the nature and various aspects of evaluation, and who evaluates the mentor's teaching activities.
- Different ways of evaluating clinically based and academically based teaching and assessment; and how mentors evaluate learning provision and assessments during practice placements. The use of models of evaluation, including heeding the findings of audits by external organisations such as the QAA and NMC.
- The likely problems of evaluation, the results of evaluations, issues ensuing from them, related consequences and subsequent actions that can be taken.
- The opportunities and scope for ongoing learning arising from the results of evaluations, mentoring RNs on specialist practice courses, and the requirement for continuing professional development in one's mentoring role as well as the mentor as a lifelong learner.

📖 Further Optional Reading

1   Kirkpatrick and Kirkpatrick's (2006) framework for evaluating training and education programmes is available from Internet websites, where they provide variable insights into this model, but a more thorough account is provided in the Kirkpatrick

and Kirkpatrick book. Implementation of the model is also discussed in the context of practice teaching in the *Practice Teaching in Healthcare* (Gopee, 2010) book.

- Kirkpatrick, D.L. and Kirkpatrick, J.D. (2006) *Evaluating Training Programs: The Four Levels*, 3rd edn. San Francisco, CA: Berrett-Koehler Publishers.

2 For an identification of sources of mentoring activities that can be presented as evidence/portfolio evidence at triennial reviews, see:

- Murray, C., Rosen, L. and Staniland, K. (eds) (2010) *The Nurse Mentor and Reviewer Update Book*. Maidenhead: McGraw-Hill Education.

To access further resources related to this chapter, visit the companion website at https://study.sagepub.com/gopee

Further Thoughts – A Journey Just Beginning

Mentoring is a career-long journey, whether it's to do with mentoring learners of one's own healthcare profession, or of allied health professions, medical students, or healthcare assistants. On the one hand, it is a journey that begins soon after your preceptee status ends. One of the strengths of nursing, midwifery and SCPHNs is the holistic approach that other healthcare professionals intend, endeavour and at times succeed in taking in their day-to-day practice. Some clinical settings have students all the time, others occasionally, but the actions that mentors take stay in the minds of healthcare professionals for several years, as they shape their careers and quality of patient care. The mentor's actions are therefore seminal in shaping the attitudes of practitioners for years to come.

On the other hand, as Rogers and Freiberg (1994: 375) indicate, 'not all journeys are trouble-free … but the process alone makes us a bit wiser. Gaining wisdom comes not with time or age, but from living the challenges of life, learning from our mistakes, and building on experiences.' This book on mentoring was designed to achieve the objectives outlined in the introductory section, which are predominantly to examine the knowledge and understanding necessary for effective and mutually beneficial mentoring, and the NMC's (2008a) standards for mentors. The knowledge and skills acquired can be built on by further pursuing the topic area as part of your own action plan. They could play a significant role along your career path, be it as a more senior clinical practitioner or in part- or full-time educational roles. What are the next steps that you'd like to take when you have obtained your mentor qualification?

Glossary

action research   Scientifically designed research that is conducted while in the process of implementing a new activity or a change

associate mentor   The NMC indicates that each student on practice placement must have a named mentor, and in this book the term associate mentor is used to signify any RN/RM who supports the named mentor

clinical interventions   Any action taken by healthcare professionals to improve the health of patients or service users, or to enhance their health and prevent health problems

clinical learning environment (CLE)   The practice setting as an environment where learning occurs amongst staff and students, which is valued and encouraged, along with effective care delivery. The term is used interchangeably with 'practice learning environment'

competency   The skill and associated practical knowledge required to perform a clinical intervention

educational audit   An audit that is normally conducted jointly by senior staff in a practice setting and a university academic to check whether the practice setting is suitable for healthcare students to be placed there as part of their professional learning

ethical competence   Refers to the ability of the healthcare professional to deliver safe and effective care that is based on full accountability, and whose practice and social behaviour are based on the principles of ethics and on moral values such as doing good, demonstrating respect for human rights and dignity, etc.

evidence-based practice (EBP)   Practice that is based on evidence, which can be research evidence

facilitation of learning   An idea that is different from the term teaching in that it signifies the lecturer or teacher structuring activities that enable students to learn by themselves, as individuals or in groups, as different from directly teaching them. The concept can be applied to acquiring healthcare knowledge base, but can also be applied to supervised learning in skills laboratories

forcefield analysis   An analysis that entails exploring a proposed change by analysing the factors that are indicating the need for the change, and the factors that are hindering the implementation of the change

healthcare organisations   NHS Acute Trusts, primary care, private hospitals, nursing homes, etc. involved in providing care and treatment

healthcare provider   Healthcare organisations in the public or independent sector that provide care and treatment to individuals with health problems

informal learning   Learning that occurs ad hoc, often based on being opportunistic and learning as opportunities arise

intuitive knowledge   Refers to personal and professional knowledge that is based on intuition and sensing, but which may not have an underpinning demonstrable reasoning or scientific evidence on which the knowledge is based.

learning pathway   A structured plan of learning based on patient journeys

link lecturer   A university lecturer who singly or as part of a team of lecturers is the named academic contact whom staff in specific practice settings can contact for information, clarification, etc. about student matters

patients or service users   The two terms are used interchangeably to signify anyone who uses or receives health or social care from healthcare organisations

person–centred care   Is an approach to practice that is underpinned by such values as respect for the person, for individuals' rights and a culture of empowerment to the patient

practice learning   Learning that occurs during practice placements

practice teacher   A specialist or advanced practice nurse who has successfully completed a course in preparation for the role of supervising registered nurses (RNs) who are students on specialist or advanced practice courses

preceptorship   A role allocated to an appropriately experienced healthcare professional for the supervision of the professional development of a newly qualified registrant in the practice setting

pre-registration   This term is used interchangeably with pre-qualifying and pre-service professional education to signify health or social care profession students' education programmes that lead to students becoming eligible to have their names entered on the NMC or HCPC professional register

registrants   Refers to qualified healthcare professionals on either the Nursing and Midwifery Council's (NMC) or Health and Care Professions Council's (HCPC) professional register

supernumerary status   Health profession students are deemed supernumerary if they are not part of the paid workforce in a practice setting, but are expected to engage in learning healthcare knowledge and skills by participating in care of patients or service users

References

Adam, D. and Taylor, R. (2014) 'Compassionate care: empowering students through nurse education', *Nurse Education Today*, 34 (9): 1242–5.

Adelman-Mullally, T., Mulder, C.K., McCarter-Spalding, D.E., Hagler, D.A., Gaberson, K.B., Hanner, M.B., Oermann, M.H., Speakman, E.T., Yoder-Wise, P.S. and Young, P.K. (2013) 'The clinical nurse educator as leader', *Nurse Education in Practice*, 13 (1): 29–34.

Anderson, E.E. (2009) 'Learning pathways in contemporary primary care settings – student nurses' views', *Nurse Education Today*, 29 (8): 835–9.

Andrews, M., Brewer, M., Buchan, T., Denne, A., Hammond, J., Hardy, G., Jacobs, L., McKenzie, L. and West, S. (2010) 'Implementation and sustainability of the nursing and midwifery standards for mentoring in the UK', *Nurse Education in Practice*, 10 (5): 251–5.

Argyle, M. (1994) *The Psychology of Interpersonal Behaviour*, 5th edn. London: Penguin.

Ausubel, D., Novak, J. and Hanesian, H. (1978) *Educational Psychology: A Cognitive View*. New York: Rinehart & Winston.

Bahn, D. (2001) 'Social learning theory: its application in the context of nurse education', *Nurse Education Today*, 21 (2): 110–17.

Bailey, M.E. and Tuohy, D. (2009) 'Student nurses' experiences of using a learning contract as a method of assessment', *Nurse Education Today*, 29 (7): 758–62.

Baldwin, A., Mills, J., Birks, M. and Budden, L. (2014) 'Role modelling in undergraduate nursing education: an integrative literature review', *Nurse Education Today*, 34 (6): e18–e26.

Bandura, A. (1986) *Social Foundations of Thought and Action: A Social-Cognitive Theory*. Englewood Cliffs, NJ: Prentice-Hall.

Bandura, A. (1997) *Self-Efficacy: The Exercise of Control*. New York: W.H. Freeman.

Barnett, J.E. (2008) 'Mentoring, boundaries, and multiple relationships: opportunities and challenges', *Mentoring & Tutoring: Partnership in Learning*, 16 (1): 3–16.

Baron, S. (2009) 'Evaluating the patient journey approach to ensure health care is centred on patients', *Nursing Times*, 105 (22): 20–3.

Barr, H. (2003) 'Inter-professional issues and work-based learning', in J. Burton and N. Jackson (eds), *Work-Based Learning in Primary Care*. Oxford: Radcliffe Medical.

Barton, T.D. (2006) 'Clinical mentoring of nurse practitioners: the doctors' experience', *British Journal of Nursing*, 15 (15): 820–4.

Benner, P. (2001) *From Novice to Expert: Excellence and Power in Clinical Nursing Practice*. London: Addison-Wesley.

Berger, P. and Luckmann, T. (1967) *The Social Construction of Reality*. Middlesex: Penguin Books.

Bergsteiner, H., Avery, G.C. and Neumann, R. (2010) 'Kolb's experiential learning model: critique from a modelling perspective', *Studies in Continuing Education*, 32 (1): 29–46.

Biggs, J. and Tang, C. (2011) *Teaching for Quality Learning at University*, 4th edn. Maidenhead: Open University Press.

Billay, D.B. and Yonge, O. (2004) 'Contributing to the theory development of preceptorship', *Nurse Education Today*, 24 (7): 566–74.

Binnie, A. and Titchen, A. (1999) *Freedom to Practice: The Development of Patient-Centred Nursing*. Edinburgh: Butterworth-Heinemann.

Bloom, B. (1956) *Taxonomy of Educational Objectives: The Classification of Educational Goals, Handbook One: Cognitive Domain*. London: Longman.

Bondy, K.N. (1983) 'Criterion-referenced definitions for rating scales in clinical evaluation', *Journal of Nursing Education*, 22 (9): 376–82.

Boud, D. (1991) *Implementing Student Self-Assessment (HERDSA Green Guide No. 5)*. Australian Capital Territory: Higher Education Research and Development Society of Australasia.

Boud, D., Keogh, R. and Walker, D. (eds) (1985) *Reflection: Turning Experience into Learning*. London: Kogan Page.

Bowker, P., French, D., Atkin, S.L., Patmore, J.E., Walton, C. and Aye, M. (2005) 'Financing a diabetes network: care pathway based costing model for Type 1 diabetes mellitus', *Diabetic Medicine*, 23 (Supp. 2): 107.

Bradshaw, A. (1997) 'Defining "competency" in nursing (Part 1): a policy review', *Journal of Clinical Nursing*, 6 (5): 347–54.

Bray, L., O'Brien, M.R., Kirton, J., Zubairu, K. and Christiansen, A. (2014) 'The role of professional education in developing compassionate practitioners: a mixed methods study exploring the perceptions of health professionals and pre-registration students', *Nurse Education Today*, 34 (3): 480–6.

British Association for Counselling and Psychotherapy (BACP) (2013) *Ethical Framework for Good Practice in Counselling & Psychotherapy*. Available at: http://www.bacp.co.uk/admin/structure/files/pdf/9479_ethical%20framework%20jan2013.pdf (accessed 2 January 2014).

Brooke, J. and Ham, A. (2003) 'Coaching managers to become better team leaders', *Strategic Communication Management (SCM)*, 7 (2): 4–27.

Brown, J., Bullock, D. and Grossberg, S. (1999) 'How the basal ganglia use parallel excitatory and inhibitory learning pathways to selectively respond to unexpected rewarding cues', *Journal of Neuroscience*, 19 (23): 10502–11.

Brown, L. (2005) 'Ethics in clinical education', in M. Rose and D. Best (eds), *Transforming Practice through Clinical Education, Professional Supervision and Mentoring*. Edinburgh: Elsevier Churchill Livingstone.

Brown, L. (ed.-in-chief) (2002) *Shorter Oxford English Dictionary*, 5th edn. Oxford: Oxford University Press.

Brown, T., Williams, B., McKenna, L., Palermo, C., McCall, L., Roller, L., Hewitt, L., Molloy, L., Baird, M. and Aldabah, L. (2011) 'Practice education learning environments:

the mismatch between perceived and preferred expectations of undergraduate health science students', *Nurse Education Today*, 31 (8): e22–8.

Bruner, J. (1960) *The Process of Education*. Cambridge, MA: Harvard University Press.

Bryar, R.M. and Griffiths, J.M. (eds) (2003) *Practice Development in Community Nursing*. London: Arnold.

Buring, S.M., Bhushan, A., Broeseker, A., Conway, S., Duncan-Hewitt, W., Hansen, L. and Westberg, S. (2009) 'Interprofessional education: definitions, student competencies, and guidelines for implementation', *American Journal of Pharmaceutical Education*, 73 (4): 59.

Burnard, P. and Chapman, C. (1990) *Nurse Education: The Way Forward*. London: Scutari Press.

Care Quality Commission (CQC) (2014) *A Fresh Start for the Regulation and Inspection of Adult Social Care*. Available at: www.cqc.org.uk/sites/default/files/documents/20131013_cqc_afreshstart_2013_final.pdf (accessed 9 July 2014).

Carlisle, C., Calman, L. and Ibbotson, T. (2009) 'Practice-based learning: the role of practice education facilitators in supporting mentors', *Nurse Education Today*, 29 (7): 715–21.

Carlson, E. and Idvall, E. (2014) 'Nursing students' experiences of the clinical learning environment in nursing homes: a questionnaire study using the CLES + T evaluation scale', *Nurse Education Today*, 34 (7): 1130–4.

Carnwell, R., Baker, S., Bellis, M. and Murray, R. (2007) 'Managerial perceptions of mentor, lecturer practitioner and link tutor roles', *Nurse Education Today*, 27 (8): 923–32.

Carper, B. (1978) 'Fundamental patterns of knowing in nursing', *Advances in Nursing Science*, 1 (1): 13–23.

Centre for Advancement of Interprofessional Education (CAIPE) (2014) *Defining IPE – Interprofessional Education*. Available at: http://caipe.org.uk/about-us/defining-ipe/ (accessed 4 May 2014).

Chan, D.S.K. and Ip, W.Y. (2007) 'Perceptions of hospital learning environment: a survey of Hong Kong nursing students,' *Nurse Education Today*, 27 (7): 677–84.

Chartered Institute of Personnel and Development (2013) *Coaching and Mentoring – Resource Summary*. Available at: www.cipd.co.uk/hr-resources/factsheets/coaching-mentoring.aspx (accessed 25 August 2014).

Chartered Society of Physiotherapy (CSP) (2002) *Curriculum Framework for Qualifying Programmes in Physiotherapy*. Available at: http://www.csp.org.uk/publications/curriculum-framework-qualifying-programmes-physiotherapy (accessed 19 March 2014).

Chartered Society of Physiotherapy (2014) *Accreditation of Clinical Educators (ACE) Scheme*. Available at: http://www.csp.org.uk/professional-union/careers-development/practice-educators/accreditation-clinical-educators-ace-scheme (accessed 3 January 2014).

Chelimsky, E. and Shadish, W. (1997) *Evaluation for the 21st Century: A Handbook*. London: Sage Publications.

Child, J. and Langford, E. (2011) Exploring the learning experiences of nursing students with dyslexia. *Nursing Standard*, 25 (40): 39–46.

Clarke, J.B. (1999) 'Evidence-based practice: a retrograde step? The importance of pluralism in evidence generation for the practice of healthcare', *Journal of Clinical Nursing*, 8 (1): 89–94.

Cochrane Collaboration (2013) *Systematic Reviews*. Available at: http://www.cochrane.org/about-us/evidence-based-health-care (accessed 12 April 2014).

Coleman, M. and Glover, D. (2010) *Educational Leadership and Management*. Maidenhead: Open University Press.

College of Occupational Therapists (COT) (2013) *Preceptorship Handbook for Occupational Therapists*, 3rd edn. London: COT.

College of Operating Department Practitioners (CODP) (2009) *Standards, Recommendations and Guidance for Mentors and Practice Placements: Supporting Pre-Registration Education in Operating Department Practice Provision*. Available at: https://www3.shu.ac.uk/hwb/placements/OperatingDepartmentPractitioners/documents/CODPstandards formentorship.pdf (accessed 4 May 2014).

College of Social Work (2012) *Practice Educator Professional Standards for Social Work*. Available at: www.tcsw.org.uk/uploadedFiles/TheCollege/_CollegeLibrary/Reform_resources/Practice-EducatorProfessional%28edref11%29.pdf (accessed 15 December 2014)

Collinson, G. (2000) 'Encouraging the growth of the nurse entrepreneur', *Professional Nurse*, 15 (6): 365–7.

Connor, M. and Pokora, J. (2012) *Coaching and Mentoring at Work: Developing Effective Practice*, 2nd edn. Maidenhead: Open University Press.

Crombie, A., Brindley, J., Harris, D., Marks-Maran, D. and Thompson, T.M. (2013) 'Factors that enhance rates of completion: what makes students stay?', *Nurse Education Today*, 33 (11): 1282–7.

Cross, K.D. (1996) 'An analysis of the concept facilitation', *Nurse Education Today*, 16 (5): 350–5.

Currie, K., Biggam, J., Palmer, J. and Corcoranm, T. (2012) 'Participants' engagement with and reactions to the use of on-line action learning sets to supports advanced nursing role development', *Nurse Education Today*, 32 (3): 267–272

Curtis, K., Horton, K. and Smith, P. (2012) 'Student nurse socialisation in compassionate practice: a Grounded Theory study', *Nurse Education Today*, 32 (7): 790–5.

Curzon, L.B. and Tummons, J. (2013) *Teaching in Further Education: An Outline of Principles and Practice*, 7th edn. London: Bloomsbury Academic.

Dale, A.E. (2006) 'Determining guiding principles for evidence-based practice', *Nursing Standard*, 20 (25): 41–6.

Daloz, L.A. (1989) *Effective Teaching and Mentoring: Realizing the Transformational Power of Adult Learning Experiences*. San Francisco, CA: Jossey-Bass.

Darling, L.A.W. (1984) 'What do nurses want in a mentor?', *Journal of Nursing Administration*, 14 (10): 42–4.

Darling, L.A.W. (1985) 'What to do about toxic mentors?', *Journal of Nursing Administration*, 15 (5): 43–4.

Davies, S. and Priestley, M.J. (2006) 'A reflective evaluation of patient handover practices', *Nursing Standard*, 20 (21): 49–52.

Davis, L., Taylor, H. and Reyes, H. (2014) 'Lifelong learning in nursing: a Delphi study', *Nurse Education Today*, 34 (3): 441–5.

de la Harpe, B. and Radloff, A. (2000) 'Informed teachers and learners: the importance of assessing the characteristics needed for lifelong learning', *Studies in Continuing Education*, 22 (2): 169–82.

de Luc, K. (2000) 'Care pathways: an evaluation of their effectiveness', *Journal of Advanced Nursing*, 32 (2): 485–96.

DeBrew, J.K. and Lewallen, L.P. (2014) 'To pass or to fail? Understanding the factors considered by faculty in the clinical evaluation of nursing students', *Nurse Education Today*, 34 (4): 631–6.

Department of Health (DH) (1990) *NHS and Community Care Act.* London: HMSO.

Department of Health (1999) *Making a Difference: Strengthening the Nursing, Midwifery and Health Visiting Contribution to Health and Health Care.* Available at: http://webarchive. nationalarchives.gov.uk/+/www.dh.gov.uk/en/Publicationsandstatistics/Publications/ PublicationsPolicyAndGuidance/DH_4007977 (accessed 21 April 2014).

Department of Health (and English National Board for Nursing, Midwifery and Health Visiting) (2001a) *Preparation of Mentors and Teachers: A New Framework of Guidance.* Available at: www.nmc-uk.org/Documents/Archived%20Publications/ENB%20 Archived%20Publications/Preparation%20of%20Mentors%20and%20Teachers%20 January%202001.PDF (accessed 6 January 2015).

Department of Health (and English National Board for Nursing, Midwifery and Health Visiting) (2001b) *Placements in Focus: Guidance for Education in Practice for Health Care Professions.* Available at: http://www.nmc-uk.org/Documents/Archived%20 Publications/ENB%20Archived%20Publications/Placements%20in%20focus%20-%20 ENB%20January%202001.PDF (accessed 23 April 2014).

Department of Health (2001c) *Working Together – Learning Together: A Framework for Lifelong Learning for the NHS.* Available at: http://webarchive.nationalarchives.gov. uk/+/www.dh.gov.uk/en/publicationsandstatistics/publications/publicationspolicy-andguidance/dh_4009558 (accessed 13 December 2014).

Department of Health (2002a) *Liberating the Talents: Helping Primary Care Trusts and Nurses to Deliver the NHS Plan.* Available at: http://webarchive.nationalarchives.gov.uk/+/www. dh.gov.uk/en/Publicationsandstatistics/Publications/PublicationsPolicyAndGuidance/ DH_4007473 (accessed 21 April 2014).

Department of Health (2002b) *PL CNO (2002) 5: Implementing the NHS Plan – Ten Key Roles for Nurses.* Available at: http://webarchive.nationalarchives.gov.uk/+/www.dh.gov. uk/en/Publicationsandstatistics/Lettersandcirculars/Professionalletters/ Chiefnursingofficerletters/DH_4004780?PageOperation=email (accessed 24 April 2014).

Department of Health (2004a) *The NHS Knowledge and Skills Framework (NHS KSF) and the Development Review Process.* Available at: http://webarchive.nationalarchives.gov. uk/+/www.dh.gov.uk/en/publicationsandstatistics/publications/publicationspolicy-andguidance/dh_4090843 (accessed 21 April 2014).

Department of Health (2004b) *Agenda for Change: What Will It Mean for You? A Guide for Staff.* Available at: http://www.dhsspsni.gov.uk/scu-agendachange-staffguide.pdf (accessed 21 April 2014).

Department of Health (2006) *Modernising Nursing Careers: Setting the Direction.* Available at: http://www.dhsspsni.gov.uk/modernising_nursing_careers-2.pdf (accessed 4 May 2014).

Department of Health (2007) *Patient Pathways: What is a Patient Pathway?* Available at: http://webarchive.nationalarchives.gov.uk/+/www.dh.gov.uk/en/Healthcare/ Primarycare/Treatmentcentres/DH_4097263 (accessed 21 April 2014).

Department of Health (2008) *National Service Framework for Long-Term Neurological Conditions: National Support for Local Implementation 2008.* Available at: http:// webarchive.nationalarchives.gov.uk/20130107105354/http:/www.dh.gov.uk/ prod_consum_dh/groups/dh_digitalassets/@dh/@en/documents/digitalasset/ dh_084580.pdf (accessed 4 May 2014).

Department of Health (2009) *Local Routes: Guidance for Developing Alcohol Treatment Pathways.* Available at: http://www.champspublichealth.com/writedir/fa98dh_110422.pdf (accessed 21 April 2014).

Department of Health (2010a) *Preceptorship Framework for Newly Registered Nurses, Midwives and Allied Health Professionals.* Available at: http://webarchive.nationalarchives.gov.uk/+/www.dh.gov.uk/en/Publicationsandstatistics/Publications/Publications PolicyAndGuidance/DH_114073 (accessed 4 May 2014).

Department of Health (2010b) *Health Technology Assessment Programme.* London: Department of Health.

Department of Health (2012a) *Health and Social Care Act 2012.* Available at: http://www.legislation.gov.uk/ukpga/2012/7/contents/enacted (accessed 13 January 2014).

Department of Health (2012b) *Compassion in Practice: Nursing, Midwifery and Care Staff: Our Vision and Strategy.* Available at: http://www.england.nhs.uk/wp-content/uploads/2012/12/compassion-in-practice.pdf (accessed 20 January 2014).

Department of Health (2012c) *Liberating the NHS: Developing the Healthcare Workforce from Design to Delivery.* Available at: https://www.gov.uk/government/uploads/system/uploads/attachment_data/file/216421/dh_132087.pdf (accessed 12 April 2014).

Department of Health (2013a) *The Education Outcomes Framework.* Available at: http://dera.ioe.ac.uk/18104/1/Education_outcomes_framework.pdf (accessed 13 January 2014).

Department of Health (2013b) *The NHS Constitution for England.* Available at: https://www.gov.uk/government/publications/the-nhs-constitution-for-england (accessed 5 April 2014).

Donabedian, A. (1988) 'The quality of care: how can it be assessed?', *American Journal of Public Health*, 260 (12): 1743–8.

Donaldson, J.H. and Carter, D. (2005) 'The value of role modelling: perceptions of undergraduate and diploma nursing (adult) students', *Nurse Education in Practice*, 5 (6): 353–9.

Donaldson, J.H. and Gray, M. (2012) 'Systematic review of grading practice: is there evidence of grade inflation?', *Nurse Education in Practice*, 12 (2): 101–14.

Dougherty, L. and Lister, S. (eds) (2011) *The Royal Marsden Hospital Manual of Clinical Nursing Procedures – Online Edition: For Hospitals and NHS Trusts*, 8th edn. Available at: http://www.royalmarsdenmanual.com/view/onlineNhs.html (accessed 19 March 2014).

Downey, M. (2003) 'Effective coaching: lessons from the coaches' coach', in G. Byrne [2007], 'Guest editorial: Unlocking potential – coaching as a means to enhance leadership and role performance in nursing', *Journal of Clinical Nursing*, 16 (11): 1987–8.

Duane, B.T. and Satre, M.E. (2014) 'Utilizing constructivism learning theory in collaborative testing as a creative strategy to promote essential nursing skills', *Nurse Education Today*, 34 (1): 31–4.

Duers, L.E. and Brown, N. (2009) 'An exploration of student nurses' experiences of formative assessment', *Nurse Education Today*, 29 (6): 654–9.

Duffin, C. (2003) 'Trusts miss deadline for staff development plans', *Nursing Standard*, 17 (16): 6.

Duffin, C. (2005) 'Pre-registration education to undergo major review', *Nursing Standard*, 19 (26): 4.

Duffy, K. (2003) *Failing Students: A Qualitative Study of Factors that Influence the Decisions Regarding Assessment of Students' Competence in Practice*. Available at: http://www.nmc-uk.org/Documents/Archived%20Publications/1Research%20papers/Kathleen_Duffy_Failing_Students2003.pdf (accessed 18 March 2014).

Durham, W.J., Kingston, P. and Sykes, C. (2012) 'Implementing a sign-off mentor preparation workshop: a tripartite approach', *Nurse Education Today*, 32 (3): 273–7.

Eades, J., Hill, K. and Craig, J. (2005) 'The shadowing experience of nursing students', *Nursing Standard*, 20 (12): 48–51.

Eller, L.S., Lev, E.L. and Feurer, A. (2014) 'Key components of an effective mentoring relationship: a qualitative study', *Nurse Education Today*, 34 (5); 815–20.

Equality Challenge Unit (2012) *Equality Act 2010: Implications for Colleges and HEIs*. Available at: http://www.ecu.ac.uk/publications/equality-act-2010-revised (accessed 17 December 2014).

Evans, D. (2003) 'Hierarchy of evidence: a framework for ranking evidence evaluating healthcare interventions', *Journal of Clinical Nursing*, 12 (1): 77–84.

Falchikov, N. (1986) 'Product comparisons and process benefits of collaborative peer group and self-assessment', *Assessment and Evaluation in Higher Education*, 11 (2): 146–66.

Faugier, J. (2005a) 'Reality check', *Nursing Standard*, 19 (19): 14–15.

Faugier, J. (2005b) 'Developing a new generation of nurse entrepreneurs', *Nursing Standard*, 19 (30): 49–53.

Field, J. (1999) 'Participation under the magnifying glass', *Adults Learning*, 11 (3): 10–13.

Fitts, P.M. and Posner, M.I. (1973) *Human Performance*. London: Prentice-Hall.

Fleming, S., Mckee, G. and Huntley-Moore, S. (2011) 'Undergraduate nursing students' learning styles: a longitudinal study', *Nurse Education Today*, 31 (5): 444–9.

Foster, H., Ooms, A. and Marks-Maran, D. (2015) 'Nursing students' expectations and experiences of mentorship', *Nurse Education Today*, 35 (1): 18–24.

Francis, R. (2013) *Report of the Mid Staffordshire NHS Foundation Trust Public Inquiry* (Francis Report). Available at: http://www.midstaffspublicinquiry.com/report (accessed 11 April 2014).

Freire, P. (1996) *Pedagogy of the Oppressed*. London: Penguin.

Fretwell, J.E. (1980) 'An inquiry into the ward learning environment', *Nursing Times*, 76 (16): 69–75.

Fulton, J., Bøhler, A., Hansen, G.S., Kauffeldt, A., Welander, E., Santos, M.R., Reis, M., Thorarinsdottir, K. and Ziarko, E. (2007) 'Mentorship: an international perspective', *Nurse Education Today*, 7 (6): 399–406.

Furlong, J. and Maynard, T. (1995) *Mentoring Student Teachers*. London: Routledge.

Gagné, R. (1983) *The Conditions of Learning and Theory of Instruction* (4th edn). New York: Holt, Rinehart & Winston.

Gainsbury, S. (2010) 'Mentors passing students despite doubts over ability', *Nursing Times*, 106 (16): 1–3.

Gallagher, A. and Wainwright, P. (2005) 'The ethical divide', *Nursing Standard*, 20 (7): 22–5.

Garbett, R. and McCormack, B. (2002) 'A concept analysis of practice development', *Journal of Research in Nursing*, 7 (2): 87–100.

Garside, J., Nhemachena, J.Z., Williams, J. and Topping, A. (2009) 'Repositioning assessment: giving students the "choice" of assessment methods', *Nurse Education in Practice*, 9 (2): 141–8.

Garvey, B., Stokes, P. and Megginson, D. (2014) *Coaching and Mentoring: Theory and Practice*, 2nd edn. London: SAGE.

Ghazi, F. and Henshaw, L. (1998) 'How to keep student nurses motivated', *Nursing Standard*, 13 (8): 43–8.

Gibbs, G. (1988) *Improving the Quality of Student Learning*. Bristol: Technical Education Services.

Gilmour, J.A., Kopeiki, A. and Douché, J. (2007) 'Student nurses as peer-mentors: collegiality in practice', *Nurse Education in Practice*, 7 (1): 36–43.

Goldsmith, J., Clarke, B. and Cross, S. (2009) 'The art of learning to teach interprofessionally', *Practice Nursing*, 20 (8): 414–16.

Gopee, N. (2000) 'Self-assessment and the concept of the lifelong learning nurse', *British Journal of Nursing*, 9 (11): 724–9.

Gopee, N. (2001) 'The role of peer assessment and peer review in nursing', *British Journal of Nursing*, 10 (2): 115–21.

Gopee, N. (2002a) 'Human and social capital as facilitators of lifelong learning in nursing', *Nurse Education Today*, 22 (8): 608–16.

Gopee, N. (2002b) 'Demonstrating critical analysis in academic assignments', *Nursing Standard*, 16 (35): 45–52.

Gopee, N. (2005) 'Facilitating the implementation of lifelong learning in nursing', *British Journal of Nursing*, 14 (14): 761–7.

Gopee, N. (2010) *Practice Teaching in Healthcare*. London: Sage Publications.

Gopee, N. and Deane, M. (2013) 'Strategies for successful academic writing: institutional and non-institutional support for students', *Nurse Education Today*, 33 (12): 1624–31.

Gopee, N. and Galloway, J. (2014) *Leadership and Management in Healthcare*, 2nd edn. London: Sage Publications.

Gopee, N., Tyrell, A., Raven, S., Thomas, K. and Hari, T. (2004) 'Effective clinical learning in primary care settings', *Nursing Standard*, 18 (37): 33–7.

Gov.uk (2013) *Health Education England Mandate*. Available at: https://www.gov.uk/government/publications/health-education-england-mandate (accessed 13 January 2014).

Gov.uk (2014) *NHS Outcomes Framework 2014 to 2015*. Available at: https://www.gov.uk/government/publications/nhs-outcomes-framework-2014-to-2015 (accessed 13 January 2014).

Gover, S. (2010) 'Triennial review workshops facilitated by practice education facilitators'. Paper presented at Royal College of Nursing Education Forum 'Partners in Practice' Conference, 26–27 February, Blackpool.

Gray, J.A.M. (2001) *Evidence-Based Health Care: How to Make Policy and Management Decisions*, 2nd edn. Edinburgh: Churchill Livingstone.

Gray, M.A. and Smith, L.N. (2000) 'The qualities of an effective mentor from the student nurse's perspective: findings from a longitudinal qualitative study', *Journal of Advanced Nursing*, 32 (6): 1542–9.

Greenhalgh, T. (2014) *How to Read a Paper: The Basics of Evidence-Based Medicine*, 5th edn. Oxford: Wiley-Blackwell.

Griffiths, L., Worth, P., Scullard, Z. and Gilbert, D. (2010) 'Supporting disabled students in practice: a tripartite approach', *Nurse Education in Practice*, 10 (3): 132–7.

Guba, E.G. and Lincoln, Y.S. (1989) *Fourth Generation Evaluation*. London: Sage.

Gutteridge, R. and Dobbins, K. (2010) 'Service user and carer involvement in learning and teaching: a faculty of health staff perspective', *Nurse Education Today*, 30 (6): 509–14.

Haidar, E. (2007) 'Coaching and mentoring nursing students', *Nursing Management*, 14 (8): 32–35.

Hall, K.M., Draper, R.J., Smith, L.K. and Bullough, Jr, R.V. (2008) 'More than a place to teach: exploring the perceptions of the roles and responsibilities of mentor teachers', *Mentoring & Tutoring: Partnership in Learning*, 16 (3): 328–45.

Hallin, K. and Danielson, E. (2009) 'Being a personal preceptor for nursing students: registered nurses' experiences before and after introduction of a preceptor model', *Journal of Advanced Nursing*, 65 (1): 161–74.

Handy, C. (1989) *Age of Unreason*. London: Business Books.

Harrison, J., Dymoke, S. and Pell, T. (2006) 'Mentoring beginning teachers in secondary schools: an analysis of practice', *Teaching and Teacher Education*, 22 (8): 1055–67.

Harvey, G., Loftus-Hills, A., Rycroft-Malone, J., Titchen, A., Kitson, A., McCormack, B. and Seers, K. (2002) 'Getting evidence into practice: the role and function of facilitation', *Journal of Advanced Nursing*, 37 (6): 577–88.

Hawkins, P. and Shohet, R. (2012) *Supervision in the Helping Professions*, 4th edn. Milton Keynes: Open University Press.

Health and Care Professions Council (HCPC) (2012a) *Standards of Education and Training Guidance*. Available at: http://www.hpc-uk.org/assets/documents/1000295 FStandardsofeducationandtrainingguidance-fromSeptember2009.pdf (accessed 3 January 2014).

Health and Care Professions Council (2012b) *Your Guide to Our Standards for Continuing Professional Development*. Available at: http://www.hpc-uk.org/assets/documents/ 10003B70Yourguidetoourstandardsofcontinuingprofessionaldevelopment.pdf (accessed 3 January 2014).

Health and Care Professions Council (2013) *About Registration: Professions*. Available at: http://www.hpc-uk.org/aboutregistration/professions/ (accessed 3 January 2014).

Health Education England (HEE) (2014a) *Our LETBs*. Available at: http://hee.nhs.uk/ about/our-letbs/ (accessed 25 January 2014).

Health Education England (2014b) *Education Commissioning for Quality*. Available at: http://yh.hee.nhs.uk/education-commissioning-for-quality/ (accessed: 25 August 2014).

Hean, S., Clark, J.M., Adams, K., Humphris, D. and Lathlean, J. (2006) 'Being seen by others as we see ourselves: the congruence between the in-group and outgroup perceptions of health and social care students', *Learning in Health and Social Care*, 5 (1): 10–22.

Heaslip, V. and Scammell, J.M.E. (2012) 'Failing underperforming students: the role of grading in practice assessment', *Nurse Education in Practice*, 12 (2): 95–100.

Heirs, B. and Farrell, P. (1986) *The Professional Decision Thinker*. London: Sidgwick & Jackson.

Hemingway, P. and Brereton, N. (2009) *What is a Systematic Review?* Available at: http:// www.medicine.ox.ac.uk/bandolier/painres/download/whatis/syst-review.pdf (accessed 2 May 2014).

Henderson, A., Cooke, M., Creedy, D.K. and Walker, R. (2012) 'Nursing students' perceptions of learning in practice environments: a review', *Nurse Education Today*, 32 (3): 299–302.

Henderson, A., Creedy, D., Boorman, R., Cooke, M. and Walker, R. (2010) 'Development and psychometric testing of the Clinical Learning Organisational Culture Survey (CLOCS)', *Nurse Education Today*, 30 (7): 598–602.

Heron, J. (1989) *Six Category Intervention Analysis: Human Potential Research Project*, 2nd edn. Guildford: University of Surrey.

Hinton, J. (2009) 'Mentorship: the experiences of a tutor in a pre-registration operating department practice education programme', *Journal of Perioperative Practice*, 19 (7): 221–4.

Hodgson, A.K. and Scanlan, J.M. (2013) 'A concept analysis of mentoring in nursing leadership', *Open Journal of Nursing*, 3 (2013): 389–94; also available at: http://dx.doi.org/10.4236/ojn.2013.35052 (http://www.scirp.org/journal/ojn/) (accessed 5 July 2014).

Holland, K. and Lauder, W. (2012) 'A review of evidence for the practice learning environment: enhancing the context for nursing and midwifery care in Scotland', *Nurse Education in Practice*, 12 (1): 60–4.

Holt, J., Coates, C., Cotterill, D., Eastburn, S., Laxton, J., Young, C. and Mistry, H. (2010) 'Identifying common competences in health and social care: an example of multi-institutional and inter-professional working', *Nurse Education Today*, 30 (3): 264–70.

Honey, P. and Mumford, A. (2000) *The Learning Styles Helper's Guide*. Maidenhead: Peter Honey.

Hood, K., Cant, R., Baulch, J., Gilbee, A., Leech, M., Anderson, A. and Davies, K. (2014) 'Prior experience of inter-professional learning enhances undergraduate nursing and healthcare students' professional identity and attitudes to teamwork', *Nurse Education in Practice*, 14 (2): 117–122.

Hughes, C. (1999) 'The dire in self-directed learning', *Adults Learning*, 11 (2): 7–9.

Hughes, L. and Marsh, T. (2006) *Creating an Interprofessional Workforce: An Education and Training Framework for Health and Social Care. Executive Summary*. Available at: http://caipe.org.uk/silo/files/cipw-exec-summary.pdf (accessed 4 May 2014).

Hughes, S.J. and Quinn, F.M. (2013) *Quinn's Principles and Practice of Nurse Education*, 6th edn. Andover: Cengage Learning EMEA.

Hunt, J. (1997) 'Towards evidence-based practice', *Nursing Management*, 4 (2): 14–17.

Hunt, L.A., McGee, P., Gutteridge, R. and Hughes, M. (2012) 'Assessment of nurses in practice: a comparison of theoretical and practical assessment results in England', *Nurse Education Today*, 32 (4): 351–5.

Hutchings, A. and Sanders, L. (2001) 'Developing a learning pathway for student nurses', *Nursing Standard*, 15 (40): 38–41.

Hutchison, T. and Cochrane, J. (2014) 'A phenomenological study into the impact of the sign-off mentor in the acute hospital setting', *Nurse Education Today*, 34 (6): 1029–33.

Huybrecht, S., Loeckx, W., Quaeyhaegens, Y., De Tobel, D. and Mistiaen, W. (2010) 'Mentoring in nursing education: perceived characteristics of mentors and the consequences of mentorship', *Nurse Education Today*, 31 (3): 274–8.

Institute of Directors (2014) *Executive Coaching*. Available at: http://www.iod.com/developing/executive-coaching (accessed 4 May 2014).

Institute of Healthcare Improvement (IHI) (2014) *Plan–Do–Study–Act (PDSA) Worksheet*. Available at: http://www.ihi.org/resources/pages/tools/plandostudyactworksheet.aspx (accessed 27 April 2014).

James, S., D'Amore, A. and Thomas, T. (2011) 'Learning preferences of first year nursing and midwifery students: utilising VARK', *Nurse Education Today*, 31 (4): 417–23.

Jarvis, P. (1995) *Adult and Continuing Education*. London: Croom Helm.

Jarvis, P. and Gibson, S. (1997) *The Teacher Practitioner and Mentor*, 2nd edn. Cheltenham: Stanley Thornes.

Jeffs, T. (2003) 'Quest for knowledge begins with a recognition of shared ignorance', *Adults Learning*, 14 (6): 28.

Johansson, U., Kaila, P., Ahlner-Elmqvist, M., Leksell, J. and Isoaho, H. (2010) 'Clinical learning environment, supervision and nurse teacher evaluation scale: psychometric evaluation of the Swedish version', *Journal of Advanced Nursing*, 66 (9): 2085–93.

Jokelainen, M., Turunen, H., Tossavainen, K., Jamookeeah, D. and Coco, K. (2011) 'A systematic review of mentoring nursing students in clinical placements', *Journal of Clinical Nursing*, 20 (19–20): 2854–67.

Joyce, B., Calhoun, E. and Hopkins, D. (2009) *Models of Learning: Tools for Teaching*, 3rd edn. Maidenhead: Open University Press.

Kane, A. and Gooding, C. (2009) *Reasonable Adjustments in Nursing and Midwifery: A Literature Review*. Available at: http://www.nmc-uk.org/Documents/ResearchPapers/Reasonable%20adjustments%20literature%20review.pdf (accessed 4 May 2014).

Kelton, M.F. (2015) 'Clinical coaching – An innovative role to improve marginal nursing students' clinical practice', *Nurse Education in Practice*. DOI:10.1016/j.nepr.2014.06.010.

Kendall-Raynor, P. (2007) 'Nurse cleared in supervision case is to face NMC', *Nursing Standard*, 21 (17): 9.

Kerry, T. and Mayes, A.S. (eds) (1995) *Issues in Mentoring*. London: Routledge/Open University.

Kirkpatrick, D.L. and Kirkpatrick, J.D. (2006) *Evaluating Training Programs: The Four Levels*, 3rd edn. San Francisco, CA: Berrett-Koehler Publishers.

Knowles, M.S., Holton, E.F. and Swanson, R.A. (2011) *The Adult Learner*, 7th edn. Oxford: Butterworth-Heinemann.

Koh, L.C. (2010) 'Academic staff perspectives of formative assessment in nurse education', *Nurse Education in Practice*, 10 (4): 205–9.

Kohler, W. (1925) 'The mentality of apes', in E. Smith, S. Nolen-Hoeksema and B. Fredrickson (eds) (2003), *Atkinson and Hilgard's Introduction to Psychology*, 14th edn. London: Thomson/Wadsworth.

Kolb, D. (1984) *Experiential Learning: Experience as the Source of Learning and Development*. London: Prentice-Hall.

Kopp, P. (2001) 'Fit for practice – 6.1: what is evidence-based practice?', *Nursing Times*, 97 (22): 47–50.

Kouzes, J.M. and Posner, B.Z. (2012) *The Leadership Challenge*, 5th edn. San Francisco, CA: Jossey-Bass.

Kramer, M. (1974) *Reality Shock: Why Nurses Leave Nursing*. St Louis, MO: Mosby.

Krathwohl, D.R. (2002) 'A revision of Bloom's *Taxonomy*: an overview', *Theory into Practice*, 41 (4): 212–18.

Krathwohl, D., Bloom, B. and Masia, B. (1999) *A Taxonomy of Educational Objectives: The Classification of Education Goals, Handbook 2: Affective Domain*, 2nd edn. Harlow: Longman.

Lait, J., Suter, E. and Deutschlander, S. (2011) 'Inter-professional mentoring: enhancing students' clinical learning', *Nurse Education in Practice*, 11 (3): 211–15.

Lakasing, E. and Francis, H. (2005) 'The crisis in student mentorship', *Primary Health Care*, 15 (4): 40–1.

Lang, N. (1976) 'Issues in quality assurance in nursing', in American Nurses' (ed.) Association *Issues in Evaluation Research*. Kansas City, MO: American Nurses Association.

Lankshear, A. (1990) 'Failure to fail: the teacher's dilemma', *Nursing Standard*, 4 (20): 35–7.

Lave, J. and Wenger, E. (1998) *Communities of Practice: Learning, Meaning and Identity*. Cambridge: Cambridge University Press.

Lee, N. (2011) 'An evaluation of CPD learning and impact upon positive practice change', *Nurse Education Today*, 31 (4) 390–5.

Lewin, K. (1951) *Field Theory in Social Science*. London: Harper & Row.

Liefer, D. (2002) 'Do you have a plan?', *Nursing Standard*, 16 (41): 14–17.

Lindberg, J.B., Hunter, M.L. and Kruszewski, A.Z. (1998) *Introduction to Nursing: Concepts, Issues and Opportunities*, 3rd edn. Philadelphia, PA: Lippincott.

Livneh, C. and Livneh, H. (1999) 'Continuing professional education among educators: predictors of participation in learning activities', *Adult Education Quarterly*, 49 (2): 91–106.

Lloyd, N. (1999) 'BJTR and interdisciplinary practice: moving forward', *British Journal of Therapy and Rehabilitation*, 6 (12): 573.

Lloyd-Jones, N., Hutchings, S. and Hobson, S.H. (2007) 'Interprofessional learning in practice for pre-registration health care: interprofessional learning occurs in practice – is it articulated or celebrated?', *Nurse Education in Practice*, 7 (1): 11–17.

Long, A., Kneafsey, R., Ryan, J. and Howard, J. (2001) *Exploring the Role and Contribution of the Nurse in the Multi-Professional Rehabilitation Team (Research Highlights 45)*. Available at: http://www.nmc-uk.org/Documents/Archived%20Publications/ENB%20Archived%20Publications/ENB_ARCHIVED_PUBLICATION_Research%20Highlights%2045%20February%202001.PDF (accessed 14 January 2014).

Luckhaupt, E., Chin, M.H., Mangione, C.M., Phillips, R.S., Bell, D., Leonard, A.C. and Tsevat, J. (2005) 'Mentorship in academic general internal medicine: results of a survey of mentors', *Journal of General Internal Medicine*, 20 (11): 1014–18.

Lunyk-Child, O.L., Crooks, D., Ellis, P.J., Ofosu, C., O'Mara, L. and Rideout, E. (2001) 'Self-directed learning: faculty and student perceptions', *Journal of Nursing Education*, 40 (3): 116–23.

Madden, C. and Mitchell, V. (1993) *Professions, Standards and Competence: A Survey of Continuing Education for the Professions*. Bristol: Department for Continuing Education, University of Bristol.

Mallik, M. and McGowan, B. (2007) 'Issues in practice based learning in nursing in the United Kingdom and the Republic of Ireland: results from a multi-professional scoping exercise', *Nurse Education Today*, 27 (1): 52–9.

Marks-Maran, D., Ooms, A., Tapping, J., Muir, J., Phillips, S. and Burke, L. (2013) 'A preceptorship programme for newly qualified nurses: a study of preceptees' perceptions', *Nurse Education Today*, 33 (11): 1428–1434.

Marshall, J.E. (2012) 'Developing midwifery practice through work-based learning: an exploratory study', *Nurse Education in Practice*, 12 (5) 273–8.

Marton, F., Hounsell, D. and Entwistle, N. (eds) (1997) *The Experience of Learning*, 2nd edn. Edinburgh: Scottish Academic Press.

Maslow, A.H. (1987) *Motivation and Personality*, 3rd edn. London: Harper & Row.

Maxwell, R.J. (1984) 'Quality assurance in health care', *British Medical Journal*, 288 (6428): 1470–2.

McArthur, G.S. and Burns, I. (2008) 'An evaluation, at the 1-year stage, of a 3-year project to introduce practice education facilitators to NHS Tayside and Fife', *Nurse Education Today*, 8 (3): 149–55.

McCarthy, B. and Murphy, S. (2008) 'Assessing undergraduate nursing students in clinical practice: do preceptors use assessment strategies?', *Nurse Education Today*, 28 (3): 301–13.

McCarthy, J. and Rose, P. (2010) *Values-Based Health and Social Care: Beyond Evidence-Based Practice*. London: Sage Publications.

McCormack, B., Manley, K. and Titchen, A. (2013) *Practice Development in Nursing and Healthcare*. Oxford: Wiley-Blackwell.

McGill, I. and Beatty, L. (1998) 'Continuing professional development', in C.M. Downie and P. Basford (eds), *Teaching and Assessing in Clinical Practice*. London: University of Greenwich.

McGivney, V. (2003) *Adult Learning Pathways: Through Routes or Cul-de-Sac*. Leicester: National Institute of Adult Continuing Education (NIACE).

McGregor, D. (1987) *The Human Side of Enterprise*. London: Penguin.

McKimm, J., Jollie, C. and Hatter, M. (2007) *Mentoring: Theory and Practice*. Available at: http://www.faculty.londondeanery.ac.uk/e-learning/feedback/files/Mentoring_Theory_and_Practice.pdf (accessed 14 January 2014).

Mead, D. (2011) 'Views of nurse mentors about their role', *Nursing Management*, 18 (6): 18–23.

Megginson, D. and Clutterbuck, D. (2005) *Techniques for Coaching and Mentoring*. Oxford: Elsevier.

Megginson, D., Clutterbuck, D., Garvey, B., Stokes, P. and Garrett-Harris, R. (2006) *Mentoring in Action: A Practical Guide*. London: Kogan Page.

Miller, C., Ross, N. and Freeman, M. (1999) *The Role of Collaborative/Shared Learning in Pre- and Post-Registration Education in Nursing, Midwifery and Health Visiting (Research Highlights 39)*. Available at: http://www.nmc-uk.org/Documents/Archived%20Publications/ENB%20Archived%20Publications/ENB_ARCHIVED_PUBLICATION_Research%20Highlights%2039%20July%201999.PDF (accessed 14 January 2014).

Mooney, H. (2009) 'Lack of support for nurse entrepreneurs may hold back practice innovation', *Nursing Times*. Available at: http://www.nursingtimes.net/whats-new-in-nursing/lack-of-support-for-nurse-entrepreneurs-may-hold-back-practice-innovation/1981253.article (accessed date: 24 April 2014).

Moore, L. (2010) Work-based learning and the role of managers', *Nursing Management*, 17 (5): 26–9.

Morris, J. and Maynard, V. (2007) 'The value of an eidence based practice module to skill development', *Nurse Education Today*, 27 (6): 534–541

Morrison, S., Boohan, M., Moutray, M. and Jenkins, J. (2004) 'Developing pre-qualification interprofessional education', *Nurse Education in Practice*, 4 (1): 20–9.

Mott Macdonald and Nursing and Midwifery Council (2013) *Quality Assurance Handbook*. Available at: http://www.nmc.mottmac.com/Portals/0/QA_Handbook_A4_version_2013-14_FINAL_V3.pdf (accessed 26 March 2014).

Mulholland, J., Scammell, J., Turnock, C. and Gregg, B. (2006) *Making Practice-Based Learning Work: Final Report*. Newcastle-upon-Tyne: Northumbria University.

Murray, C., Rosen, L. and Staniland, K. (eds) (2010) *The Nurse Mentor and Reviewer Update Book*. Maidenhead: McGraw-Hill Education.

National Committee of Inquiry into Higher Education (NCIHE) (1997) *Higher Education in the Learning Society (The Dearing Report)*. Norwich: HMSO.

National Institute for Health and Care Excellence (NICE) (2014a) *Safe Staffing for Nursing in Adult Inpatient Wards in Acute Hospitals*. Available at: www.nice.org.uk/guidance/sg1/resources/guidance-safe-staffing-for-nursing-in-adult-inpatient-wards-in-acute-hospitals-pdf (accessed 1 September 2014).

National Institute for Health and Care Excellence (2014b) *NICE Pathways: Mapping our Guidance*. Available at: http://pathways.nice.org.uk/ (accessed 17 December 2014).

National Institute for Health and Care Excellence (2014c) *Quality, Innovation, Productivity and Prevention (QIPP)*. Available at: www.evidence.nhs.uk/qipp (accessed 2 May 2014).

National Nursing Research Unit (King's College London) (2014) *Sustaining and Assuring the Quality of Student Nurse Mentorship: What are the Challenges?* Available at: www.kcl.ac.uk/nursing/research/nnru/policy/By-Issue-Number/Policy-Issue-43.pdf. (accessed 3 January 2015).

Neary, M. (2000a) *Teaching, Assessing and Evaluation for Clinical Competence*. Cheltenham: Stanley Thornes.

Neary, M. (2000b) 'Responsive assessment of clinical competence (Part 1)', *Nursing Standard*, 15 (9): 34–6.

Newton, J.M., Billett, S. and Ockerby, C.M. (2009) 'Journeying through clinical placements: an examination of six student cases', *Nurse Education Today*, 29 (6): 630–4.

Newton, J.M., Jolly, B.C., Ockerby, C.M. and Cross, W.M. (2010) 'Clinical learning environment inventory: factor analysis', *Journal of Advanced Nursing*, 66 (6): 1371–81.

NHS Education for Scotland (2014a) *Flying Start NHS*. Available at: http://www.flying start.scot.nhs.uk/ (accessed 22 March 2014).

NHS Education for Scotland (2014b) *Practice Education Facilitator and Care Home Education Facilitator*. Available at: http://www.nes.scot.nhs.uk/media/2570814/pef_chef_report_final_11.3.14.pdf (accessed 27 June 2014).

NHS Employers (2011) *European Working Time Directive*. Available at: http://www.nhs employers.org/PlanningYourWorkforce/MedicalWorkforce/EWTD/Pages/EWTD. aspx (accessed 14 January 2014).

NHS England (2014a) *NHS Revalidation – Responding to Concerns Glossary (A-Z)*. Available at www.england.nhs.uk/revalidation/ro/resp-con/a-z/ (accessed 14 December 2014).

NHS England (2014b) *About Us*. Available at: http://www.england.nhs.uk/about/ (accessed 30 April 2014).

NHS England (2014c) *Compassion in Practice: Our Culture of Compassionate Care*. Available at: http://www.england.nhs.uk/nursingvision/ (accessed 13 January 2014).

NHS England National Quality Board (NQB) (2014) *How to Ensure the Right People, with the Right Skills, Are in the Right Place at the Right Time: A Guide to Establishing Nursing,*

Midwifery and Care Staffing Capacity and Capability. Available at: http://www.england.nhs.uk/wp-content/uploads/2013/11/nqb-how-to-guid.pdf (accessed 3 July 2014).

NHS Improving Quality (NHS IQ) (2013) *Providing Care Closer to Home for Frail and Older People.* Available at: http://www.nhsiq.nhs.uk/resource-search/case-studies/7ds-pan-gwent.aspx (accessed 6 April 2014).

Nicklin, P. and Kenworthy, N. (eds) (2000) *Teaching and Assessing in Nursing Practice: An Experiential Approach,* 3rd edn. London: Baillière Tindall.

Norman, I.J., Watson, R., Murrells, T., Calman, L. and Redfern, S. (2002) 'The validity and reliability of methods to assess the competence to practise of pre-registration nursing and midwifery students', *International Journal of Nursing Studies,* 39 (2): 123–244.

Nursing and Midwifery Council (NMC) (2004a) *Reporting Unfitness to Practise: A Guide for Employers and Managers.* Available at: http://www.elderabuse.org.uk/Documents/Other%20Orgs/NMC%20guide%20on%20complaining%20about%20nurses%20employers.pdf (accessed 4 May 2014).

Nursing and Midwifery Council (2004b) *Standards of Proficiency for Specialist Community Public Health Nurses.* London: Nursing and Midwifery Council.

Nursing and Midwifery Council (2004c) *Supporting Nurses and Midwives through Lifelong Learning.* London: Nursing and Midwifery Council.

Nursing and Midwifery Council (2005a) *NMC Consultation on Proposals Arising from a Review of Fitness for Practice at the Point of Registration.* London: NMC.

Nursing and Midwifery Council (2005b) *NMC Approved Standard for Practice Teachers. NMC Circular 39/2005.* Available at: http://www.nmc-uk.org/Documents/Circulars/2005circulars/NMC%20circular%2039_2005.pdf (accessed 4 January 2014).

Nursing and Midwifery Council (2006a) *Preceptorship Guidelines, NMC Circular 21/2006.* Available at: http://www.nmc-uk.org/Documents/Circulars/2006circulars/NMC%20circular%2021_2006.pdf (accessed 5 May 2014).

Nursing and Midwifery Council (2006b) *Responses to the NMC Consultation on Proposals Arising from a Review of Fitness for Practice at the Point of Registration: Final Report.* Available at: www.nmc-uk.org/Documents/Consultations/NMC%20Consultations%20-%20ftp%20at%20the%20point%20of%20registration%20-%20final%20report.doc (accessed 6 January 2015).

Nursing and Midwifery Council (2007a) *Ensuring Continuity of Practice Assessment through the Ongoing Achievement Record, NMC Circular 33/2007.* Available at: http://www.nmc-uk.org/Documents/Circulars/2007circulars/NMC%20circular%2033_2007.pdf (accessed 19 April 2014).

Nursing and Midwifery Council (2007b) *Sign-Off Status and Preceptorship for Practice Teacher Students, NMC Circular 27/2007.* Available at: http://www.nmc-uk.org/Documents/Circulars/2007circulars/NMC%20circular%2027_2007.pdf (accessed 4 May 2014).

Nursing and Midwifery Council (2007c) *Guidance for the Introduction of the Essential Skills Clusters for Pre-registration Nursing Programmes.* Available at: http://www.nmc-uk.org/Documents/Circulars/2007circulars/NMC%20Circular07_2007%20Annexe%201.pdf (accessed 12 April 2014).

Nursing and Midwifery Council (2008a) *Standards to Support Learning and Assessment in Practice.* London: Nursing and Midwifery Council.

Nursing and Midwifery Council (2008b) *The Code: Standards of Conduct, Performance and Ethics for Nurses and Midwives.* London: Nursing and Midwifery Council.

Nursing and Midwifery Council (2009a) *Standards for Pre-registration Midwifery Education.* Available at: http://www.nmc-uk.org/Documents/NMC-Publications/nmcStandards forPre_RegistrationMidwiferyEducation.pdf (accessed 14 January 2014).

Nursing and Midwifery Council (2009b) *Additional Information to Support Implementation of NMC Standards to Support Learning and Assessment in Practice.* Available at: http://www.nmc-uk.org/Documents/Standards/NMC-Additional-information-for-Support-learning-and-assessment-in-practice-2008.pdf (accessed 4 May 2014).

Nursing and Midwifery Council (2010a) *Standards for Pre-Registration Nursing Education.* Available at: http://standards.nmc-uk.org/Pages/Welcome.aspx (accessed 15 April 2014).

Nursing and Midwifery Council (2010b) *Extract from Directive 2005/36/EC of the European Parliament and of the Council of 7 September 2005 on the Recognition of Professional Qualifications.* Available at: http://standards.nmc-uk.org/Documents/Annexe1_EU_Directive_2005_20100916.pdf (accessed 12 March 2014).

Nursing and Midwifery Council (2010c) *Sign-Off Mentor Criteria, NMC Circular 05/2010.* Available at: http://www.nmc-uk.org/Documents/Circulars/2010circulars/NMCcircular05_2010-1.pdf (accessed 30 April 2014).

Nursing and Midwifery Council (2010d) *Record Keeping: Guidance for Nurses and Midwives.* Available at: http://www.nmc-uk.org/Documents/NMC-Publications/NMC-Record-Keeping-Guidance.pdf (accessed 3 May 2014).

Nursing and Midwifery Council (2011) *The PREP Handbook.* Available at: http://www.nmc-uk.org/Educators/Standards-for-education/The-Prep-handbook/ (accessed 1 April 2014).

Nursing and Midwifery Council (2013a) *Quality Assurance Framework: For Nursing and Midwifery Education and Local Supervising Authorities.* Available at: http://www.nmc-uk.org/Educators/Quality-assurance-of-education/Quality-assurance-framework (accessed 6 January 2014).

Nursing and Midwifery Council (2013b) *NMC Council Agrees a Model of Revalidation for Nurses and Midwives.* Available at: http://www.nmc-uk.org/media/Latest-news/NMC-agrees-a-model-of-revalidation-for-nurses-and-midwives/ (accessed 25 January 2014).

Nursing and Midwifery Council (2013c) *Raising Concerns: Guidance for Nurses and Midwives.* Available at: http://www.nmc-uk.org/Documents/NMC-Publications/NMC-Raising-and-escalating-concerns.pdf (accessed 1 April 2014).

Nursing and Midwifery Council (2014) *Revalidation.* Available at: http://www.nmc-uk.org/Nurses-and-midwives/Revalidation/ (accessed 15 April 2014).

Nursing and Midwifery Council (2015) *The Code: Professional Standards of Practice and Behaviour for Nurses and Midwives.* Available at: www.nmc-uk.org/Documents/NMC-Publications/NMC-Code-A5-FINAL.pdf (accessed: 30 January 2015).

O'Driscoll, M.F., Allan, H.T. and Smith, P.A. (2010) 'Still looking for leadership: who is responsible for student nurses' learning in practice?', *Nurse Education Today*, 30 (3): 212–17.

Office of Public Sector Information (OPSI) (2001) *Special Educational Needs and Disability Act 2001.* Available at: http://www.legislation.gov.uk/ukpga/2001/10/contents (accessed 5 May 2014).

Office of Public Sector Information (2005) *Disability Discrimination Act 2005.* Available at: http://www.legislation.gov.uk/ukpga/2005/13/contents (accessed 5 May 2014).

Open University (2001) *Assessing Practice in Nursing and Midwifery: K320 Workbook 3.* Milton Keynes: Open University Press.

Orton, H. (1981) 'Ward learning climate and student nurse response', *Nursing Times*, 77 (17): 65–8.

Orton, H.D., Prowse, J. and Millen, C. (1993) *Charting the Way to Excellence (Ward Learning Climate Project)*. Sheffield: Sheffield Hallam University.

Overill, S. (1998) 'A practical guide to care pathways', *Journal of Integrated Care*, 2: 93–8.

Page, S. (2001) 'Demystifying practice development', *Nursing Times*, 97 (22): 36–7.

Paice, E., Heard, S. and Moss, F. (2002) 'How important are role models in making good doctors', *British Medical Journal*, 325 (7366): 707–10.

Palfreyman, S., Tod, A. and Doyle, J. (2003) 'Comparing evidence-based practice of nurses and physiotherapists', *British Journal of Nursing*, 12 (4): 246–53.

Pallen, N. and Timmins, F. (2002) 'Research-based practice: myth or reality? A review of the barriers affecting research utilisation in practice', *Nurse Education in Practice*, 2 (2): 99–108.

Parker, J. (2010) *Effective Practice Learning in Social Work (Transforming Social Work Practice Series)*, 2nd edn. Exeter: Learning Matters.

Passmore, H. and Chenery-Morris, S. (2014) 'Exploring the value of the tripartite assessment of students in pre-registration midwifery education: a review of the evidence', *Nurse Education in Practice*, 14 (1): 92–7.

Pedler, M., Burgoyne, J. and Boydell, T. (1997) *The Learning Company: A Strategy for Sustainable Development*. London: McGraw-Hill.

Peters, R.S. (1966) *Ethics and Education*. London: George Allen & Unwin.

Peters, R.S. (1973) *The Philosophy of Education (Oxford Readings in Philosophy)*. Oxford: Oxford University Press.

Phillips, T., Schostak, J. and Tyler, J. (2000) *Practice and Assessment: An Evaluation of the Assessment of Practice at Diploma, and Degree and Post-Graduate Level in Pre- and Post-Registration Nursing and Midwifery Education (Research Highlight 43)*. Available at: http://www.nmc-uk.org/Documents/Archived%20Publications/ENB%20Archived%20Publications/ENB_ARCHIVED_PUBLICATION_research_highlight_43.PDF (accessed 14 January 2014).

Piaget, J. (1962) 'The stages of intellectual development of the child', in I. Roth (ed.), *Introduction to Psychology*. Milton Keynes: Lawrence Erlbaum Associates Ltd (LEA)/ Open University.

Pirrie, A., Wilson, V., Harden, R.M. and Elsegood, J. (1998) 'Multiprofessional education: Part Two – promoting cohesive practice in healthcare (Association for Medical Education in Europe (AMEE) Guide No. 12)', *Medical Teacher*, 20 (5): 409–16.

Pollard, C. and Hibbert, C. (2004) 'Expanding student learning using patient pathways', *Nursing Standard*, 19 (2): 40–3.

Price, A. and Price, B. (2009) 'Role modelling practice with students on clinical placements', *Nursing Standard*, 24 (11): 51–6.

Price, B. (2007) 'Practice-based assessment: strategies for mentors', *Nursing Standard*, 21 (36): 49–56.

Price, B. (2010) 'Disseminating best practice through teaching', *Nursing Standard*, 24 (27): 35–41.

Proctor, B. (2001) 'Training for the supervision alliance: attitude, skills and intention', in J. Cutcliffe, T. Butterworth and B. Proctor (eds), *Fundamental Themes in Clinical Supervision*. London: Routledge.

Quality Assurance Agency for Higher Education (QAA) (2001) *Guidelines for HE Progress Files*. Available at: http://www.qaa.ac.uk/Publications/informationAndGuidance/Pages/Guidelines-for-HE-Progress-Files.aspx (accessed 26 March 2014).

Quality Assurance Agency for Higher Education (2006a) *Outcomes from Institutional Audit Work-based and Placement Learning, and Employability*. Available at: www.qaa.ac.uk/en/Publications/Documents/Outcomes-institutional-audit-Work-based-placement-learning-employability.pdf (accessed 13 December 2014).

Quality Assurance Agency for Higher Education (2006b) *Code of Practice for the Assurance of Academic Quality and Standards in Higher Education, Section 6: Assessment of Students*. Available at: http://www.qaa.ac.uk/Publications/InformationAndGuidance/Pages/Code-of-practice-Section-6.aspx (accessed 4 January 2014).

Quality Assurance Agency for Higher Education (2008) *The Framework for Higher Education Qualifications in England, Wales and Northern Ireland*. Available at: http://www.qaa.ac.uk/Publications/InformationAndGuidance/Pages/The-framework-for-higher-education-qualifications-in-England-Wales-and-Northern-Ireland.aspx (accessed 4 January 2014.

Quality Assurance Agency for Higher Education (2010) *Code of Practice for the Assurance of Academic Quality and Standards in Higher Education, Section 3: Disabled Students*. Available at: http://www.qaa.ac.uk/Publications/InformationAndGuidance/Pages/Code-of-practice-Section-3.aspx (accessed 4 January 2014).

Quality Assurance Agency for Higher Education (2014) *Higher Education Review*. Available at: http://www.qaa.ac.uk/InstitutionReports/types-of-review/higher-education-review/Pages/default.aspx (accessed 5 May 2014).

Race, P. (2010) *Making Learning Happen: A Guide for Post-Compulsory Education*, 2nd edn. London: Sage Publications.

Ramsden, P. (2003) *Learning to Teach in Higher Education*, 2nd edn. London: Routledge Falmer.

Rattray, J.E., Paul, F. and Tully, V. (2006) 'Partnership working between a higher education institution and NHS Trusts: developing an acute and critical care module', *Nursing in Critical Care*, 11 (3): 111–17.

Reeves, S. and Pryce, A. (1998) 'Emerging themes: an exploratory research project of an interprofessional education module for medical, dental and nursing students', *Nurse Education Today*, 18 (7): 534–41.

Roberts, D. (2010) 'Vicarious learning: a review of the literature', *Nurse Education in Practice*, 10 (1): 13–16.

Roberts, P., Priest, H. and Bromage, C. (2001) 'Selecting and utilising data sources to evaluate health care education', *Nurse Researcher*, 8 (3): 15–29.

Rogers, A. and Horrocks, H. (2010) *Teaching Adults*, 4th edn. Maidenhead: Open University Press/McGraw-Hill Education.

Rogers, C. (1983) *Freedom to Learn in the 80s*. Columbus, OH: Charles Merrill.

Rogers, C. and Freiberg, H.J. (1994) *Freedom to Learn*, 3rd edn. Upper Saddle River, NJ: Pearson Education.

Rogers, E.M. (2003) *Diffusion of Innovations*, 5th edn. New York: Free Press.

Rooke, N. (2014) 'An evaluation of nursing and midwifery sign off mentors, new mentors and nurse lecturers' understanding of the sign off mentor role', *Nurse Education in Practice*, 14 (1): 43–8.

Rotem, A. and Hart, G. (1995) 'The clinical learning environment: nurses' perceptions of professional development in clinical settings', *Nurse Education Today*, 15 (1): 3–10.

Rowntree, D. (1987) *Assessing Students: How Shall We Know Them?* London: Kogan Page.

Roxburgh, M., Conlon, M. and Banks, D. (2012) 'Evaluating hub-and-spoke models of practice learning in Scotland, UK: a multiple case study approach', *Nurse Education Today*, 32 (7): 782–9.

Royal College of Nursing (RCN) (2002) *Helping Students Get the Best from Their Practice Placements (A Royal College of Nursing Toolkit)*. London: Royal College of Nursing.

Royal College of Nursing (2004) *The Future Nurse: Evidence of the Impact of Registered Nurses*. London: Royal College of Nursing.

Royal College of Nursing (2005) *Maxi Nurses: Nurses Working in Advanced and Extended Roles Promoting and Developing Patient-Centred Healthcare*. London: Royal College of Nursing.

Royal College of Nursing (2006) *Practice Development*. London: Royal College of Nursing.

Royal College of Nursing (2007) *Guidance for Mentors of Nursing Students and Midwives: An RCN Toolkit*. London: Royal College of Nursing.

Royal College of Nursing (2012) *Quality with Compassion: The Future of Nursing Education* (Willis Report). Available at: http://www.williscommission.org.uk/recommendations (accessed 11 January 2014).

Saarikoski, M., Isoaho, H., Warne, T. and Leino-Kilpi, H. (2008) 'The nurse teacher in clinical practice: developing the new sub-dimension to the clinical learning environment and supervision (CLES) scale', *International Journal of Nursing Studies*, 45 (8) 1233–7

Sackett, D.L., Rosenburg, W., Gray, J.M., Haynes, R.B. and Richardson, S.W. (1996) 'Evidence-based medicine: what it is and what it isn't', *BMJ*, 312 (7023): 71–2.

Sackett, D.L., Strauss, S.E., Richardson, S.W., Rosenburg, W. and Haynes, R.B. (2000) *Evidence-Based Medicine: How to Practice and Teach EBM*, 2nd edn. Edinburgh: Churchill Livingstone.

Salmon, D. and Jones, M. (2001) 'Shaping the inter-professional agenda: a study examining qualified nurses' perceptions of learning with each other', *Nurse Education Today*, 21 (1): 18–25.

Scammell, B. (1990) *Communication Skills*. Basingstoke: Macmillan.

Schon, D. (1995) *The Reflective Practitioner: How Professionals Think in Action*. Aldershot: Arena.

Scottish Government (2014) *Flying Start NHS*. Available at: http://www.flyingstart.scot.nhs.uk/ (accessed 21 April 2014).

Scullion, P. (2002) 'Effective dissemination strategies', *Nurse Researcher: Qualitative Approaches*, 10 (1): 65–7.

Scullion, P.A. (2010) 'Models of disability: their influence in nursing and potential role in challenging discrimination', *Journal of Advanced Nursing*, 66 (3): 697–707.

Sharp, M. (2000) 'The assessment of incompetence: practice teachers' support needs when working with failing DipSW students', *Journal of Practice Teaching*, 2 (3): 5–18.

Simpson, J. and Weiner, E. (1989) *The Oxford English Dictionary*, 2nd edn. Oxford: Oxford University Press.

Sines, D., Harris, D., Firth, J. and Boden, L. (2006) 'Applied leadership: ensuring fitness for practice', *Nursing Management*, 13 (8): 28–31.

Skinner, B.F. (1971) *Beyond Freedom and Dignity*. New York: Alfred Knopf.

Smith, J. and Rudd, C. (2010) 'Implementing the productive ward management programme', *Nursing Standard*, 24 (31): 45–8.

Society and College of Radiographers (2014) *Education Approval and Accreditation*. Available at: http://www.sor.org/learning/education-accreditation/education-approval-and-accreditation (accessed 23 March 2014).

Spouse, J. (2001a) 'Bridging theory and practice in the supervisory relationship: a sociocultural perspective', *Journal of Advanced Nursing*, 33 (4): 512–22.

Spouse, J. (2001b) 'Work-based learning in healthcare environments', *Nurse Education in Practice*, 1 (1): 12–18.

Steinaker, N.W. and Bell, M.R. (1979) *The Experiential Learning: A New Approach to Teaching and Learning*. New York: Academic Press.

Stevens, D. (2003) 'The practice educator in specialist community practice', *Journal of Community Nursing*, 17 (2): 30–1.

Stewart, S. and Carpenter, C. (2009) 'Electronic mentoring: an innovative approach to providing clinical support', *International Journal of Therapy and Rehabilitation*, 16 (4): 199–206.

Stickley, T. (2011) 'From SOLER to SURETY for effective non-verbal communication', *Nurse Education in Practice*, 11 (6): 395–8.

Stickley, T., Stacey, G., Pollock, K., Smith, A., Betinis, J. and Fairbank, S. (2010) 'The practice assessment of student nurses by people who use mental health services', *Nurse Education Today*, 30 (1): 20–5.

Stuart, C.C. (2013) *Mentoring, Learning and Assessment in Clinical Practice: A Guide for Nurses, Midwives and Other Health Professionals*, 3rd edn. Edinburgh: Churchill Livingstone.

Sullivan, E.J. (2012) *Effective Leadership and Management in Nursing*, 8th edn. London: Prentice Hall International; and Upper Saddle River, NJ: Pearson Education.

Sundler, A.J., Björk, M., Bisholt, B., Ohlsson, U., Engström, A.K. and Gustafsson, M. (2014) 'Student nurses' experiences of the clinical learning environment in relation to the organization of supervision: a questionnaire survey', *Nurse Education Today*, 34 (4): 661–6.

Sykes, C., Urquhart, C. and Foster, A. (2014) 'Role of the Practice Education Facilitator (PEF): the Cambridgeshire model underpinned by a literature review of educational facilitator roles', *Nurse Education Today*, 34 (11): 1395–97.

Tee, S.R., Owens, K., Plowright, S., Ramnath, P., Rourke, S., James, C. and Bayliss, J. (2010) 'Being reasonable: supporting disabled nursing students in practice', *Nurse Education in Practice*, 10 (4): 216–21.

Tennant, M. (2005) *Psychology and Adult Learning*, 3rd edn. London, Routledge.

Thiroux, J. and Krasemann, K. (2014) *Ethics, Theory and Practice*, 11th edn. Harlow: Pearson Education Limited.

Thomas, L. (2005) 'An inspiration to all', *Nursing Standard*, 19 (24): 27.

Thompson, C. (1998) 'Testing our intuition', *Nursing Standard*, 12 (27): 18.

Thompson, C., McCaughan, D., Cullum, N., Sheldon, T. and Raynor, P. (2002) 'The value of research in clinical decision-making', *Nursing Times*, 98 (42): 30–4.

Timmins, F. (2002) 'The usefulness of learning contracts in nurse education: the Irish perspective', *Nurse Education in Practice*, 2 (3): 190–6.

Titchen, A. (2003) 'The practice development diamond', Paper presented at the RCN Annual International Nursing Research Conference, 10–12 April, UMIST, Manchester.

Tobin, M.J. (2004) 'Mentoring: seven roles and some specifics', *American Journal of Respiratory and Critical Care Medicine*, 170 (2): 114–117.

United Kingdom Central Council for Nursing, Midwifery and Health Visiting (UKCC) (1999) *Fitness for Practice*. Available at: http://www.nmc-uk.org/Documents/ Archived%20Publications/UKCC%20Archived%20Publications/Fitness%20for%20 Practice%20and%20Purpose%20The%20UKCC%20Commission%20for%20 Nursing%20and%20Midwifery%20Education%20Report%20September%201999. PDF (accessed 14 January 2014).

van Eps, M., Cooke, M., Creedy, D. and Walker, R. (2006) 'Student evaluations of a year-long mentorship program: a quality improvement initiative', *Nurse Education Today*, 26 (6): 519–24.

van Wijngaarden, J.D.H., Dirks, M., Dippel, D.W.J., Minkman, M. and Niessen, L.W. (2006) 'Towards effective and efficient care pathways: thrombolysis in acute ischaemic stroke', *Qjm*, 99 (4): 267–72.

Viney, R. and McKimm, J. (2010) 'Mentoring', *British Journal of Hospital Medicine*, 71 (2): 106–9.

Waddington, K. and Marsh, L. (1998) 'Work-based learning in a multigrade, multiskilled group: an action research perspective', *Managing Clinical Nursing*, 2 (4): 101–4.

Wallace, M. (1999) *Lifelong Learning: PREP in Action*. Edinburgh: Churchill Livingstone.

Walsh, M. and Ford, P. (1989) *Nursing Rituals, Research and Rational Actions*. Oxford: Heinemann Nursing.

Ward, C. and McCormack, B. (2000) 'Creating an adult learning culture through practice development', *Nurse Education Today*, 20 (4): 259–66.

Ward, L., Fenton, K. and Maher, L. (2010) 'The high impact actions for nursing and midwifery 3: staying safe, preventing falls', *Nursing Times*, 106 (29): 12–13.

Warne, T., Johansson, U., Papastavrou, E., Tichelaar, E., Tomietto, M., Van den Bossche, K., Moreno, M.F.V. and Saarikoski, V.M. (2010) 'An exploration of the clinical learning experience of nursing students in nine European countries', *Nurse Education Today*, 30 (8): 809–15.

Waskett, C. (2010) 'Clinical supervision using the 4S model 1: considering the structure and setting it up', *Nursing Times*, 106 (16): 12–14.

Waters, D., Clarke, M., Ingall, A.H. and Dean-Jones, M. (2003) 'Evaluation of a pilot mentoring programme for nurse managers', *Journal of Advanced Nursing*, 42 (5): 516–26.

Watson, J.B. (1978) 'The great psychologists: from Aristotle to Freud', in E. Smith, S. Nolen-Hoeksema and B. Fredrickson (eds) (2003), *Atkinson and Hilgard's Introduction to Psychology*, 14th edn. London: Thomson/Wadsworth.

Webb, C. and Shakespeare, P. (2008) 'Judgements about mentoring relationships in nurse education', *Nurse Education Today*, 28 (5): 563–71.

White, J. (2007) 'Supporting nursing students with dyslexia in clinical practice', *Nursing Standard*, 21 (19): 35–42.

Wilkinson, J. (1999) 'A practical guide to assessing nursing students in clinical practice', *British Journal of Nursing*, 8 (4): 218–22.

Wilkinson, J.E., Rushmer, R.K. and Davies, H.T.O. (2004) 'Clinical governance and the learning organization', *Journal of Nursing Management*, 12 (2): 105–13.

Williams, B., Perillo, S. and Brown, T. (2015) 'What are the factors of organisational culture in health care settings that act as barriers to the implementation of evidence-based practice? A scoping review', *Nurse Education Today*, 35 (2): e34–e41.

Williamson, G. (2009) 'Student support on placement: the student experience and staff perceptions of the implementation of placement development team', *The 2009 RCN International Nursing Research Conference: Book of Abstracts* (section 9.1.3): 107.

Wood, S. (2005) 'The experiences of a group of pre-registration mental health nursing students', *Nurse Education Today*, 25 (3): 189–96.

Wright, S. (1990) *Building and Using a Model of Nursing*. London: Edward Arnold.

Wright, S.M. and Carrese, J.A. (2002) 'Excellence in role modelling: insight and perspectives from the pros', *Canadian Medical Association Journal*, 167 (6): 638–43.

Young, P., Moore, E., Griffiths, G., Raine, R., Stewart, R., Cownie, M. and Frutos-Perez, M. (2010) 'Help is just a text away: the use of short message service texting to provide an additional means of support for health care students during practice placements', *Nurse Education Today*, 30 (2): 118–23.

Index